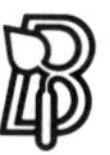

AAS
Agents and Actions Supplements
Vol. 38/II

Series Editors
K. Brune, Erlangen
M. J. Parnham, Bonn

Recent Progress on Kinins

Pharmacological and Clinical Aspects
of the Kallikrein-Kinin System

Part I

Proceedings of the International Conference "Kinin 91 Munich",
held in Munich, September 8–14, 1991

Edited by

G. Bönner
H. Fritz
Th. Unger
A. Roscher
K. Luppertz
(Technical Editor)

Birkhäuser Verlag
Basel · Boston · Berlin

Volume Editors' Addresses:

Editors:

PD Dr. Gerd Bönner
Krankenhaus Köln Merheim
Medizinische Klinik
Ostmerheimer Strasse 200
D–5000 Köln 91

Prof. Dr. Hans Fritz
Abteilung für Klinische Chemie
und Klinische Biochemie in der
Chirurgischen Klinik Innenstadt
der Universität München
Nussbaumstrasse 20
D–8000 München 2

Prof. Dr. Thomas Unger
Deutsches Institut für
Bluthochdruckforschung e.V.
Im Neuenheimer Feld 366
D–6900 Heidelberg 1

Prof. Dr. Adelbert Roscher
Dr. von Haunersches Kinderspital
der Universität München
Lindwurmstrasse 4
D–8000 München 40

Technical Editor:

Dr. Karin Luppertz
Abteilung für Klinische Chemie
und Klinische Biochemie in der
Chirurgischen Klinik Innenstadt
der Universität München
Nussbaumstrasse 20
D–8000 München 2

A CIP catalogue record for this book is available from the Library of Congress, Washington D.C., USA

Deutsche Bibliothek Cataloging-in-Publication Data

Recent progress on kinins. – Basel ; Boston ; Berlin : Birkhäuser.
  (Agents and actions : Supplements ; Vol. 38)
  ISBN 3-7643-2816-9 (Basel . . .)
  ISBN 0-8176-2816-9 (Boston)
NE: International Conference Kinin <1991, München>; Agents and actions / Supplements
2. Pharmacological and clinical aspects of the kallikrein kinin system.
  Pt. 1 (1992)

**Pharmacological and clinical aspects of the kallikrein kinin
system** : proceedings of the International Conference "Kinin 91
Munich", held in Munich, September 8–14, 1991 / ed. by
G. Bönner . . . – Basel ; Boston ; Berlin : Birkhäuser.
  (Agents and actions : Supplements ; Vol. 38)
NE: Bönner, Gerd [Hrsg.]
Pt. 1 (1992)
  (Recent progress on kinins ; 2)
  ISBN 3-7643-2818-5 (Basel . . .)
  ISBN 0-8176-2818-5 (Boston)

Product Liability: The publisher can give no guarantee for information about drug dosage and administration contained in this book. In each individual case the respective user must check its accuracy by consulting other medical and pharmaceutical literature.

The use of registered names, trademarks, etc. in this publication does not imply, even in the absence of a specific statement, that such names are exempt from the relevant protective laws and regulations and therefore free for general use.

© 1992 Birkhäuser Verlag
  P.O. Box 133
  4010 Basel/Switzerland

Printed in Germany on acid-free paper, directly from the authors' camera-ready manuscripts.

ISBN 3-7643-2816-9 (Vol. 38 (Set))   ISBN 0-8176-2816-9 (Vol. 38 (Set))
ISBN 3-7643-2817-7 (Vol. 38/I)   ISBN 0-8176-2817-7 (Vol. 38/I)
ISBN 3-7643-2818-5 (Vol. 38/II)   ISBN 0-8176-2818-5 (Vol. 38/II)
ISBN 3-7643-2819-3 (Vol. 38/III)   ISBN 0-8176-2819-3 (Vol. 38/III)

CONTENTS

Cellular Actions of Kinins

Functional Aspects of Kallikreins or Proteinases, Kininogens and Kallikrein or Proteinase Inhibitors

Coagulation and Fibrinolysis

Kinins, Kinin Receptors and Kinin Receptor Antagonists

Cellular Actions of Kinins

BRADYKININ STIMULATES Ca^{2+} ENTRY VIA NITRENDIPINE-SENSITVE Ca^{2+} CHANNELS IN CULTURED HUMAN FIBROBLASTS

Leora Baumgarten and Mitchel Villereal

Department of Pharmacological and Physiological Sciences,
University of Chicago, 947 E. 58th Street, Chicago IL, 60637

Summary: Bradykinin stimulates Ca^{2+} entry in cultured human fibroblasts via nitrendipine-sensitive Ca^{2+} channels in cultured human fibroblasts. The Ca^{2+} entering via this pathway does not contribute directly to the elevation of cytosolic Ca^{2+}, but rather appears to be specifically taken up into an internal Ca^{2+} pool.

INTRODUCTION

We first demonstrated bradykinin to be mitogenic in cultured human fibroblasts approximately ten years ago (1). Since that time, there have been a number of publications supporting the mitogenicity of bradykinin in this cell system. Also, during this time period, a number of publications have appeared on the signalling pathways utilized by bradykinin in fibroblasts. These studies have shown that bradykinin can activate phospholipase C to cause breakdown of phosphatidylinositol producing $Ins(1,4,5)P_3$ and DAG (2,3), to activate adenylate cyclase and guanylate cyclase producing cAMP and cGMP (4,5) and to activate phospholipase A_2 (6). Many studies also have been performed to investigate the role of bradykinin in controlling intracellular Ca^{2+}. In recent years, we have focused much of our energy on the study of this last process. While there are a number of studies describing the role of bradykinin in mobilizing intracellular Ca^{2+} stores, through the release of $Ins(1,4,5)P_3$, much less is understood about the role of bradykinin in controlling Ca^{2+} entry pathways or Ca^{2+} channels.

When fibroblasts are stimulated with a high dose of bradykinin (10-100 nM) we observe that the Ca^{2+} response is biphasic (7). The initial phase is a transient peak which rapidly declines to the secondary plateau phase of the response. In the absence of extracellular Ca^{2+} we obtain only the rapid transient phase, indicating that the plateau phase is the result of an influx of extracellular Ca^{2+}. Initially we assumed that the plateau phase would result from the activation of a single Ca^{2+} channel by way of a second mes.mt senger process activated by bradykinin. However, as we investigated this process in more detail we soon found the situation to be much more complex. We have data which is consistent with the activation of multiple Ca^{2+} channels by bradykinin, some of which contribute to the plateau phase and some of which do not. In this manuscript we describe the activation of a nitrendipine-sensitive, L-type channel by bradykinin.

METHODS

To investigate the Ca^{2+} responses stimulated by addition of bradykinin, we have utilized two complementary approaches. The first is the measurement of $^{45}Ca^{2+}$ influx into populations of fibroblasts (see ref. 8 for details). The second technique utilizes an image analysis system coupled to a fluorescence microscope which allows us to monitor the fura 2 signal from a field of 30-40 fibroblasts and to analyze the signal on an individual cell basis (see ref. 9 for details).

RESULTS AND DISCUSSION

Recent patch clamp studies demonstrated that an L-type, dihydropyridine-sensitive Ca^{2+} channel exists in cultured fibroblasts. We were interested in determining whether an L-type Ca^{2+} channel is activated when human fibroblasts are stimulated by BK and if so, what role this channel plays in the subsequent Ca^{2+} signal. Our prediction was that such a channel might play a significant role in the maintenance of the plateau phase of the Ca^{2+} response.

Initial $^{45}Ca^{2+}$ influx experiments demonstrated that depolarization of fibroblasts by incubation in a high K^+ medium stimulates $^{45}Ca^{2+}$ influx almost 3-fold. This stimulation can be blocked by nitrendipine, a high affinity dihydropyridine which is an antagonist for L-type Ca^{2+} channels (Table 1). We also observed that the addition of Bay K 8644, an L channel agonist would enhance the effect of depolarization so that together the two treatments produced a greater than 6-fold increase of $^{45}Ca^{2+}$ influx over basal levels (Table I). This stimulation was inhibited by the presence of nitrendipine.

We next looked at the effect of high K^+ and Bay K 8644 on the $[Ca^{2+}]_i$ levels in fura-2 loaded fibroblasts. Our expectation was that this treatment, which produces very high levels of $^{45}Ca^{2+}$ influx, would produce a large sustained increase in $[Ca^{2+}]_i$. To our suprise, the increase in $[Ca^{2+}]_i$ accompanying a greater than 6-fold increase in $^{45}Ca^{2+}$ influx was only a modest 50-75 nM over the basal levels of around 50 nM (figure 1). The modest increase in $[Ca^{2+}]_i$ was indeed blocked by nitrendipine, suggesting that an L-type Ca^{2+} channel was probably involved.

Table 1. Effect of membrane depolariztion and Bay K 8644 on ^{45}Ca^{2+} influx in the presence and absence of nitrendipine

	Ca^{2+} flux (nmol/g prot/min)	
	control	+ nitrendipine
5 mM K^{+}	160	142
20 mM K^{+}	466	163
5 mM K^{+} + Bay K	400	174
20 mM K^{+} + Bay K	1072	198

^{45}Ca^{2+} influx was measured over a 5 minute time period during which time uptake is linear. Bay K 8644 and nitrendipine were present at a dose of 1 uM. This data is representative of 10 similar experiments.

Since the above data confirmed the existence of a nitrendipine-sensitive Ca^{2+} channel in our human fibroblasts, we next investigated whether bradykinin would activate this channel. Initial experiments were performed by measuring ^{45}Ca^{2+} influx. We observed that addition of bradykinin would stimulate a 5-fold increase in Ca^{2+} influx over basal levels and that approximately half of the ^{45}Ca^{2+} influx was blocked by a maximum dose of nitrendipine (8). Since the K$_i$ of the nitrendipine inhibition was 2 nM, the influx of Ca^{2+} appears to be via an L-type channel or one with similar characteristics. The observation that only half of the bradykinin-stimulated ^{45}Ca^{2+} influx was blocked at maximum doses of nitrendipine was an indication that multiple Ca^{2+} channels may be activated by bradykinin addition.

Following these ^{45}Ca^{2+} influx studies we began to investigate the role of the nitrendipine-sensitive Ca^{2+} channel in the bradykinin-stimulated Ca^{2+} response. We returned to the image analysis system to explore whether addition of nitrendipine would block all or at least part of the bradykinin-stimulated plateau phase of the Ca^{2+} response. To our surprise, the addition of maximum doses of nitrendipine had no effect on the bradykinin-stimulated Ca^{2+} response (figure 2). Thus, even though addition of bradykinin stimulates a nitrendipine-sensitive ^{45}Ca^{2+} influx which is 3-fold the basal flux, there is no apparent nitrendipine-sensitive change in the bradykinin-stimulated cytosolic free Ca^{2+} concentration as measured by fura-2.

The observation that a 3-fold stimulation of Ca^{2+} influx via nitrendipine-sensitive Ca^{2+} channels by bradykinin does not contribute to the cytosolic Ca^{2+} signal

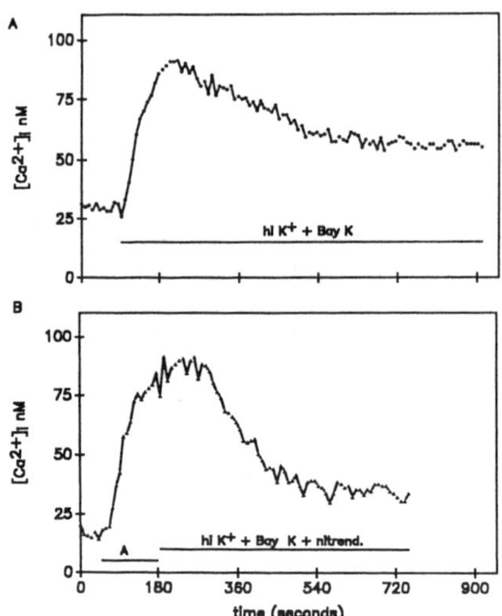

Figure 1. High K^+, Bay K 8644 induced elevation in $[Ca^{2+}]_i$. Each trace shown is from an individual cell in a field of cells and is a typical response. Initially the cells are perfused with Hepes-HBSS, during the time indicated by the bar the media is switched to: A) 30 mM K^+ Hepes-HBSS + 100 nM Bay K 8644, B) 30 mM K^+ Hepes-buffered HBSS + 100 nM Bay K 8644, and then subsequently the media is switched to 100 nM nitrendipine in addition to 30 mM K^+ and 100 nM Bay K 8644.

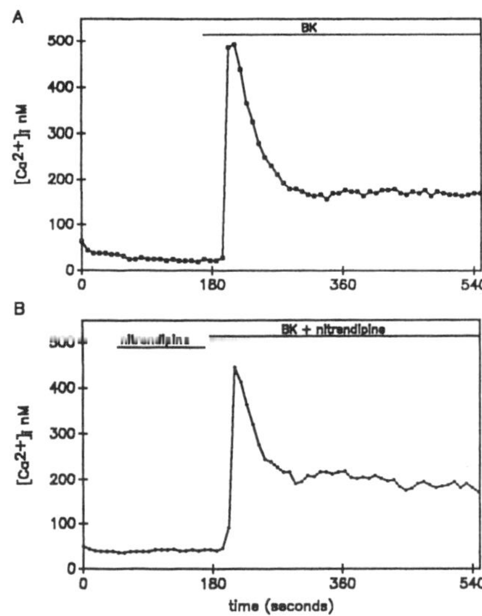

Figure 2. BK-stimulated change in $[Ca^{2+}]_i$ in the presence and absence of nitrendipine. Each trace shown is from an individual cell in a field of cells and represents a typical response. A) Cells are initially perfused with Hepes-HBSS, then at the time indicated by the bar cells are stimulated with 10 ng/ml BK. B) Cells are initially perfused with Hepes-HBSS, then pretreated with 100 nM nitrendipine and subsequently stimulated with 10 ng/ml BK in the continued presence of 100 nM nitrendipine.

made us go back and reconsider the observation that a 6-fold stimulation of Ca^{2+} influx by high K$^+$ and Bay K 8644 produced only a modest rise in [Ca^{2+}]$_i$. Where is this very large influx of Ca^{2+} going if it is not going into the cytoplasm to produce an increase in [Ca^{2+}]$_i$ as measured by fura-2? A consideration of the two methods for measuring Ca^{2+} entry tells us that ^{45}Ca^{2+} influx measures entry of Ca^{2+} into both the cytosol and into intracellular stores while measurement by fura-2 records only that Ca^{2+} in the cytosol, since fura-2 is not present in the Ca^{2+} pools. Thus, it is possible that the large influx of Ca^{2+} measured by ^{45}Ca^{2+} influx somehow finds its way into intracellular storage sites without contributing to a substantial rise in the cytosolic free Ca^{2+} concentration. Previous models have been suggested in which direct loading of intracellular Ca^{2+} stores might occur without the Ca^{2+} entering into the general cytoplasm (10,11). The variation of these models that we prefer is the one in which Ca^{2+} entering through these channels would find itself in a relatively restricted region of the cytoplasm in close proximity to the internal Ca^{2+} pools. Most of the entering Ca^{2+} would then be pumped into the stores and would never make it into the general cytoplasm and therefore would not be seen by fura-2.

We tested this hypothesis by measuring the entry of a divalent cation which could enter through L-type Ca^{2+} channels but would not serve as a substrate for the Ca^{2+} ATPase present on the membranes of the internal Ca^{2+} pools. We chose to look at Ba^{2+} influx. Ba^{2+} will interact with fura-2 in much the same manner as Ca^{2+} and cause a similar shift in the spectrum of the Ca^{2+} dye. Thus, a measurement of the 340/380 ratio of fura-2 can be used to monitor the influx of Ba^{2+}. These experiments were performed in Ca^{2+}-free medium so that the signal recorded in the cell is a composite of the transient release of intracellular Ca^{2+}, which is over in about 1 minute, and the more sustained influx of Ba^{2+}. We observed that in control cells there was very little Ba^{2+} influx but when cells were stimulated with bradykinin there was a fairly linear increase in the Ba^{2+} concentration in the cytosol (figure 3).

neither pumped out of the cell or into intracellular storage sites (12,13). Thus, we were in a position to ask the critical question of whether the nitrendipine-sensitive Ca^{2+} channels would contribute to the cytosolic divalent level when the uptake of the divalent into intracellular stores was prevented. The answer is that this channel does contribute dramatically to the cytosolic levels of Ba^{2+} in the absence of its being pumped into intracellular organelles. Blockage of the nitrendipine-sensitive channels blocks about half of the bradykinin-stimulated increase in cytosolic Ba^{2+} levels (control slope of 0.25 vs nitrendipine-treated slope of 0.1 in figure 3), a proportion which is highly consistent with the percentage of nitrendipine-sensitive ^{45}Ca^{2+} influx stimulated by bradykinin.

Thus, on the basis of the evidence that we have to date, we hypothesize that

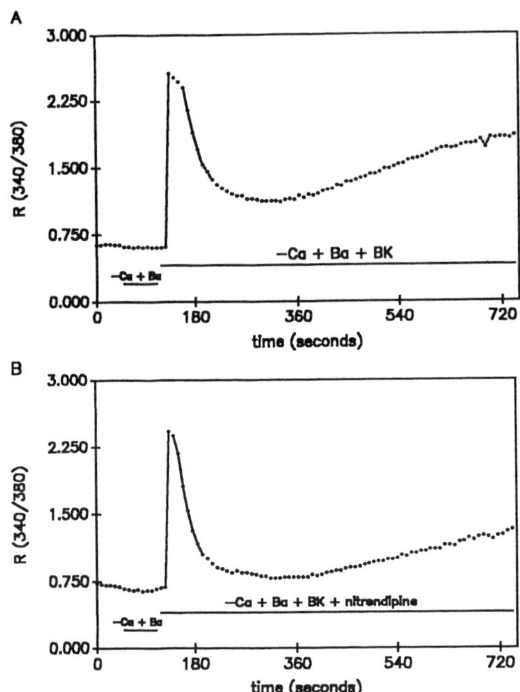

Figure 3. Nitrendipine inhibition of BK-stimulated Ba^{2+}-influx, as seen with fura-2. Each trace shown is from an individual cell in a field of cells and represents a typical response. A) Cells are initially perfused with Hepes-HBSS, then at the time indicated by the bar, cells are switched to calcium-free media containing 2 mM $BaCl_2$. Subsequently cells are stimulated with 25 ng/ml BK. B) essentially as in A except that cells are stimulated with 25 ng/ml BK plus 100 nM nitrendipine.

there are L-type Ca^{2+} channels in the plasma membrane of fibroblasts which are regulated by bradykinin. The Ca^{2+} which enters via these channels is preferentially taken up into intracellular storage sites with very little of it available to elevate the general cytosolic free Ca^{2+} concentration. There are two explanations for why the high K^+ plus Bay K 8644 activation of these channels gives a small elevation of the fura-2 signal while the bradykinin stimulation of these channels gives no measurable fura-2 signal. First, the 6-fold stimulation with high K^+ + Bay K 8644 may be sufficient to overwhelm the pumping capacity of the internal stores and thereby cause a small elevation of $[Ca^{2+}]_i$, while the 3-fold stimulation of influx via this channel produced by bradykinin may be insufficient to overwhelm this pumping capacity. Alternatively, bradykinin may serve to activate the pumping capacity of the internal stores so that virtually all of the entering Ca^{2+} is taken up whereas in the case of the high K^+ + Bay K 8644 stimulation some fraction of the Ca^{2+} may overcome the pumping capacity and enter the general cytoplasm. The latter of these possibilities seems the more likely since we find that addition of high K^+ + Bay K 8644 during the plateau phase of the bradykinin response produces no further elevation of the plateau (data not shown). If it were a matter of the channels not being fully activated by bradykinin, then addition of high K^+ + Bay K 8644 should produce more influx and thus an elevation of the Ca^{2+} plateau phase. This data implies that, when bradykinin is present, even a 6-fold increase in $^{45}Ca^{2+}$ influx is not sufficient for the Ca^{2+} entering via L-type channels to elevate the general cytoplasmic free calcium concentration.

CONCLUSION

We propose that there are L-type Ca^{2+} channels present in fibroblasts and that these channels can be activated by bradykinin. The physiological role of these channels is not clear at present. They do not contribute to the general rise in $[Ca^{2+}]_i$ seen following bradykinin stimulation but rather appear to allow Ca^{2+} to enter into internal Ca^{2+} pools.

ACKNOWLEDGEMENTS

We would like to thank Kathy Toscas for her excellent technical assisstance on this project. This work was supported by NIH grant GM-28359 and Training grant GM-07151.

REFERENCES

1.   Owen NE and Villereal ML. Lys-bradykinin stimulates Na^+ influx and DNA synthesis in cultured human fibroblasts. Cell 1983; 32:979-985.

2.   Jamieson GA and Villereal ML. Mitogen-stimulated release of inositol phosphates in human fibroblasts. Arch. Biochem. Biophys. 1987; 252:478-486.

3.   Etscheid BG, Albert K, Villereal ML, and Palfrey HC. Transduction of the bradykinin response in human fibroblasts: long-lasting elevation of diacylglycerol level and its correlation with protein kinase C activation. Cell Regulation 1991; 2:229-239.

4.   Fahey JV, Ciosek CP and Newcombe DS. Human synovial fibroblasts: the relationships between cyclic AMP, bradykinin and prostaglandins. Agents and Actions 1977; 7:255-264.

5.   Snider RM and Richelson, E. J. Bradykinin receptor-mediated cyclic GMP formation in a nerve cell population (murine neuroblastoma clone N1E-115). Neurochem. 1984; 43:1749-1754.

6.   Hong SL and Deykin D. The activation of phosphatidylinositol-hydrolyzing phospholipase A2 during prostaglandin synthesis in transformed mouse BALB/3T3 cells. J. Biol. Chem. 1981; 256:5215-5219.

7.   Byron KL, Babnigg, G and Villereal ML. Bradykinin-induced Ca^{2+} entry, release and refilling of intracellular Ca^{2+} stores: Relationships revealed by image analysis of individual human fibroblasts. J. Biol. Chem. 1992; 267:108-118.

8.   Baumgarten LB, Toscas K and Villereal, ML. Dihydropyridine-sensitive L-type Ca^{2+} channels in human foreskin fibroblasts cells: Characterization of activation with the growth factor lys-bradykinin. J. Biol. Chem. (in press).

9.   Byron KL and Villereal ML. Mitogen-induced Ca^{2+} changes in individual human fibroblasts: Image analysis reveals asynchronous responses which are characteristic for different mitogens. J. Biol. Chem 1989; 264:18234-18239.

10.   Putney JW. A model for receptor-regulated calcium entry. Cell Calcium 1986; 7:1-12.

11.   Merritt JE and Rink TJ. Regulation of cytosolic free calcium in fura-2 loaded rat parotid acinar cells. J. Biol. Chem 1987; 262:17362-17369.

12.   Kwan CY and Putney JW. Uptake and intracellular sequestration of divalent cations in resting and methacholine-stimulated mouse lacrimal acinar cells. J. Biol. Chem. 1990; 265:678-684.

13.   Byron KL Signal tranduction and regulation of intracellular calcium in human fibroblasts. Ph.D. Disertation, University of Chicago 1990.

$[Ca^{2+}]_i$ EFFECTS OF BRADYKININ B_2 RECEPTOR ACTIVATION IN PC12 CELLS

F. Grohovaz, D. Zacchetti, P. D'Andrea, P. Lorenzon and J. Meldolesi

"B. Ceccarelli" & CNR Cytopharmacol. Ctrs, Dept Pharmacology and S. Raffaele Institute, University of Milano, Italy

SUMMARY: In PC12 cells, activation of B2 receptors by bradykinin promotes an elevation of cytosolic Ca^{2+} by two mechanisms: IP3 mediated release of Ca^{2+} from intracellular stores and stimulation of multiple Ca^{2+} influx pathways. Since these events can have different kinetics and spatial localizations they can induce diversified effects in different cell areas.

INTRODUCTION

Elevation of the cytosolic free Ca^{2+} concentration $([Ca^{2+}]_i)$, from a resting level of about 10^{-7} M to values in the micromolar range, regulates a host of cellular functions in eukaryotic cells. Studies on PC12 cell populations have demonstrated that bradykinin (BK) activation of B_2 receptors (coupled to polyphosphoinositide (PPI) hydrolysis) promotes an increase of $[Ca^{2+}]_i$ by two separate mechanisms: a transient release from intracellular stores and a sustained influx across the plasmalemma (1). These mechanisms were further investigated by fura-2 imaging microscopy of individual NGF-differentiated PC12 cells, and by cuvette spectrofluorimetry of recently isolated PC12 clones.

MATERIALS AND METHODS

PC12 cells were cultured according to conventional procedures. Before the $[Ca^{2+}]_i$ experiments they were first serum deprived for 24 hours and then treated with 50 ng/ml mouse 2.5S NGF, for one day in the same serum free medium and for an additional week in complete medium.

Cell clones were isolated from the parent line after transfection with the pMV7 vector containing the neomycin resistence gene (2). Experiments were carried out in a standard KRH medium (1).

For $[Ca^{2+}]_i$ measurements, cells were loaded for 45 min at 37°C with 0.5-4 uM fura-2AM in the KRH medium supplemented with 5% FCS, washed and further incubated to allow deesterification of the dye.

Fura-2 loaded cell suspensions were supplemented with 250 uM sulfinpyrazone (to prevent dye leakage) and transferred to a thermostatted cuvette (37°C) mantained under continuous stirring in a Perkin Elmer LS5B fluorimeter.

Single cell fluorescence analyses were performed by a digital video-imaging system (3).   Pairs of images at 350 and 385 nm excitation wavelenght were stored digitally. After background and calibration images were similarly acquired at the two wavelenghts, $[Ca^{2+}]_i$ concentration was calculated pixel by pixel on pairs of corresponding 350 and 385 nm images according to Grynkiewicz et al (4).

RESULTS AND DISCUSSION

In order to identify the sources of the [Ca^{2+}]$_i$ increases, experiments were carried out in which BK was initially applied to cells bathed in a Ca^{2+}-free, EGTA(1mM)-containing, medium and Ca^{2+} was restored to its physiological concentration $\approx$2 min later. Figure 1 shows the [Ca^{2+}]$_i$ changes induced by BK (100nm), administered according to the protocol described above, in an NGF-differentiated PC12 cell. Both release from intracellular stores and influx occurred, causing [Ca^{2+}]$_i$ elevations of comparable size and different kinetics. This type of result, however, was not the rule. In fact the study of hundreds of cells revealed that individual responses to BK are highly heterogeneous and often consist of either release from intracellular stores or influx only (3). This result indicate the coexistance of multiple clones in the analysed PC12 population. When a single cell was exposed to repeated pulses

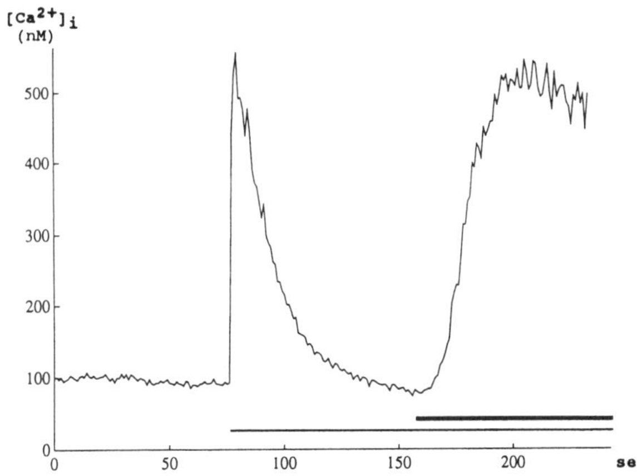

Figure 1. Temporal plot of [Ca^{2+}]$_i$ changes induced by BK in a NGF-differentiated PC12 cell. The thin bar mark the presence of BK and the thick bar the presence of [Ca2+]o.

of BK, administered according to the above protocol with 20 min washes in complete medium between the stimulations, the $[Ca^{2+}]_i$ response pattern was maintained. In contrast, when other agonists (CCh and ATP), similarly inducing PPI hydrolysis, were applied in sequence, the release/influx ratios showed considerable variation (Table I).

Table I. Release/influx ratios in five PC12 cells exposed in sequence to the indicated agonists.

Cell	1	2	3	4	5
Bradykinin	0.5	7	2.5	1	2
Carbachol	1	-	i	-	-
ATP	2	1	3	i	4

Values given are ratios between peak responses elicited according to the Ca^{2+} free-Ca^{2+} reintroduction protocol. Subsequent treatments were intercalated by 20 min washes in standard KRH medium.
- : no response ; i : influx only

These observations suggest that the activation of Ca^{2+} release and influx are not steps of the same signal cascade initiated by PPI hydrolysis, but are differently controlled by each receptor (3). This notion is further strenghtened by recent evidence suggesting that the B_2 receptor can activate plasma membrane channels by interactions mediated by specific G proteins (5). On the other hand a peculiar control of B_2 receptors on PPI transmembrane signaling was already observed (6), consisting in a reinforcement of both PPI hydrolysis and $[Ca^{2+}]_i$ responses induced by application of insulin or other growth factors on BK-(but neither ATP nor CCh) primed PC12 cells.

The existence of two rapidly exchanging Ca^{2+} release mechanisms, one activated by InsP3 and the other by caffeine/ryanodine (Cf/Ry), raises questions about their possible functional interconnection, following BK stimulation. Experiments with agonists selective for the two channel types were performed on a PC12 isolated clone, sensitive to caffeine. The results revealed that, in PC12, IP3 and Cf/Ry-operated channels are coexpressed in a single intracellular organelle (7), in contrast to other cell types where they appear segregated in two physically distinct Ca^{2+} stores. The physiological significance of the colocalization of IP3 and Cf/Ry channels in a unique store is obscure. According to different models, the periodic increases in the concentration of cytosolic Ca^{2+} ($[Ca^{2+}]_i$ oscillations), observed in many cells, requires two distinct stores (8, 9). In this respect it is of interest to notice that in PC12 cells $[Ca^{2+}]_i$ oscillations have never been observed. In contrast, in

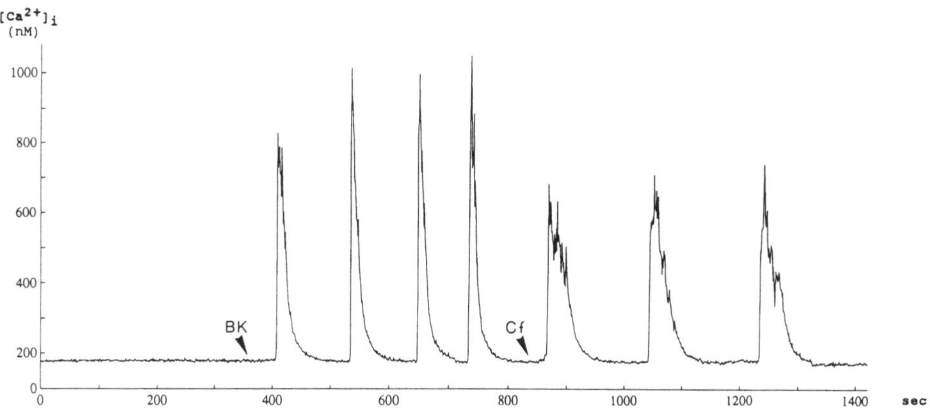

Figure 2. $[Ca^{2+}]_i$ oscillations evoked by 5 pM BK in a silent chromaffin cell. Addition of 2 mM caffeine modifies the pattern of single transients.

chromaffin cells, where the IP3 and Cf/Ry channels are reported to reside in separate stores, low doses of BK are able to induce $[Ca^{2+}]_i$ oscillations and caffeine modulates the kinetics of these repetitive spikes (Fig.2).

In view of the various mechanisms by which BK induces Ca^{2+} elevations in the cytosol, the possibility of different $[Ca^{2+}]_i$ distribution patterns, after application of the peptide, has been considered. Imaging results indicate that IP3-induced release from intracellular stores had the tendency to specifically occur in the soma of differentiated PC12 cells. Conversely, the receptor-mediated Ca^{2+} entry is mostly confined to the neurite like structures.

In conclusion, the direct measurement of $[Ca^{2+}]_i$ at subcellular level provides direct evidence of the activation of this intracellular messenger by BK. In addition, the intracellular topology of the $[Ca^{2+}]_i$ changes suggests that the effects of the peptide do not necessarily affect the whole cell but can probably induce diversified events in different cell areas.

ACKNOWLEDGEMENTS

We thank Guido Fumagalli, Cristina Fasolato, Emilio Clementi and Tullio Pozzan for their excellent collaboration in part of the studies summarized here. The work was supported by grants of the Consiglio Nazionale delle Ricerche, Target Project Biotechnology and Special Project Biology and Pathology of Ca^{2+}.

REFERENCES

1. Fasolato C, Pandiella A, Meldolesi J and Pozzan T. Generation of inositol phosphates, cytosolic Ca^{2+}, and ionic fluxes in PC12 cells treated with bradykinin. J Biol Chem 1988; 263:17350-17359.

2. Schweitzer E S and Kelly R B. Selective packaging of human growth hormone into synaptic vesicles in a rat neuronal (PC12) cell line. J Cell Biol 1985; 101:667-676.

3. Grohovaz F, Zacchetti D, Clementi E, Lorenzon P, Meldolesi J and Fumagalli G. $[Ca^{2+}]_i$ imaging in PC12 cells: multiple response patterns to receptor activation reveal new aspects of transmembrane signaling. J Cell Biol 1991; 113:1341-1350.

4. Grynkiewicz G, Poenie M and Tsien R Y. A new generation of Ca^{2+} indicators with greatly improved fluorescence properties. J Biol Chem 1985; 260:3440-3450.

5. Clementi E, Scheer H, Zacchetti D, Fasolato C, Pozzan T and Medolesi J. Receptor-activated Ca^{2+} influ⁎. Two independently regulated mechanisms of influx stimulation coexist in neurosecretory PC12 cells. J Biol Chem 1992; in press.

6. Pandiella A and Meldolesi J. Reinforcement of signal generation at B_2 bradykinin receptors by insulin, epidermal growth factors, and other growth factors. J Biol Chem 1989; 264: 3122-3130.

7. Zacchetti D, Clementi E, Fasolato C, Lorenzon P, Zottini M, Grohovaz F, Fumagalli G, Pozzan T and Meldolesi J. Intracellular Ca^{2+} pools in PC12 cells. J Biol Chem 1991; 266:20152-20158.

8. Berridge M J. Cytoplasmic calcium oscillations: a two pool model. Cell Calcium 1991; 12:63-72.

9. Meyer T and Streyer L. Calcium spiking. Ann Rev Biophys Byophis Chem 1991; 20:153-174.

AAS 38/II
Recent Progress on Kinins
© 1992 Birkhäuser Verlag Basel

MODULATION OF KININ RESPONSES IN HUMAN SYNOVIUM BY INTERLEUKIN-1

Joan M. Bathon, John E. Croghan, Daniel W. Goldman,
Donald W. MacGlashan and David Proud

The Johns Hopkins University School of Medicine,
Department of Medicine, Baltimore, MD, U.S.A.

SUMMARY: Bradykinin (BK) is a weak stimulus for prostaglandin E_2 (PGE_2) release in untreated human synovial cells, but a potent stimulus in interleukin-1 (IL-1) pretreated cells. The mechanism(s) by which IL-1 induces responsiveness of synovial cells to BK appears to be multifactorial. IL-1 not only upregulates the number of kinin receptors on these cells, but may also upregulate a calcium-dependent process involved in the synthesis of prostaglandins.

INTRODUCTION

Kinins have been implicated in the pathogenesis and/or propagation of inflammatory diseases of the joint, such as rheumatoid arthritis, by virtue of their abilities to induce vasodilation, edema and pain. Indeed, kinins have been demonstrated in the joint fluids of a variety of inflammatory joint diseases (1-3), and injection of bradykinin into canine joints induces an acute inflammatory response (3). It has been suggested that the proinflammatory properties of kinins are mediated, in part, by their ability to induce prostaglandin release from a variety of target cells and tissues (4-6). We have previously shown that, in contrast to its effect on other cell types, BK is an ineffective stimulus for PGE_2 release in untreated human synovial cells, but a potent one in IL-1 pretreated cells (7). The ability of IL-1 to induce responsiveness to BK showed relative physiological specificity for BK and lysylbradykinin (LBK), as evidenced by the lack of response of IL-1 pretreated cells to a variety of other peptide and nonpeptide, receptor-mediated agonists. In contrast, the nonreceptor-mediated, nonphysiologic agonist, calcium ionophore A23187, mimicked the response of BK, in that it was an ineffective stimulus for PGE_2 response in untreated cells but a potent stimulus in IL-1 treated cells.

These observations suggest that the mechanism by which IL-1 induces kinin responsiveness in human synovial cells is multifactorial. First, given the specificity of the enhanced responsiveness among receptor-mediated peptide agonists for kinins, we hypothesized that IL-1 may selectively upregulate the number or affinity of kinin receptors on synovial cells. Since kinin receptors have not been previously examined on any articular cells, we characterized the number, affinity and subtype of specific kinin binding sites on synovial cells and examined the effect of IL-1 on these parameters. Secondly, given the ability of IL-1 to synergize with A23187, we hypothesized that IL-1 may alter a calcium-dependent process involved in kinin-induced prostaglandin synthesis. IL-1 could either directly raise cytosolic calcium levels $[Ca^{2+}]_i$ or indirectly alter the ability of BK to raise $[Ca^{2+}]_i$. Alternatively, because prostaglandin synthesis is dependent upon one or more calcium-dependent enzymes, IL-1 may induce de novo synthesis of one of these enzymes, the activation of which would then occur following a BK-induced rise in $[Ca^{2+}]_i$. We have examined, therefore, the ability of BK to raise cytosolic calcium levels $[Ca^{2+}]_i$ in human synovial cells, as well as the specificity of this effect among other peptide and nonpeptide agonists. In addition, we have examined the effect of IL-1 pretreatment on agonist induced changes in $[Ca^{2+}]_i$.

MATERIALS AND METHODS

Synovial specimens were obtained from patients with rheumatoid arthritis (RA) and osteoarthritis (OA) at the time of surgical joint replacement. Homogenous, fibroblast-like populations of synovial cells were obtained by digestion with collagenase or growth from explants, as previously described (7), and grown to confluence in DMEM/20% FCS. Receptor binding experiments were performed in fourth passage cells in six-well culture dishes. PGE_2 and $[Ca^{2+}]_i$ experiments were performed in second to sixth passage cells in 24-well culture dishes.

Kinin binding studies were performed at 4°C on intact, confluent cells that had been previously treated with recombinant IL-1α (0.1 ng/ml) or vehicle for 24 hrs. Cells were washed with ice-cold isomolar PIPES buffer (pH 7.4) containing (g/l) PIPES, 7.7; NaCl, 6.4; KCl, 0.37; glucose, 1.0; and supplemented with 0.1% BSA, 0.1% sodium azide, bacitracin (0.1 mM), captopril (0.1 mM) and phosphoramidon (0.01 mM). The binding assay was initiated by the addition of [3H]BK (0.1-300 nM) in the presence or absence of 3 μM unlabeled BK. The incubation was terminated by washing with PIPES buffer. The cells were lifted with 0.25% trypsin and the radioactivity counted. Specific binding of [3H]BK was calculated by subtracting nonspecific binding (determined in the presence of 3 μM unlabeled BK) from total binding. Saturation studies of [3H]BK binding were analyzed by the nonlinear curve fitting program LIGAND (Elsevier-Biosoft, NY).

For $[Ca^{2+}]_i$ measurements, cells were loaded with Fura-2 AM (4 μM) for 60 min, washed and exposed to agonist for 3 min in calcium-containing buffer. Fluorescence intensities at 352 and 380 nm were monitored and recorded before and after stimulation, as previously described (8). Data were applied to the Tsien formula (9) to calculate cytosolic free calcium concentration. For PGE_2 experiments, cells were washed and exposed to agonist for 30 min. Supernatants were collected and assayed for PGE_2 by radioimmunoassay.

RESULTS

Binding of [^{3}H]BK to intact human synovial cells. Specific binding of [^{3}H]BK to human synovial cells was observed and was saturated at a concentration of 10 nM (Fig. 1). Scatchard transformation of the binding data from individual experiments yielded linear plots (data not shown). Concurrent analysis of all eight experiments using the LIGAND program was performed and data were best fit to a one-site model, yielding a K_d of 2.3 nM and B_{max} of 58 $\pm$ 9 fmol/10^6 cells (mean $\pm$ S.E.M.; range, 21-94 fmol/10^6 cells), corresponding to 34,000 $\pm$ 5,000 binding sites per cell. The specificity of the kinin binding site was examined by evaluating the potency of a series of peptide agonists and antagonists in displacing [^{3}H]BK (1 nM) from synovial cells. The following rank order potency was constructed (IC_{50}, nM): Hoe 140 (D-Arg^o-Hyp^3-Thi^5-D-Tic^7-Oic^8-BK), 3; LKB, 5; BK, 8; NPC 567 (D-Arg^o[Hyp^3, D-Phe^7]BK), 100; Des(Arg^9)BK, >1000; Leu^8-Des(Arg^9)BK, >1000; substance P, >1000; angiotensin II, >1000; neurokinins A and B, >1000. The ability of the B_2 receptor antagonists, Hoe 140 and NPC 567, and the lack of efficacy of the B_1 receptor antagonist, Leu^8-des(Arg^9)BK, in displacing [^{3}H]BK from synovial cells indicate the synovial cell binding site to be of the B_2 class of kinin receptors.

The effect of IL-1 on binding of [^{3}H]BK to human synovial cells was next evaluated. After establishing that IL-1 treatment (0.1 ng/ml for 24 hrs) did not alter the percentage of nonspecific binding to [^{3}H]BK, saturation binding studies on matched cells, that had been pretreated with IL-1 or vehicle, were performed. IL-1 treatment was associated consistently with a 1.5 2.0 fold increase in specific binding (Fig. 1). Scatchard analyses of data from individual experiments in IL-1 treated cells yielded linear plots similar to those for untreated cells (data not shown) and concurrent analysis of binding data from all IL-1 treated cells were again best fit to a one site model. Both individual and concurrent analysis by LIGAND of the five matched experiments indicated that the enhanced specific binding of [^{3}H]BK to IL-1 treated cells could be explained by an increase in B_{max} rather than a change in K_d. Thus, the average B_{max} for untreated vs. IL-1 treated cells were 53 $\pm$ 4 and 104 $\pm$ 24 fmol/10^6 cells, respectively ($p < .05$, Wilcoxon signed rank), whereas average K_d measured 1.8 and 1.3 nM, respectively (p value NS).

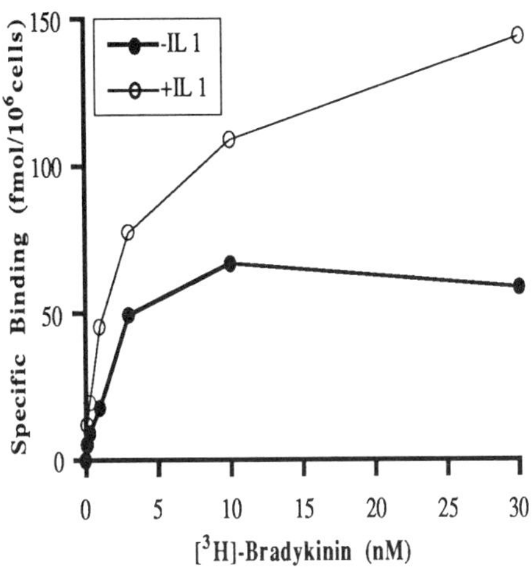

Fig. 1. Specific binding of [3H]BK to monolayers of synovial cells. Cells were pretreated with 0.1 ng/ml of IL-1 or control medium for 24 hrs. Binding of [3H]BK was performed as described in "Methods".

Functional characteristics of the kinin receptor on synovial cells.

PGE2 Production. Because we have already established that IL-1 treated, but not untreated, synovial cells respond to BK by releasing PGE2, we limited our evaluation of PGE2 responses to peptide agonists and antagonists to IL-1 treated cells. The specificity and rank order potencies of peptides in stimulating or inhibiting PGE2 release correlated well with their abilities to displace [3H]BK from synovial cells. Thus, BK and LBK were potent stimuli for PGE2 release (ED$_{50}$'s of 0.5 and 1.0 nM, respectively), while des(Arg^9)BK, substance P, angiotensin II and neurokinins A and B were ineffective stimuli (ED$_{50}$'s all >1000 nm) . Consistent with binding data indicating the synovial cell kinin receptor to be of the B$_2$ subtype, Hoe 140 was a potent inhibitor of BK-induced PGE2 release while Leu^8-des(Arg^9)BK was not (IC$_{50}$'s, 20 nM and >1000 nm, respectively).

Changes in [Ca^{2+}]$_i$. The ability of BK to raise [Ca^{2+}]$_i$, and the effect of IL-1 treatment on this response, was also evaluated. Baseline [Ca^{2+}]$_i$ in untreated cells, exposed to buffer alone, was 169 ± 14 nM (n=22). In contrast to its ineffectiveness in stimulating PGE2 release from untreated synovial cells, BK was a potent inducer of increased levels of [Ca^{2+}]$_i$ in these cells (ED$_{50}$ 1 nM; net maximal response 1.2 μM [Ca^{2+}]$_i$; n=4). LBK was equipotent to BK in inducing a rise in [Ca^{2+}]$_i$, while micromolar concentrations of des(Arg^9)BK, substance P and the nonpeptide agonist, platelet activating factor (PAF), were ineffective in this regard (Fig. 2).

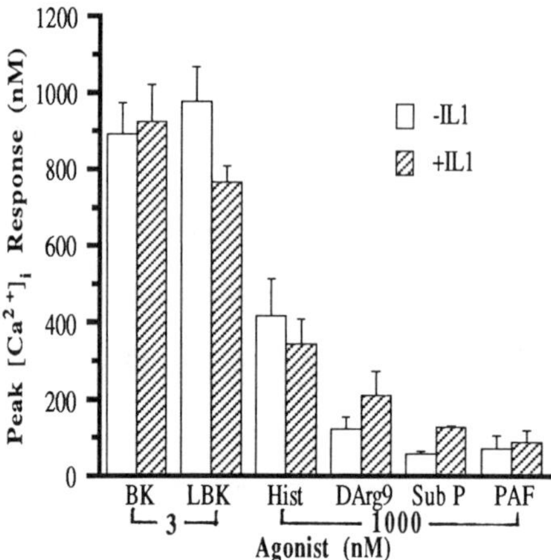

Fig. 2. Effect of peptide and nonpeptide agonists on synovial cell [Ca^{2+}]$_i$. Cells were pretreated with 0.1 ng/ml of IL-1 or vehicle for 24 hrs, washed and exposed to agonist (3 nM or 1 μM) for 3 min. [Ca^{2+}]$_i$ levels were measured as described in "Methods". Baseline [Ca^{2+}]$_i$ was subtracted from peak response and data expressed as net peak response.

Among the non-kinin, physiological stimuli examined, only histamine was capable of inducing a rise in [Ca^{2+}]$_i$, but this was modest and achieved only at micromolar concentration. Cells that were chronically exposed to IL-1 (24 hrs) exhibited slightly higher baseline [Ca^{2+}]$_i$ (214 ± 14 nM), compared to untreated cells (p < .0001, n=22). However, as shown in Fig. 2, they responded to BK, LBK, des(Arg^9)BK, histamine, substance P and PAF in a magnitude and manner similar to that of untreated cells. Consistent with a receptor-mediated event, the BK mediated increase in [Ca^{2+}]$_i$ was completely abolished by the B$_2$ kinin receptor antagonist, Hoe 140 (IC$_{50}$, 10 nM). Finally, a positive correlation (linear regression analysis, p < 0.05) between the ability of an agonist to induce PGE$_2$ production from, and to raise [Ca^{2+}]$_i$ in, synovial cells was observed. Thus, BK, at nanomolar concentration, was a potent stimulus for both PGE$_2$ and [Ca^{2+}]$_i$ increases while histamine, even at micromolar concentration, was only a weak stimulus for both parameters.

DISCUSSION

In these studies, we have demonstrated the presence, and upregulation by IL-1, of kinin receptors on cultured human synovial cells and have elucidated the role of these receptors in BK-mediated calcium and PGE$_2$ responses. BK is a potent stimulus for prostaglandin release from a variety of cells and tissues but is effective in this regard in human synovial cells only after pretreatment with IL-1. We were surprised, therefore, to identify a kinin binding site on these cells whose subtype (B_2), number (B_{max}, 34,000 binding sites per cell or 58 ± 9 fmol/10^6 cells) and affinity (K_d, 2.3 nM) were quite similar to those described for kinin receptors in other cells and tissues whose physiological responses to BK are not dependent upon IL-1 pretreatment (4-6). Although binding of BK to its receptor on untreated synovial cells was not associated with PGE_2 release, this site did appear to mediate BK-induced PGE_2 release from IL-1 treated cells, as evidenced by the similarity in values for BK's ED_{50} (0.5 nM) and K_d of binding, and by the similarity in rank order potencies of peptides for displacement of [^{3}H]BK and inhibition of PGE_2 production from synovial cells.

We hypothesized that one mechanism by which IL-1 may enhance kinin-induced PGE_2 release from synovial cells is by upregulation of kinin receptors on these cells. We have confirmed this hypothesis by the observation that IL-1 treatment of synovial cells induces a 1.5 - 2.0 fold increase in kinin receptor number, while no change in affinity is observed. This ability of IL-1 to upregulate kinin receptors could have broad implications for a variety of disease states, since it provides a mechanism whereby kinin responsiveness is amplified locally by products of the environmental milieu. This relatively modest increase in kinin receptor number is unlikely in synovial cells, however, to be the sole mechanism by which IL-1 promotes BK-induced PGE_2 release. Even without IL-1 treatment, synovial cells display approximately 36,000 binding sites per cell, a number in other cell types that is clearly sufficient to mediate physiological responses (10-12).

We hypothesized, therefore, that in addition to its effect of kinin receptors, IL-1 also alters a calcium-dependent process involved in kinin-induced prostaglandin synthesis. In accord with this hypothesis, the relative potency of an agonist in inducing PGE_2 production from synovial cells would be dependent upon its ability to raise $[Ca^{2+}]_i$ and, thereby, to activate a calcium-dependent enzyme involved in prostaglandin synthesis. IL-1 pretreatment could promote such an effect by directly raising $[Ca^{2+}]_i$ or by enhancing BK's capacity to raise $[Ca^{2+}]_i$. Alternatively, IL-1 may have no effect on $[Ca^{2+}]_i$, but may induce de novo synthesis of a prostaglandin-generating enzyme that is itself calcium-dependent (e.g., phospholipase A_2) or of an alternate enzyme that, although not calcium dependent (e.g., cyclooxygenase), acts in concert with the calcium-dependent enzyme activated by BK (e.g., phospholipase A_2) to synthesize prostaglandins. In these studies, we have confirmed the potent ability of kinins, but not a variety of other receptor-mediated peptide and nonpeptide agonists, to raise $[Ca^{2+}]_i$ in untreated human synovial cells. IL-1 pretreatment was associated with only a slight elevation in baseline $[Ca^{2+}]_i$ and, furthermore, did not alter the specificity or magnitude of the BK-induced calcium response, confirming that IL-1 and BK act at different sites to achieve their synergistic response. Finally, the potency of an agonist in inducing PGE_2 release from IL-1 treated synovial cells correlated well with its ability to elevate $[Ca^{2+}]_i$ in these cells. These data support the concept that an acute increase in $[Ca^{2+}]_i$ is not enough, in and of itself, to stimulate PGE_2 release from human synovial cells but that de novo synthesis of one or more prostaglandin-generating enzymes is a prerequisite. Current studies are aimed at the identification of the specific prostaglandin-generating enzyme(s) activated by BK and upregulated by IL-1.

REFERENCES

1.   Melmon KL, Webster ME, Goldfinger SE, Seegmiller JE. The presence of a kinin in inflammatory synovial effusions from arthritides of varying etiologies. Arthritis Rheum. 1967; 10:13-20.

2.   Jasani MK, Katori M, Lewis GP. Intracellular enzymes and kinin enzymes in synovial fluid in joint diseases. Ann Rheum Dis 1969; 28:497-511.

3.   Eisen V. Plasma kinins in synovial exudates. Br J Exp Pathol 1970; 51:322-327.

4.   Goldstein RH, Polgar P. The effect and interaction of bradykinin and prostaglandins on protein and collagen production by lung fibroblasts. J Biol Chem 1982; 257:8630-8633.

5.   Bareis DL, Manganiello VC, Hirata F, Vaughan M, Axelrod J. Bradykinin stimulates phospholipid methylation, calcium influx, prostaglandin formation and cAMP accumulation in human fibroblasts. Proc Natl Acad Sci USA 1983; 80:2514-2518.

6.   McIntyre TM, Zimmerman GA, Satoh K, Prescott SM. Cultured endothelial cells synthesize both platelet-activating factor and prostacyclin in response to histamine, bradykinin and adenosine triphosphate. J Clin Invest 1985; 76:271-280.

7.   Bathon JM, Proud D, Krackow K, Wigley FM. Preincubation of human synovial cells with IL-1 modulates prostaglandin E_2 release in response to bradykinin. J Immunol 1989; 143:579-586.

8.   MacGlashan DW Jr. Single-cell analysis of Ca^{++} changes in human lung mast cells: graded vs. all-or-nothing elevations after IgE-mediated stimulation. J Cell Biol 1989; 109:123-134.

9.   Grynkiewicz GM, Poenie M, Tsien RY. A new generation of Ca^{2+} indicators with greatly improved fluorescent properties. J Biol Chem 1985; 260:34040-3450.

10.   Innis RB, Manning DC, Stewart JM, Snyder SH. [3H]Bradykinin receptor binding in mammalian tissue membranes. Proc Natl Acad Sci USA 1981; 78:2630-2634.

11.   Roscher AA, Manganiello VC, Jelesma CL, Moss J. Receptors for bradykinin in intact cultured human fibroblasts. J Clin Invest 1983; 72:626-635.

12.   Snider RM, Richelson E. Bradykinin receptor-mediated cyclic GMP formation in a nerve cell population (murine neuroblastoma clone N1E-115). J Neurochem 1984; 43:1749-1754.

AAS 38/II
Recent Progress on Kinins
© 1992 Birkhäuser Verlag Basel

SIGNAL TRANSDUCTION PATHWAYS OF BK2 RECEPTOR IN THE RENAL GLOMERULUS AND MESANGIAL CELLS : A MINI REVIEW

J.P. Girolami, C. Emond and J.L. Bascands

INSERM U 133, Institut Louis Bugnard, Faculté de Médecine Rangueil, 31062 Toulouse Cedex, France

SUMMARY: Using binding techniques we identified specific B2 kinin binding sites showing a pharmacological profile similar in glomeruli and in mesangial cell. Scatchard analysis revealed two classes of binding sites : a very-high-affinity site (Kd =0.44 nM) and a high affinity site (Kd=6.3nM). Activation of the BK receptor of mesangial cells is associated with i) a transient dose-dependent increase in inositol 1,4,5 Triphosphate, ii) a biphasic rise in cytosolic free calcium, iii) a progressive secretion of PGE2, iv) an inhibition of the PGE2-stimulated increase of cAMP formation. All these effects were prevented by B2 antagonists. This multiple signal transduction pathway could suggest either heterogeneity in the BK receptor of the mesangial cell or different biological responses to be identified. Taken together, the results indicate that BK, at least in cultured cells, acts as a contractile effector, however, the physiological significance of a kinin receptor in the glomerulus remains to be elucidated.

INTRODUCTION

Nonapeptide bradykinin (BK) is a potent vasodilator, natriuretic and diuretic peptide (1). Such different properties suggest a wide variety in the mechanisms of action. In the kidney, the main locations of BK-binding sites are along the cortical and medullary tubules (2). It is likely that these collecting sites are involved in the diuretic and natriuretic effects of BK. On the other hand BK exhibit potent effects on glomerular haemodynamics, specially the reduction of the ultrafiltration coefficient as demonstrated by micropuncture studies (3). However, this has not, as yet, been associated with any pharmacological characterisation of bradykinin binding site in the glomerulus. On the basis of these considerations we looked for the presence of specific BK receptors in renal glomerulus and in mesangial cells (MCs) as these cells are in a key position in the glomerulus and could play a role in the regulation of the glomerular filtration rate. Furthermore MC dysfunction is also associated with the development of several renal diseases. Our recent results (4-8) bring complementary evidence for the presence of a BK2-receptor in the glomerulus and in MCs in culture. The characteristics of this newly identified BK receptor are reviewed here.

DISCUSSION

Identification of renal BK receptors with radioligands

The cellular location of the renal kinin receptors remains unclear in spite of a recent autoradiography study by Manning and Snyder (9) in which ^{3}H-bradykinin was used. Other specific radio-ligand binding studies have identified bradykinin receptor-like binding sites in the kidney (10). In isolated nephron segments of the rabbit, the major sites for kinin binding are the cortical and medullary collecting tubules (3). Bradykinin receptor-like binding has also been demonstrated in rat renomedullary interstitial cells (11). However, in all these studies, only the binding sites were characterized, and not the functional counterparts. Using iodinated Tyr_0-BK we have identified a specific binding site showing B2-receptor-like characteristics in crude glomerular preparations (4). The density of this binding site was decreased during low-sodium intake and water restriction (6), suggesting a down-regulation mechanism since the level of kallikrein activity was increased. This hypothesis is partly confirmed in the ischemic kidney of two-kidney, one clip Goldblatt hypertensive rat where the density of binding sites was increased and inversely correlated with the decrease in kallikrein activity (7).

Cellular localisation

The crude glomerular membrane preparation used for these binding studiesincluded cells of different : basement membranes and membranes from epithelial, endothelial and mesangial cells. We decided to investigate the possible presence of bradykinin binding sites in mesangial cells further because they represent about one third of the glomerular cell population and also because several receptors for other vasoactive hormones have been identified in these cells (12). Using the same binding system as with crude glomerular membranes we found specific BK binding in both membrane fractions from mesangial cells and in intact adherent cells (5). Scatchard analysis revealed two classes of binding sites. The specificity of the binding is that expected from a B2 receptor. The very-high-affinity site (Kd = 0.44 ± 0.2 nM) had the lower maximum density (B max = 11.7 ± 2.3 fmol/ mg prot) and the second site which is still a high-affinity site (Kd = 6.3 ± 2.5nM) had a higher B max = 112.3 ± 12.6 fmol/ mg prot .

Signal transduction pathways

In neuronal and smooth muscle cells activation of BK receptors is associated with intracellular calcium mobilisation (13-16). On the other hand, the BK receptor in endothelial cell is associated to cGMP production (17,18). Therefore these various pathways suggest that BK receptors can be involved either in cell contraction or relaxation depending on the cell type studied.

We have recently shown that, in MCs, BK induced a dose-dependent increase in inositol 1,4,5 trisphosphate (IP3) production inhibited by D-Arg-Hyp^3-D-Phe^7-BK but not by des-Arg^9-leu^8-BK (8). The production of IP3 was transient with a maximum formation after 30 sec whereas BK-induced IP3 production in fibroblasts was progressive and long lasting (19).

As expected from the effect of BK on IP3 formation, BK induced a dose-dependent increase in free cytosolic calcium ([Ca^{2+}]i) with an ED50 close to 8 nM. The rise in [Ca^{2+}]i demonstrated a classical biphasic profile consisting in a transient increase indicating the release of Ca^{2+} from intracellular stores followed by a sustained phase indicating the influx of extracellular medium (Fig 1). When the experiments were repeated in the absence of extracellul_r Ca^{2+}, only the transient release from intracellular stores persisted (Fig 3) which confirms the involvement of extracellular Ca^{2+} in the sustained phase. However the influx of extracellular Ca^{2+} was not inhibited by the usual voltage-dependent calcium channel inhibitors such nifedipine or verapamil. Therefore, the influx of extracellular calcium induced by BK is not mediated via voltage-dependent channels but probably via an as yet un-identified receptor-operated channel. The BK-induced increase in [Ca^{2+}]i is inhibited by the B2 antagonists, D-Arg-Hyp^3-D-Phe^7-BK, Thi$^{5-8}$- D-Phe^7-BK and HOE 140 and among those tested, HOE 140 was the most potent.

Challenging MCs with BK also resulted in dose-dependent secretion of PGE2 (5). The PGE2 production was inhibited by indomethacine. This BK effect also appears specific to the activation a B2 receptor as it is inhibited by Thi$^{5-8}$- D-Phe^7-BK and D-Arg-Hyp^3-D-Phe^7-BK .

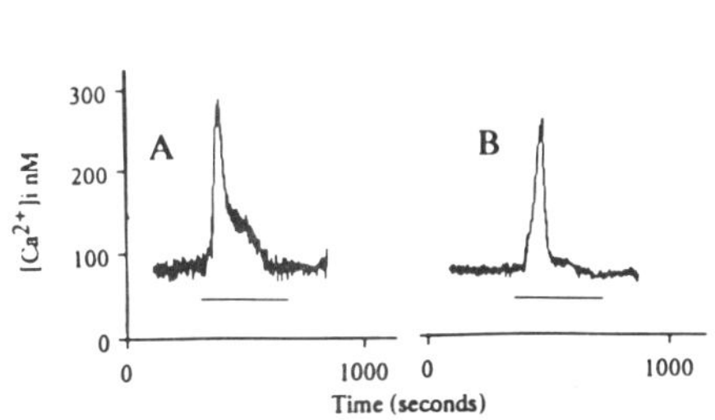

Figure 1. Effect of 10^{-7}M bradykinin on cytosolic free calcium ([Ca^{2+}]i) in monolayers of rat mesangial cells loaded with fura-2 AM in the presence (A) or absence (B) of extracellular Ca^{2+}

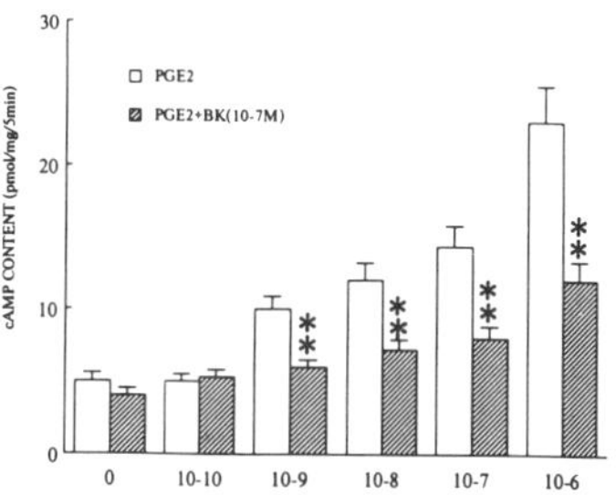

Figure 2. Effect of 10^{-7}M bradykinin on cAMP stimulation by increasing concentration of PGE2 in cultured rat mesangial cells. ** P< 0.01,when compared to the effect of PGE2 alone.

It has been suggested that the secretion of PGE2 by MCs could be interpreted a feed-back regulatory mechanism in response to a contractile agonist such as angiotensin II and arginine vasopressine (20). It is indeed well known that PGE2 acting through a Gs protein can stimulate the formation of cAMP a potent relaxant of MCs (20). We have tested this hypothesis by studing the interrelationship between PGE2 and BK on intracellular production of cAMP. As demonstrated in Fig 2, PGE2 induced a dose-dependent increase in cell cAMP content. The PGE2-induced rise in cAMP production is prevented in a dose-dependent manner by BK. The inhibitory effect of BK is completely prevented by preincubating the MCs with H7 a potent inhibitor of protein kinase C (PKC) suggesting a PKC-dependent mechanism. The same effects were confirmed using decapsulated isolated glomeruli.

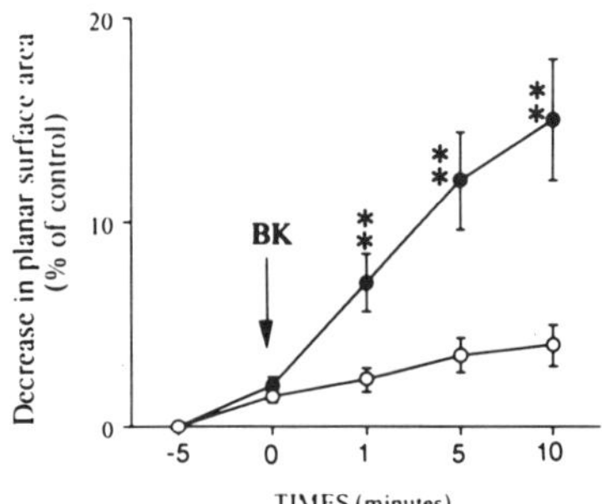

Figure 3. Effect of 10⁻⁷M bradykinin on the planar surface area of cultured rat mesangial cells estimated by image analysis . At the indicated time, the cell surface was compared to that of the same cell at the time 0 (control) and expressed as % of control. Results are mean±SE, (n=11) ; ** P< 0.01,when compared to time 0, Student' *t* test for paired samples.

Taken together, the data suggest that BK, at least, in cultured cell acts as a contractile effector. Using image analysis techniques we demonstrated that BK induced a rapid time-dependent contraction as shown in Fig 3. The reduction in average cell area was 8±3% after 1 min, and reached a 15± 5% maximum decrease after 15 min.

CONCLUSIONS AND PERSPECTIVES

In conclusion, on the basis of inhibition profiles of the antagonists tested, we bring evidence for the presence of a BK2 receptor in mesangial cells in culture. However the multiple transduction pathways summarized in Figure 4 (-i) activation of PLC, -ii) activation of PLA2, -iii) inhibition of adenylate cyclase) linked to activation of this receptor, is worth being discussed. This multiple transduction pathway suggests either a delicate cross-talk between the different signalling systems or a heterogeneity in the BK2 receptor family. These two hypotheses are presently under investigation. For the moment, however, time we cannot state, firstly, whether activation of the PLA2 pathway is a PLC-dependent mechanism as demonstrated in the fibroblast (9) and secondly, whether inhibition of the PGE2-induced cAMP increase results from a direct effect of PKC of the adenylate cyclase or on the coupling system.

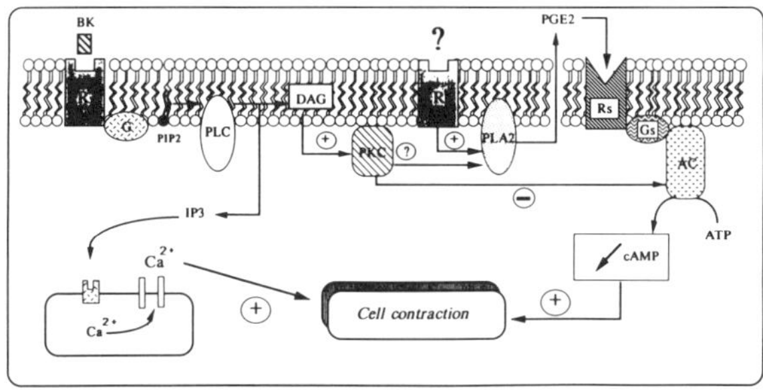

Figure 4. Signalling pathways activated by BK in rat mesangial cells.

Whether activation of the different signalling systems indicates activation of a single receptor or distinct receptors, as already suggested in fibroblasts (21), is an important point to be elucidated. It is nonetheless true that BK induces contraction of MCs in culture as well as in isolated glomeruli (Girolami, umpublished results). Furthermore the physiologcal role of this BK2 receptor in the glomerulus remains to be clarified and raises the question of the origin of endogenous BK. Considering the short biological life of kinin *in vivo*, release of kinin close to its site of action is the more likely hypothesis . It is true that these glomerular BK2 sites are upstream of the major well established site of kallikrein synthesis and release, i.e.the distal connecting tubule. Therefore, how can the generated kinins reach the glomerular sites? This would be possible if renal kallikrein was secreted at the basal surface and reached the cortical circulation via the interstitial space or via deep medullary circulation as already hypothetized (22). Also due to the nephron anatomy, a close proximity of afferent arteriole and distal granular cells revealed by kallikrein specific staining has been extensively documented and discussed (23). More recently the presence of kallikrein mRNA was demonstrated in the vascular pole of the glomerulus (24). Still more recently, the demonstration that endothelial cells in culture are able to release kinin (25) strongly suggests the existene of an endothelial kallikrein-kinin system which is consistent with previous data demonstrating a kallikrein-like enzyme in vascular walls (26,27). Therefore, although no clear-cut observations have established the presence of active kallikrein in the glomerulus, several reports indicate that the glomerular production of kinin is possible.

Beside this puitative glomerular effect, BK induced an increase in renal blood flow without any change in the filtration rate (28). These two last observations suggest that i) BK acts as a vasodilator at least at the afferent arteriole level, ii) a contraction of MCs could be interpreted as a regulatory feed-back mechanism to keep the filtration rate constant. However, this hypothesis implies that the BK2 receptor mediating the vasodilation of the afferent arteriole and the contraction of MCs, either acts through different signalling pathways, or cellular interactions. Since, in MCs, the BK2 receptor induces a biological response similar to that of contractile effectors such as angiotensin II, the teleology of the BK2 receptor in MCs may be especially important to consider under situations in which the AII receptor is poorly activated such as desensitization due to high concentration of AII or weak stimulation because of blunted AII formation during angiotensin converting enzyme inhibition therapy.

ACKNOWLEDGMENTS

The author acknowledges Professor D Regoli for the generous gift of BK analogs and the fruitfull discussions. HOE 140 was kindly provided by Hoechst A.G. The authors express their gratitude to Miss C. Pecher, Y.Cazenave for technical assistance

REFERENCES

1. Regoli D, Barabé J. Pharmacology of bradykinin and related kinins. Pharmacol Rev 1980 ; 32 : 1-46.

2. Tomita K, Pisano JJ. Binding of (3H) bradykinin in isolated nephron segments of the rabbit. Am J Physiol 1984 ; 246 : F732-F737.

3. Baylis C, Deen WM, Myers BD, Brenner BM. Effects of some vasodilator drugs on transcapillary fluid exchange in renal cortex. Am J Physiol 1976 ; 230 : 1148-1158.

4. Bascands JL, Pécher C, Cabos G, Girolami JP. B2-Kinin receptor like binding in rat glomerular membranes. Biochem Biophys Res Commun 1989 ; 154 : 99-104.

5. Emond C, Bascands JL, Pécher C, Cabos-Boutot G, Pradelles P, Regoli D, Girolami JP. Characterization of a B2-bradykinin receptor in rat renal mesangial cells. Eur J Pharmacol 1990 ; 190 : 381-392.

6. Emond C, Bascands JL, Cabos-Boutot G, Pécher C, Girolami JP. Effect of changes in sodium or water intake on glomerular B2-kinin-binding sites. Am J Physiol 1989 ; 257 : F353-F358.

7. Emond C, Bascands JL, Rakotoarivony J, Praddaude F, Bompart G, Pécher C, Ader JL, Girolami JP. Glomerular B2-kinin binding sites in two-kidney, one-clip hypertensive rats. Am J Physiol 1991 ; 260 : F626-F634.

8. Bascands JL, Emond C, Pécher C, Regoli D, Girolami JP. Bradykinin stimulates production of inositol (1,4,5) trisphosphate in cultured rat mesangial cells via B2-kinin receptor. British J Pharmacol 1991 ; 102 : 962-916.

9. Manning DC, Snyder SH. Bradykinin receptors localized by quantitative autoradiography in kidney, ureter and bladder. Am J Physiol 1989 ; 256 : F909-F915.

10. Innis R, Manning DC, Stewart JM, Snyder SH. [3H]Bradykinin receptor binding in mammalian tissues membranes. Proc Natl Acad Sci U.S.A.1981;78:2630-2634

11. Fredrick MJ, Abel FC, Righsel WA, Muirhead EE, Odya CE. B2-bradykinin receptor-like binding in rat renomedullary interstitial cells. Life Sci 1985 ; 37 : 331-338.

12. Pfeilschifter J. Cross-talk between transmembrane signalling system : a prerequisite for the delicate regulation of glomerular haemodynamics by mesangial cells. European J Clin Invest 1989 ; 19 : 347-363.

13. Reiser G, Binmöller FJ, Donié F. Mechanisms for activation and subsequent removal of cytosolic Ca^{2+} in bradykinin-stimulated neuronal and glial cell lines. Exp Cell Res 1990 ; 186 : 47-53.

14. Bleakman D, Thayer SA, Glaum SR, Miller RJ. Bradykinin-induced modulation of calcium signals in rat dorsal root ganglion neurons in vitro. Mol Pharm 1990 ; 38 : 785-796.

15. Fasolato C, Pizzo P, Pozzan T. Receptor-mediated calcium influx in PC12 cells. ATP and bradykinin activate two independent pathways. J Biol Chem 1990 ; 265 : 20351-20355.

16. Boyajian CL, Garritsen A, Cooper DMF. Bradykinin stimulates Ca^{2+} Mobilization in NCB-20 cells leading to direct inhibition of adenylylcyclase.J Biol. Chem 1991 ; 266 : 4995-5003

17. Boulanger C, Schini VB, Moncada S, Vanhoutte PM. Stimulation of cyclic GMP production in cultured endothelial cells of the pig by bradykinin, adenosine diphosphate, calcium ionophore A23187 and nitric oxide. Br J Pharmacol 1990 ; 101 : 152-156.

18. Schini VB, Boulanger C, Regoli D, Vanhoutte PM. Bradykinin stimulates the production of cyclic GMP via activation of B2 kinin receptors in cultured porcine aortic endothelial cells. J Pharmacol Exp Ther 1990 ; 252 : 581-585.

19. Burch RM, Axelrod J. Dissociation of bradykinin-induced prostaglandin formation from phosphatidylinositol turnover in Swiss 3T3 fibroblasts : evidence for G protein regulation of phospholipase A2. Proc Natl Acad Sci USA 1987 ; 84 : 6374-6378.

20. Mené P., Simonson MS., Dunn MJ. Pysiology of mesangial cell. Physiol.Rev. 1989; 69 : 1347-1411.

21. Roberts RA, Bradykinin receptors : characterization, distribution and mechanisms of signal transduction. Progress in Growth Factor Research 1989; 1 : 237-252.

22. Scicli AG, Carretero OA. Renal kallikrein-kinin system. Kidney Int. 29 : 120-130, 1986.

23. Barajas L, Powers K, Carretero OA; Scicli AG, Inagami T. Immunocytochemical localization of renin and kallikrein in rat cortex. Kidney Int. 29 : 965-970, 1986.

24. Xiong w, Chao J, Chao L. Renal kallikrein mRNA localization by in situ hybridization. Kidney Int. 35 : 1324-1329, 1989.

25. Wiemer G, Schölkens BA, Becker RHA, Busse R. Ramiprilat enhances endothelial autocoid formation by inhibiting breakdown of endothelium-derived bradykinin. Hypertension. 18 : 558-563, 1991.

26. Nolly H, Carretero OA, Scicli G. Madeddu P, Scicli AG. A kallikrein-like enzyme in blood vessels of one-kidney, one clip hypertensive rats. Hypertension. 16 : 436-440, 1990.

27. Oza NB, Schwartz JH, Giud D, Levinsky NG. Rat aortic smooth muscle cells in culture express kallikrein, kininogen, and bradykininase activity. J. Clin. Invest. 85 : 597-600, 1990.

28. Beierwaltes WH., Carretero OA, Scicli AG. Renal hemodynamics in response to a kinin analogue antagonist. Am. J. Physiol. 1988 ; 255 : F408-F414.

INFLUENCE OF DIABETES MELLITUS ON RENAL VASCULAR RESPONSES TO BRADYKININ

J. Quilley, D. Sarubbi, J.C. McGiff

Department of Pharmacology, New York Medical College, Valhalla, N.Y. 10595

SUMMARY: Streptozotocin-induced diabetes resulted in diminished vasodilator responses to bradykinin in the preconstricted isolated perfused kidney of the rat which were associated with decreased renal phospholipase A_2 activity and reduced release of PGE_2 into the renal venous effluent.

INTRODUCTION

In this study we addressed the effect of experimental diabetes on renal vasodilator responses to bradykinin as it related to phospholipase A_2 activity and release of prostaglandins. Bradykinin, as a vasodilator peptide, stimulates the release of arachidonic acid (AA), the metabolites of which may influence the resultant vascular effect (1). Moreover, diabetes has been associated with derangements of AA metabolism (2) which, in turn, may modify the responses to vasoactive hormones.

MATERIALS AND METHODS

Diabetes was induced in Male Wistar rats, age 6 weeks, with streptozotocin, 70 mg/kg i.v., and rats with blood glucose levels >350 mg/dL were used 3-4 weeks or 8-11 weeks later. Age-matched control rats received citrate buffer, pH 4.2. Following anesthesia with pentobarbitone, 65 mg/kg i.p., and midline laparotomy, the in situ right kidney was perfused at constant flow with oxygenated Kreb's buffer at 37°C. The vena cava was cannulated for collection of the renal venous perfusate and the ureter transected. Flow was adjusted to obtain a basal perfusion pressure of 70-90 mmHg and vascular tone was then elevated with phenylephrine in order to amplify vasodilator responses. Changes in perfusion pressure were recorded in response to randomized doses of bradykinin and in some experiments the renal venous effluent was collected for measurement of immunoassayable PGE_2.

In additional experiments, renal phospholipase A_2 activity was measured in subcellular fractions of the cortex, medulla and papilla by determining the release of labelled oleic acid from L-α-1-palmitoyl-2-oleoyl-[oleo-1-^{14}C]-phosphatidyl choline incubated in Tris buffer containing 5 mM $CaCl_2$ for 1h at 37°C.

RESULTS

Bradykinin (30-3000 ng) produced dose-dependent decreases in perfusion pressure in diabetic and control rat kidneys (Fig 1). However, the

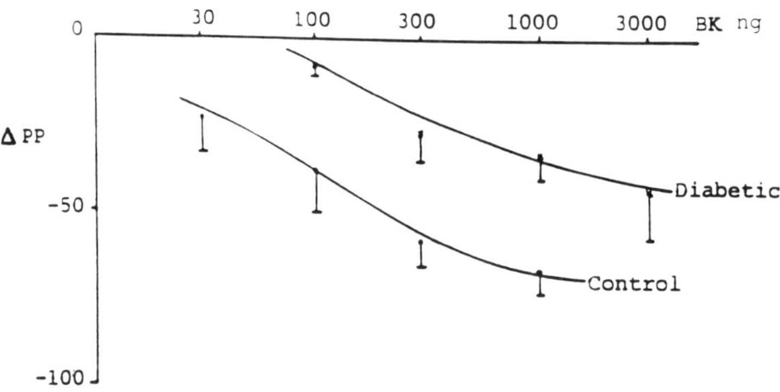

Fig 1.   BK-induced decreases in PP in kidneys from
diabetic and age-matched control rat kidneys

dose-response curve was shifted to the right for the diabetic rat kidneys, an effect independent of the duration of diabetes. Basal perfusion pressure for control and diabetic rat kidneys were 81±6 mmHg and 74±4 mmHg, respectively, whereas elevated perfusion pressures were 182±5 mmHg and 161±11 mmHg, respectively.

In rats with diabetes of 8-11 weeks duration, the release of immunoassayable PGE_2 in response to bradykinin was used as an index of AA release. Thus, we have previously shown that cyclooxygenase activity is increased in diabetic rat kidneys using conversion of exogenous AA as an index (3).

Bradykinin caused dose-dependent increases in the release of PGE_2 into the renal venous effluent of both control and diabetic rats (Fig 2). However, the stimulated release of PGE_2 was significantly less from the diabetic rat kidney and was associated with reduced phospholipase A_2 activity of the medulla and papilla (Fig 3).

DISCUSSION

This study demonstrates that renal vasodilator responses to bradykinin are reduced by diabetes which is also associated with diminished hormone-stimulated release of prostaglandins and decreased phospholipase A_2 activity. However, it has not been established whether decreased release of vasodilator AA metabolites contribute to the diminished renal vasodilator response to bradykinin which, in addition to stimulating the release of AA, also increases the release of EDRF or NO. In this regard, vasorelaxant responses to acetylcholine are also

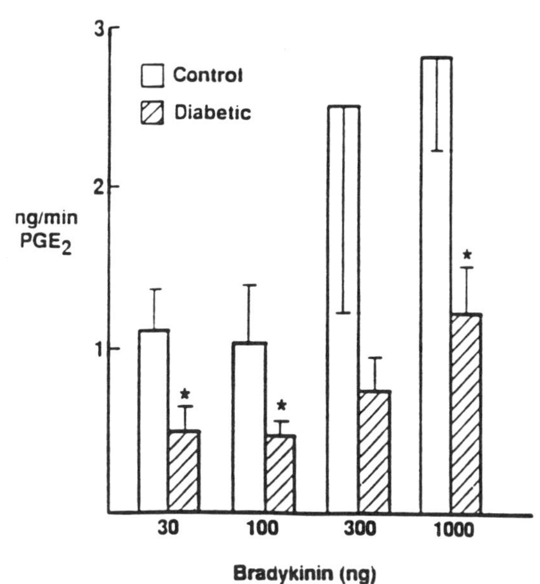

Fig 2.　BK-induced renal venous efflux of PGE_2 from kidneys of diabetic and age-matched control rats.

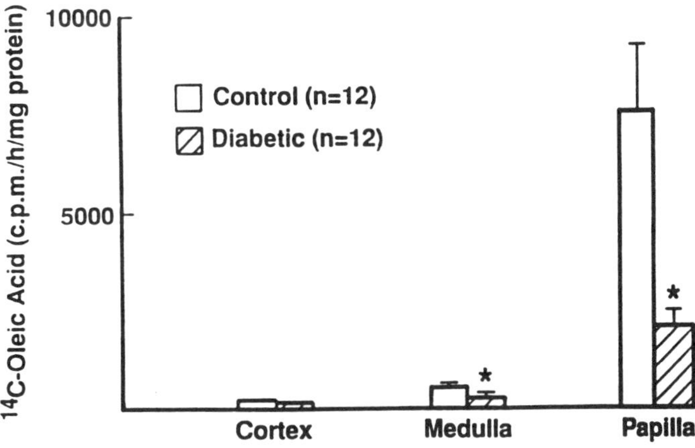

Fig. 3. Phospholipase A_2 activity in microsomal-mitochondrial fractions of renal cortex, medulla and papilla of diabetic and age-matched control rats.

diminished in diabetes (4), suggesting a defect in the synthesis or action of NO which could contribute to the reduced responsiveness to bradykinin that we have observed. Thus, the reduced vasodilation and prostaglandin release in response to bradykinin could be coincidental and reflect decreased receptor number or affinity, although the finding of reduced phospholipase A_2 activity in diabetes indicates that availability of AA would be reduced independently of changes in receptor characteristics. However, it is unlikely that reduced release of prostaglandins, which we have observed in response to other vasoactive hormones (5) contributes to the renal vasodilator effect of bradykinin in diabetic rats as indomethacin does not affect the renal vasodilator response to bradykinin in non-diabetic rats, suggesting that the response is independent of cyclooxygenase products (6). Nonetheless, a role of AA metabolites generated via other pathways cannot be excluded and is consistent with our observations that show that availability, but not conversion, of AA is reduced by diabetes.

CONCLUSION

Experimental diabetes mellitus in the rat results in impaired renal vasodilator responses to bradykinin that are associated with reduced release of prostaglandins, possibly resulting from diminished renal phospholipase A_2 activity.

ACKNOWLEDGEMENTS. This work was supported by National Institutes of Health Grants 5R01-HL-25394 and 5P01-HL-34300. We thank Jennifer Jones for typing the manuscript.

REFERENCES

1. McGiff, J.C., Quilley, J. Prostaglandins act as modulators and mediators of the vascular and renal actions of kinins. In: Role of Chemical Mediators in the Pathophysiology of Acute Illness and Injury. Edited by R. McConn, Raven Press, New York, p.37-44, 1982.

2. Quilley, J., McGiff, J.C. Arachidonic acid metabolism and urinary excretion of prostaglandins and thromboxane in rats with experimental diabetes mellitus. J. Pharmacol. Exptl. Ther. 234:211-216, 1985.

3. Quilley, J., McGiff, J.C. Renal vascular responsiveness to arachidonic acid in experimental diabetes. Br. J. Pharmacol. 100:336-340, 1990.

4. Oyama, Y., Kawasaki, H., Hutton, Y., Kanno, M. Attenuation of
    endothelium-dependent relaxation in aorta from diabetic rats. Eur. J.
    Pharmacol. 131:75-78, 1986.

5. Sarubbi, D., McGiff, J.C., Quilley, J. Renal vascular responses and
    eicosanoid release in diabetic rats. Am. J. Physiol. 257:F762-F768, 1989.

6. Cachofeiro, V., Nasjletti, A. Increased vascular responsiveness to
    bradykinin in kidneys of spontaneously hypertensive rats: effects of
    N^W-nitro-L-arginine. Hypertension 18:683-688, 1991.

AAS 38/II
Recent Progress on Kinins
© 1992 Birkhäuser Verlag Basel

BRADYKININ-MEDIATED METABOLIC EFFECTS IN ISOLATED PERFUSED RAT HEARTS

B.A. Schoelkens and W. Linz

Hoechst AG, W-6230 Frankfurt/Main, Germany

SUMMARY: Bradykinin perfusion (BK $1x10^{-12}$ to $1x10^{-8}$ mol/l) of isolated working rat hearts with postischemic reperfusion arrhythmias induced a reduction of the incidence as well as duration of ventricular fibrillation, improvement of cardiodynamics via increased left ventricular pressure, contractility, and coronary flow without changes in heart rate. These beneficial effects were accompanied by reduced activities of the cytosolic enzymes lactate dehydrogenase and creatine kinase as well as lactate output. In the myocardial tissue lactate content was reduced and the energy rich phosphates increased compared to saline perfused control hearts. Glycogen stores were also preserved. These beneficial effects of BK were concentration-dependently abolished by perfusion of the B_2 kinin receptor antagonist HOE 140 and the nitric oxide (NO) synthase inhibitor N^G-nitro-L-arginine (L-NNA).

These results suggest that improved cardiac function during and after myocardial ischemia as well as increased energy rich phophates and glycogen stores are mediated by BK and the subsequent release of NO, shifting myocardial metabolism during ischemia and reperfusion to the glucose pathway which leads to changes indicative for cardioprotection.

INTRODUCTION

The myocardium utilizes a variety of substrates for generating energy. The most significant of these are glucose, free fatty acids, lactate and pyruvate (1). It was reported that BK increased nutritional flow and glucose oxidation in normoxic isolated rat hearts (2) and it is known that glucose may be beneficial in reperfusion-induced arrhythmias (3).

To characterize BK-mediated metabolic effects in the ischemic myocardium, isolated working rat hearts were subjected to local ischemia by occlusion of the left coronary artery followed by reperfusion.

MATERIALS AND METHODS

Isolated working rat heart preparations from Wistar rats of either sex weighing 280-300 g were used in all experiments (4). They were perfused with Krebs-Henseleit buffer for an initial 20-min period (preischemic period). Thereafter, acute regional myocardial ischemia was produced by occluding the left coronary artery close to its origin for 15 min (ischemic period). The clip was then reopened, and changes during reperfusion were monitored for 30 min (reperfusion period). During the preischemic, ischemic and reperfusion period the venous effluent was sampled to determine lactate output and the activities of the cytosolic enzymes lactate dehydrogenase and creatine kinase. At the end of the experiment the hearts were stored in liquid nitrogen to measure the myocardial tissue content of lactate, glycogen, and the energy rich phosphates ATP and creatine phosphate. Via a balloon catheter placed in the left ventricle cardiodynamics such as left ventricular pressure, contractility, (dP/dt_{max}), heart rate, and coronary flow were recorded continuously. To evaluate the specificity of BK-mediated effects the new B_2 kinin receptor antagonist HOE 140 (5) was used. Furthermore the NO-synthase inhibitor L-NNA was tested to evaluate the role of NO-formation in these BK-mediated effects in isolated perfused rat hearts.

RESULTS

Perfusion with BK in concentrations of 1×10^{-12} up to 1×10^{-8} mol/l induced a marked reduction of the incidence as well as duration of ventricular fibrillation. The concentration of 1×10^{-10} mol/l which had no influence on coronary flow already attenuated reperfusion arrhythmias. In parallel with the abolition of ventricular fibrillation an improvement of cardiodynamics via increased left ventricular pressure, dP/dt_{max} and coronary flow without changes in heart rate could be observed starting with concentrations of 1×10^{-9} mol/l, when compared with the vehicle perfused control hearts. These beneficial effects were accompanied by reduced activities of the cytosolic enzymes lactate dehydrogenase and creatine kinase as well as lactate output during the ischemic and reperfusion period. In myocardial tissue BK-mediated metabolic changes occur already with concentrations of 1×10^{-12} mol/l.

Investigations on the metabolic states during different time points of our experiments demonstrated a significant decrease of glycogen, ATP and creatine phosphate, and a significant increase of lactate in myocardial tissue samples taken during the preischemic and ischemic period in comparison to tissue controls of freshly prepared preparations (Fig. 1). Perfusion of ischemic hearts with BK (1×10^{-10} mol/)l improved all mentioned metabolic parameters to values measured in the freshly prepared preparations (Fig. 1).

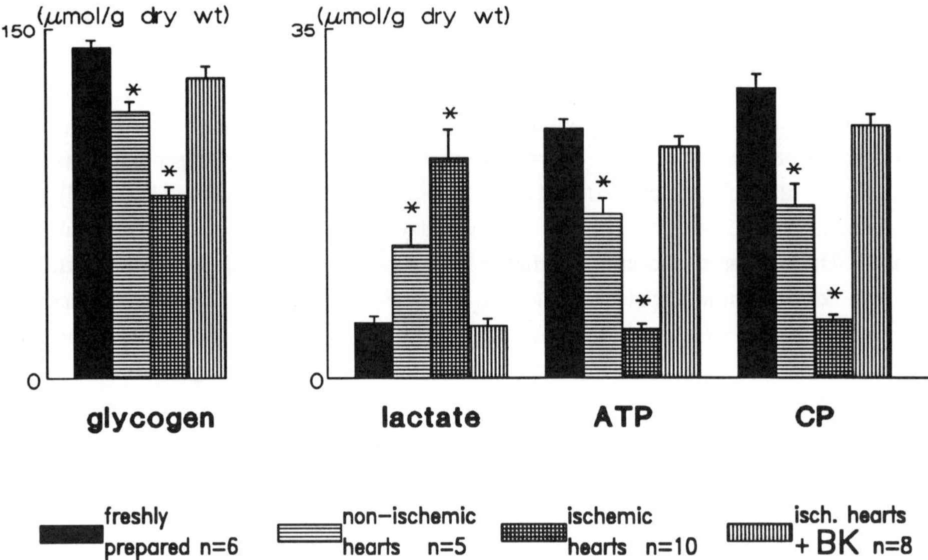

Figure 1. Effects of bradykinin (BK) perfusion ($1x10^{-10}$ mol/l) on glycogen, lactate, ATP and creatine phosphate (CP) in isolated ischemic working rat hearts in comparison to freshly prepared and non-ischemic hearts. $*p < 0.05$ vs freshly prepared hearts

Surprisingly perfusion of ischemic rat hearts with the angiotensin converting enzyme (ACE) inhibitor ramiprilat led to an almost identical fingerprint of metabolic changes, suggesting that inhibition of kininase II, synthesized by endothelial cells and localized on their luminal surface, results in attenuation of BK degradation with the subsequent metabolic changes.

Addition of the B_2 kinin receptor antagonist HOE 140 or of the NO-synthase inhibitor L-NNA to the perfusion medium abolished the BK-mediated effects in the heart (Fig. 2,3).

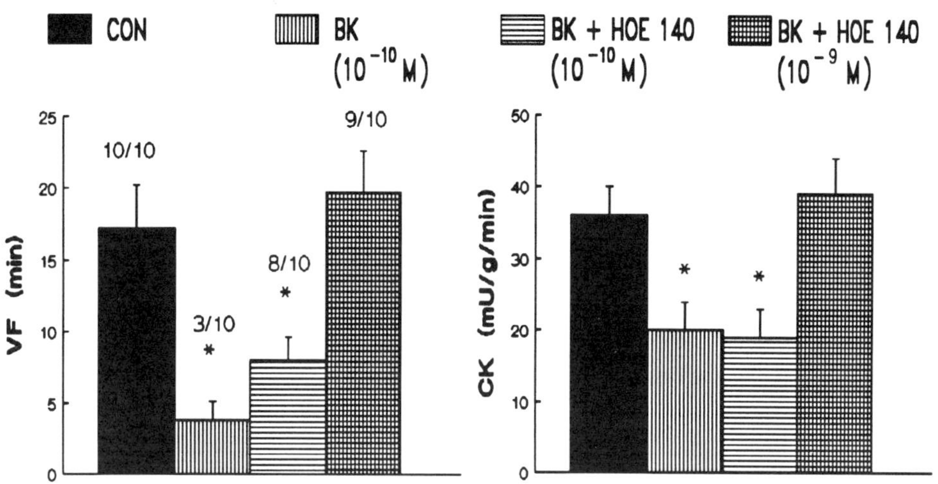

Figure 2. Effects of bradykinin (BK 1x10^{-10} mol/l) perfusion alone, and in combination with HOE 140 (1x10^{-10} and 1x10^{-9} mol/l) on ventricular fibrillations (VF) and creatine kinase (CK) release in isolated ischemic working rat hearts.
*$p < 0.05$ vs control hearts perfused with Krebs-Henseleit solution

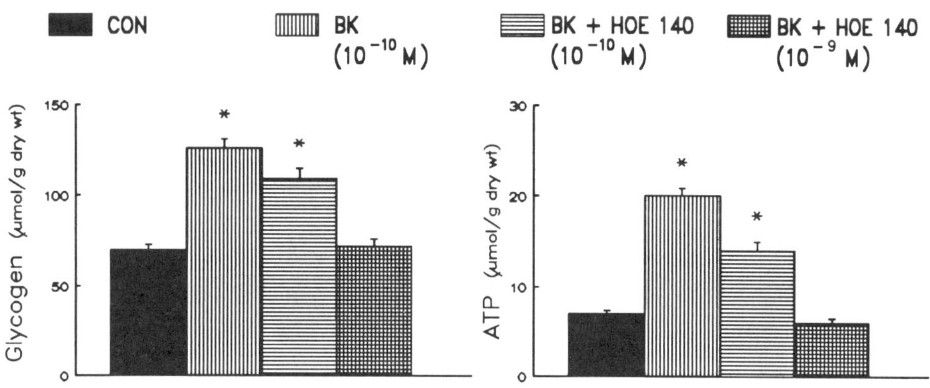

Figure 3. Effects of bradykinin (BK 1x10^{-10} mol/l) perfusion alone, and in combination with HOE 140 (1x10^{-10} and 1x10^{-9} mol/l) on glycogen and ATP stores in isolated ischemic working rat hearts. *$p < 0.05$ vs control hearts perfused with Krebs-Henseleit solution.

DISCUSSION

Earlier studies in anesthetized dogs with occlusion-reperfusion injuries showed comparable beneficial metabolic changes following intracoronary infusion of BK (6). BK in low concentrations reduced myocardial tissue lactate content and increased energy rich phosphates and glycogen stores compared to vehicle perfused control hearts. These BK-mediated metabolic changes in ischemic myocardial tissue occur with concentrations of 1×10^{-12} mol/l, which are without influence on cardiodynamic parameters. Changes in these parameters are usually observed when using concentrations of 1×10^{-9} mol/l of BK. Thus changes in metabolic parameters appear with BK-concentrations three orders of magnitude lower than those needed to induce cardiodynamic changes.

The action of higher concentrations of BK could be explained by enhanced coronary flow which stimulates cardiac afferent sympathetic nerves and increases myocardial contractility (7), and coronary hyperperfusion with concomitant enhancement of mechanical function, increased glucose transport as well as fatty acid utilization in isolated intact rat hearts (8). The action of lower concentrations of BK went along with favorable metabolic effects optimizing nutritional flow across the capillary wall which in turn leads to an elevated glucose uptake in the isolated rat hearts (2). In our studies with isolated rat hearts with postischemic reperfusion injuries, the BK-mediated effects can be coined as "cardioprotective", if one defines cardioprotection as the beneficial effects of agents on the structure, function and metabolism of the heart. An important part of this protective effect are metabolic changes, suggesting that BK is able to shift myocardial metabolism during ischemia and reperfusion to the glucose pathway, which in turn leads to changes indicative for a cardioprotective potential. Glucose protects against potassium loss during ischemia and improves the characteristics of the action potential of papillary muscles (9,10). Especially ATP originating from glycolysis may play a crucial role in membrane electrophysiology and stability of the ischemic heart (3,11). By this way isolated rat hearts perfused with glucose exhibited fewer reperfusion arrhythmias than hearts perfused with acetate or palmitate, suggesting that the substrate used before reperfusion may affect the incidence of arrhythmias during reperfusion (12).

Both BK and the ACE inhibitor produced a comparable spectrum of changes indicating at least in part a common mechanism of action. Most probably the BK effects were mediated via stimulation of B_2 kinin receptors, and the release of an endothelium-dependent relaxing factor that may be NO. Studies in cultured bovine and human endothelial cells have shown that addition of BK or the local inhibition of ACE led to increased NO formation, assessed by endothelium cyclic GMP- and prostacyclin synthesis (13). Increased cyclic GMP may improve the energy state resulting in high emergy rich phosphates in isolated rat hearts after reperfusion (14), and for prostacaclin was protective in ischemic rat hearts with postischemic reperfusion arrhythmias (15).

CONCLUSION

Perfusion with BK induced beneficial metabolic effects in isolated ischemic working rat hearts, accompanied by a reduction of postischemic ventricular arrhythmias, a reduction of the release of cytosolic enzymes and an improvement in cardiodynamics. These BK effects were probably mediated via stimulation of endothelial B_2 kinin receptors and the release of an endothelium-derived relaxing factor that may be NO.

REFERENCES

1. Scheuer J. Myocardial metabolism in cardiac hypoxia. Am J Cardiol 1967; 19:385-392.

2. Rösen P, Eckel J, Reinauer H. Influence of bradykinin on glucose uptake and metabolism studied in isolated cardiac myocytes and isolated perfused rat hearts. Hoppe Seylers Z Physiol Chem 1983; 364:431-438.

3. Bricknell OL, Opie LH. Effects of substrates on tissue metabolic changes in the isolated rat heart during underperfusion and on release of lactate dehydrogenase and arrhythmias during reperfusion. Circ Res 1978; 43:102-115.

4. Linz W, Schölkens BA, Han YF. Beneficial effects of the converting enzyme inhibitor, ramipril, in ischemic rat hearts. J Cardiovasc Pharmacol 1986; 8(Suppl 10):S91-S99.

5. Wirth K, Hock FJ, Albus U, Linz W, Alpermann HG, Anagnostopoulus H, Henke St, Breipohl G, König W, Knolle J, Schölkens BA. HOE 140 a new potent and long acting bradykinin-antagonist: in vivo studies. Br J Pharmacol 1991;102:774-777.

6. Linz W, Martorana PA, Schölkens BA. Local inhibition of bradykinin degradation in ischemic hearts. 1990; J Cardiovasc Pharmacol 15(Suppl 6):S99-S109.

7. Munch PA, Longhurst JC. Bradykinin increases myocardial contractility: relation to the Gregg phenomenon. Am J Physiol 1991; 260:R1095-R1103.

8. Miller WP, Shimamoto N, Nellis S, Liedtke AJ. Coronary hyperperfusion and myocardial metabolism in isolated and intact hearts. Am J Physiol 1987; 253:1271-1278.

9. Burke WM, Asokan SK, Moschos CB, Oldewurtel HA, Regan TJ. Effect of glucose and non-glucose perfusion on myocardial potassium ion transfer and arrhythmia during ischemia. Am J Cardiol 1969; 24:713-722.

10. MacLeod DP, Prasad K. Influence of glucose on the transmembrane action potential of papillary muscle. J Gen Physiol 1969; 53:792-815.

11. Opie LH. The glucose hypothesis: relation to acute myocardial ischemia. J Mol Cell Cardiol 1970; 1:107-116.

12. Bernier M, Hearse DJ. Reperfusion-induced arrhythmias: mechanisms of protection by glucose and mannitol Am J Physiol 1988; 254:H862-H870.

13. Wiemer G, Schölkens BA, Becker RHA, Busse R. Ramiprilat enhances endothelial autacoid formation by inhibiting breakdown of endothelium-drived bradykinin. Hypertension 1991; 18:558-563.

14. Vuorinen P, Laustiola K, Metsä-Ketelä T. The effects of cyclic AMP and cyclic GMP on redox state and ernergy state in hypoxic rat atria. Life Sci 1984; 35:155-161.

15. Linz W, Schölkens BA, Kaiser J, Just M, Bei-Yin Q, Albus U, Petry P. Cardiac arrhythmias are ameliorated by local inhibition of angiotensin formation and bradykinin degradation with the converting-enzyme inhibitor ramipril. Cardiovasc Drugs Therap 1989; 3:873-882.

INVOLVEMENT OF BRADYKININ-INDUCED $[Ca^{2+}]i$ OSCILLATIONS IN PHOSPHATIDYLCHOLINE BREAKDOWN IN K-*ras*-TRANSFORMED FIBROBLASTS

Tao Fu, Yukio Okano and Yoshinori Nozawa

Department of Biochemistry, Gifu University School of Medicine, Gifu 500, Japan

SUMMARY: Bradykinin (BK) induced a biphasic 1,2-diacylglycerol production in both K-*ras*-transformed (DT) cells and its parent NIH3T3 cells. The first phase was coincident with the transient phospho-inositide turnover and the second sustained phase was derived from hydrolysis of phosphatidylcholine (PC). In DT cells, the PC breakdown was considerably due to phospholipase C and dependent on intracellular calcium oscillations.

INTRODUCTION

The *ras* proto-oncogenes encode highly conserved, membrane-associated low molecular GTP-binding proteins which are thought to be important in the pathways regulating cell proliferation and differentiation (1). Genes with point mutations encode modified proteins (v-*ras*) which are resistant to inactivation by GTPase-activating protein (2) and causes sustained activation of unknown *ras* targets, leading to oncogenic transformation. Recently, we have found that bradykinin (BK), bombesin and fetal calf serum (FCS) induced $[Ca^{2+}]i$ oscillations in K-*ras*-transformed DT cells, but not in the parent NIH3T3 cells (3). Electrophysiological investigations revealed that BK-induced oscillations of membrane potentials were associated with $[Ca^{2+}]i$ oscillations in cells expressing transforming H-*ras* oncogene (4). On the other hand, it has been reported that v-*ras* oncogene products enhance the activity of a phospatidylcholine-specific phospholipase C (PC-PLC) (5), which produces the elevated level of DG, an endogeneous activator of protein kinase C (6), and a sustained increase in DG has been suggested to be essential to the maintenance of the transformed phenotype (7). However, the precise mechanism by which the *ras* proteins modulate the phospholipid metabolism has not yet been disclosed.

In this study, to address further the mechanism involved, we examined the effect of BK-induced $[Ca^{2+}]i$ changes on phospholipid metabolism in K-*ras*-transformed cells and discussed the role of PC breakdown in the growth signal transduction.

MATERIALS AND METHODS

Fura-2/AM and fura-2 were purchased from Dojin Laboratories (Kumamoto, Japan), BK from Sigma Chemical Co. (St. Louis, MO, USA); [methyl-^{3}H]choline chloride (85 Ci/mmol) from American Radiolabeled Chemical (St. Louis, MO, USA); [9,10-^{3}H]myristic acid (39.3Ci/mmol) was from Du Pont-New England Nuclear; silica gel LK6D from Whatman Chemical Separation Inc (Clifton, NJ, USA) and silica gel 60 plates were from Merck (Darmstadt, Germany). All other chemicals were obtained from commercial sources and were of the highest quality available.

Cell cultures. DT cells and the parent NIH3T3 cells were grown in Dulbecco's modified Eagle's medium (DMEM, Gibco, Grand Island, NY, USA) supplemented with 10% FCS. Special care was taken to maintain the cell lines at subconfluent densities at all times. For BK stimulation, cells were cultured in DMEM containing 10% FCS for 48 h and then in DMEM containing 1% FCS for another 48 h prior to adding the agonist.

Intracellular calcium assay in cell population and in single cells. $[Ca^{2+}]i$ was measured in fura-2-loaded cells as described previously (3, 8).

Extraction and analysis of choline metabolites from cells labeled with [^{3}H]choline. For the quantification of cellular choline and phosphocholine levels, the aqueous phases from methanolic extracts of [methyl-^{3}H]choline-labeled cells were fractionated by thin-layer chromatography with the following solvent system: methanol/0.5% NaCl/28% NH_3 (50:50:1, by volume) (9). The standards corresponding to the different water-soluble metabolites were cochromatographed and identified with iodine vapour.

Measurements of mass content of DG and activity of protein kinase C (PKC). The cellular DG contents and PKC activities were measured as described previously (3, 8).

RESULTS

<u>Effects of BK on phospholipid metabolism</u>

BK induced a biphasic DG production in both DT cells and the parent NIH3T3 cells; the first phase was coincident with the rapid and transient increase in inositol 1,4,5-trisphosphate (IP$_3$) and the second sustained phase, peaked at 3 min after adding BK (100 nM) and lasted for several hours, was derived from hydrolysis of PC (10).

In NIH3T3 cells, BK elicited a greater production of choline rather than phosphocholine in [^{3}H]choline-labeled cells and the significant phosphatidylethanol (PEt) formation in the presence of ethanol in the [^{3}H]myristic acid-labeled cells, suggesting that the breakdown of PC was at least in part due to the phospholipase D (PLD). Similar results were reported in BK-stimulated human fibroblasts by Blitterswijk *et al* (11). However, in DT cells, BK induced predominantly phosphocholine generation and little PEt formation, indicating the involvement of PLC-mediated PC breakdown.

When NIH3T3 cells were pretreated with an inhibitor of phosphatidic acid (PA)-phosphohydrolase propranolol (200 μM for 10 min), the second peak of DG formation induced by BK was decreased by 67.4%. Since DG kinase(s) in fibroblasts has been reported to prefer as substrate DG from phosphoinositide to that from PC, we suggest that in BK-stimulated NIH3T3 cells PC is mainly hydrolyzed by PLD. In the same condition, however, the second peak of DG formation in DT cells was not inhibited by propranolol, thus supporting a distinct pathway of PC breakdown in response to BK.

BK-induced $[Ca^{2+}]i$ oscillations in DT cells

Digital image analyses of fura-2-loaded DT cells revealed BK-induced $[Ca^{2+}]i$ oscillations, whereas the initial transient $[Ca^{2+}]i$ responses were observed in NIH3T3 cells (3). When BK-induced $[Ca^{2+}]i$ rises were examined for cell suspension, the oscillations in DT cells were detected as a sustained $[Ca^{2+}]i$ elevation following the initial $[Ca^{2+}]i$ spike. The long-lasting $[Ca^{2+}]i$ oscillations (for at least 2 h after BK-stimulation), could be terminated by removing either the agonist or the extracellular Ca^{2+} by adding EGTA from the assay media. Voltage-clamp recording of BK-stimulated DT cells revealed oscillatory inward currents which were considered to be generated by influxes of divalent cations to maintain $[Ca^{2+}]i$ oscillations in the cells (12).

Effects $[Ca^{2+}]i$ oscillations on phosphatidylcholine breakdown in DT cells

Pretreatment with EGTA (1 mM for 3 min) completely abolished the BK-induced $[Ca^{2+}]i$ oscillations as well as the second sustained DG formation in DT cells. In addition, a receptor-operated Ca^{2+} channel blocker, SK&F 96365 (13), prevented the BK-induced inward current oscillations as well as $[Ca^{2+}]i$ oscillations without affecting the unstimulated level and the initial $[Ca^{2+}]i$ spike. The blocker dose-dependently suppressed the BK-induced sustained $[Ca^{2+}]i$ elevation due to the $[Ca^{2+}]i$ oscillations and the phosphocholine generation as well as the second peak of DG production in DT cells (data not shown). However, this drug did not affect the BK-induced $[Ca^{2+}]i$ response and formation of $[^3H]$choline metabolites in NIH3T3 cells. The results suggest possible association of $[Ca^{2+}]i$ oscillations with the activation of PC-PLC in DT cells.

DISCUSSION

According to our findings obtained here, together with those of other investigators, we like to propose the hypothetical models for BK-mediated signal transduction in K-*ras*-transformed (DT) and nontransformed NIH3T3 cells (Figure 1). In NIH3T3 cells, the interaction of BK with its receptor (BK-R) stimulates hydrolysis of phosphatidylinositol 4,5-bisphosphate (PIP_2) by a GTP-binding protein-coupled PLC, thus leading to the generation of IP_3 and DG. The former facilitates Ca^{2+}-release from intracellular storage sites (14), and the latter promotes activation of PKC which may inhibit Ca^{2+} influx through the plasma membrane (3, 6). On the other hand, activation of PKC in NIH3T3 cells enhances the activity of PC-PLD to produce choline and PA. The latter product PA is further converted to DG by PA-phosphohydrolase, since propranolol an inhibitor of the

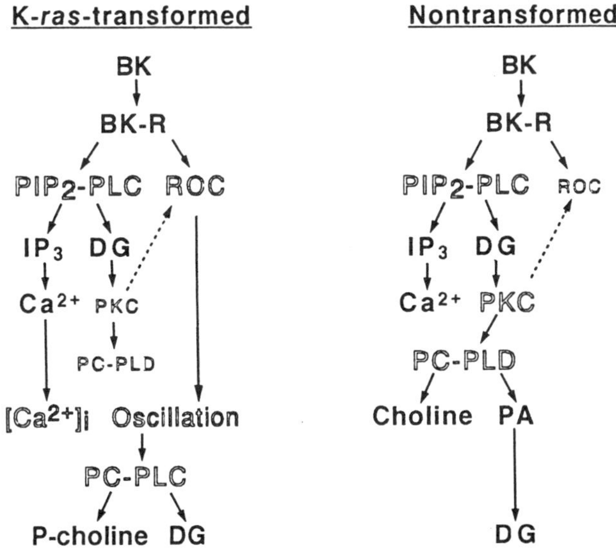

Figure 1. The hypothetical models for BK-mediated signal transduction in K-*ras*-transformed (DT) and nontransformed (NIH3T3) cells.

BK, bradykinin; BK-R, BK receptor; DG, 1,2-diacylglycerol; IP_3, inositol 1,4,5-trisphosphate; PC, phosphatidylcholine; P-choline, phosphocholine; PIP_2, phosphatidylinositol 4,5-bisphosphate; PLC, phospholipase C; PLD, phospholipase D; ROC, receptor-operated Ca^{2+} channel.

enzyme considerably reduced the sustained DG formation. Furthermore, pretreatment with a PKC inhibitor H-7 significantly inhibited both PEt formation and choline release in response to BK (10), supporting the notion that activation of PC-PLD is dependent on PKC and a subsequent feedback loop consists of PKC and PC-PLD/PA-phosphohydrolase in BK-triggered signal transduction in fibroblasts (11).

It has been reported that BK stimulates phosphoinositide turnover in DT cells to a greater extent compared with NIH3T3 cells, and that PKC is partially down-regulated due to a constitutive high level of DG in DT cells (10).

BK stimulated PC-PLD in NIH3T3 cells, whereas it failed to activate the enzyme in DT cells probably because of PKC down-regulation. We have shown that BK-induced $[Ca^{2+}]i$ oscillations were negatively modulated by PKC, suggesting that down-regulation of PKC is required for the oscillations in K-*ras*-transfected cells(3). Experiments with the extracellular Ca^{2+}-chelator and the Ca^{2+} channel blocker unraveled the close link of the Ca^{2+} signal to the PC-PLC activity. Since PC-PLC is known to be Ca^{2+}-dependent, $[Ca^{2+}]i$ oscillations are considered to cause the activation of PC-PLC.

Although the physiological significance of mitogen-induced $[Ca^{2+}]i$ oscillations have not been clarified, it would be possible that the oscillations induce activation of PC-PLC leading to sustained DG formation, which down-regulates PKC to facilitate Ca^{2+} influx through a receptor-operated Ca^{2+} channel. In addition, a close correlation was observed between occurrence of BK-induced $[Ca^{2+}]i$ oscillations and the colony-forming potency in soft agar (3). It can be thus predicted that the $[Ca^{2+}]i$ oscillations may reflect one of the malignant phenotypes of *ras*-transformed cells.

ACKNOWLEDGMENT

This study was supported in part by the research grants from the Ministry of Education, Science and Culture of Japan.

REFERENCES

[1] Barbacid M. *ras Genes*. Annu Rev Biochem 1987; 56: 779-827.

[2] McCormick F. *ras GTPase activating protein: signal transmitter and signal terminator*. Cell 1989; 56: 5-8.

[3] Fu T, Sugimoto Y, Oki T, Murakami S, Okano Y, Nozawa Y. *Calcium oscillation associated with reduced protein kinase C activities in ras-transformed NIH3T3 cells*. FEBS Lett 1991; 281: 263-6.

[4] Lang F, Friedrich M, Kahn E, Woll E, Hammerer M, Waldegger S. et al. *Bradykinin-induced oscillations of cell membrane potential in cells expressing the H-ras oncogene*. J Biol Chem 1991; 266: 4938-42.

[5] Lacal JC, Moscat J, Aaronson ST. *Novel source of 1,2-diacylglycerol elevated in cells transformed by H-ras oncogene*. Nature 1987; 330:269-71.

[6] Nishizuka Y. *The role of protein kinase C in cell surface signal transduction and tumour promotion*. Nature 1984; 308: 693-8.

[7] Macara IG. *Oncogenes, ions, and phospholipids*. Am J Physiol 1985; 248(Pt 1):C3-C11.

[8] Fu T, Okano Y, Hagiwara M, Hidaka H, Nozawa Y. *Bradykinin-induced translocation of protein kinase C in neuroblastoma NCB-20 cells: Dependence on 1,2-diacylglycerol content and free calcium*. Biochem Biophys Res Commun 1989; 162(2):1279-86.

[9] Yavin E. *Regulation of phospholipid metabolism in differentiating cell from rat brain cerebral hemispheres in culture*. J Biol Chem 1976; 251:1392-7.

[10] Fu T, Okano Y, Nozawa Y. *Differential pathways, phospholipase C and phospholipase D, of bradykinin-induced biphasic 1,2-diacylglycerol formation in NIH3T3 fibroblasts and its K-ras-transformed cells*. Biochem J in press.

[11] van Blitterswijk WJ, Hilkmann H, de Wild J, van der Bend RJ. *phospholipid metabolism in bradykinin-stimulated human fibroblasts: I. Biphasic formation of diacylglycerol from phosphatidylinositol and phosphatidylcholine, controlled by protein kinase C*. J Biol Chem 1991; 266:10337-10343.

[12] Higashida H, Hoshi N, Hashii M, Fu T, Noda M, Nozawa Y. *Ba^{2+} current oscillation evoked by bradykinin in ras-transformed fibroblasts*. Biochem Biophys Res Commun 1991; 178(2):713-7.

[13] Merritt JE, Armstrong WD, Benham CD, Hallam TJ, Jacob AJ, Leigh BK, et al. *SK&F 96365, a novel inhibitor of receptor-mediated calcium entry*. Biochem J 1990; 271:515-22.

[14] Berridge MJ, Irvine RF. *Inositol trisphosphate, a novel second messenger in cellular signal transduction*. Nature 1984; 312: 315-21.

AAS 38/II
Recent Progress on Kinins
© 1992 Birkhäuser Verlag Basel

RENAL ALTERATION AND DEVELOPMENT
OF HYPERTENSION IN DIABETIC RATS

V. Pellufo, M.A. Costa, M.G. Marina Prendes, O.L. Catanzaro

Cátedra de Fisiología, Facultad de Farmacia y Bioquimica, U.B.A. ARGENTINA.
Programa de péptidos vasodepresivos (PROSIVAD) CONICET

SUMMARY: There is a close association between diabetes and hypertension. Many studies have demonstrated an increased incidence of hypertension in the presence of diabetic nephropathy. The aim of the present work was to study the kallikrein-kinin system during the diabetic states with hypertension. In this study neonatal rats were injected with streptozotocin at two days of age. Plasma glucose, proteinuria, urinary kallikrein, blood pressure, creatinine clearance, diuresis and body weight were measured. Results: control rats vs diabetic rats. Plasma glucose (mg/dl): 0 minutes 80.2 ± 2.5 vs 105.5 ± 4.5; 60 minutes 120.4 ± 2.3 vs 220.0 ± 4.6; 120 minutes 105.0 ± 1.5 vs 140.0 ± 3.6; $p < 0.05$. Proteinuria at 8 months of age (mg/24 hs): 12.5 ± 1.6 vs 20.6 ± 2.4; $p < 0.05$. Urinary kallikrein at 8 months of age (umol/min/24 hs)/(ml/min) x 10^3: 46.9 ± 3.0 vs 28.5 ± 2.5; p 0.005. Blood pressure at 8 months of age (mm Hg): 110.0 ± 2.0 vs 132.0 ± 4.0; $p < 0.001$. Creatinine clearance at 10 months of age (ml/min): 0.46 ± 0.03 vs 0.70 ± 0.14; $p < 0.05$. Diuresis at 8 months of age (ml/24 hs): 1.55 ± 0.65 vs 10.30 ± 1.44, $p < 0.001$. The early modifications of kallikrein-kinin system in the diabetes states may contribute to development hypertension with modifications in the hemodynamics renal function.

INTRODUCTION

It has been demonstrated that diabetes is usually related to circulatory and renal disturbances. Besides it is associated with a higher hypertension incidence (1, 2).

Previous works carried out in this laboratory showed that the kallikrein-kinin system was altered in hypertensive non-insulin-dependent diabetic rats (pharmacological model induced by the administration of streptozotocin) (3).

Renal kallikrein is a serine protease located at the distal tubule which induces natriuresis and diuresis. It is also associated to a higher glomerular filtration rate and renal plasma flow (4).

The aim of the present work was to investigate the renal functionality and the kallikrein-kinin system during the development of hypertension in diabetic rats up to 10 months of age.

MATERIALS AND METHODS

Wistar strain male rats were used. Animals were injected with streptozotocin (100 mg/kg body weight, sc) at two days of age, developing non-ketotic diabetes at about 7 weeks of age.

Diabetes was characterized in all animals by the glucose tolerance test performed at the age of 3, 6 and 8 months.

Systolic arterial pressure (SAP) was measured by an indirect method based upon the cannulation of the tail artery.

Urinary samples (24 hs) were collected with metabolic cages and the following determinations were performed:

-    Proteins: Lowry method (5)
-    Creatinine: kinetic method (6)
-    Kallikrein and prekallikrein: were determined by enzymatic activity determination of active kallikrein using a chromogenic substrate (S2266 Kabi).

When the animals reached the age of 3 months they were divided into three groups:

-    Control rats
-    Diabetic rats
-    Diabetic rats with hypertension.

Later, the second group also developed hypertension therefore only two groups were considered.

Results were expressed as $X \pm$ SEM. Statistical analysis was performed by means of "t" test, $p < 0.05$ were considered statistically significant.

RESULTS

Diabetic rats showed an alteration of the glucose tolerance test compared with the controls, this modification was observed up to the end of the study.

Animals showed an increase in systolic arterial pressure (SAP) at 3 months of age, returning it to normal values 3 months later (Table 1). However another increase in systolic arterial pressure was observed when animals were 8 months of age, but this increase remained up to the end of the study (10 months): 8 months of age BP (mm Hg) 110.0 ± 2.0 (C.R) vs 132.0 ± 4.0 (D.R), p < 0.001; 10 months of age 112.0 ± 3.0 (C.R) vs 138.0 ± 9.0 (D.R), p < 0.05 (Fig. 1).

Table 1. Results obtained in rats at 3 months of age

	Control rats	Diabetic rats	Diabetic rats with hypertension
Arterial Blood Pressure (mm Hg)	109 ± 3	110 ± 7	134 ± 5 (**)
Urinary Protein (mg/24 hrs)	3.44 ± 0.41	7.69 ± 0.68 (**)	6.07 ± 0.98 (*)
Urinary Esterase (E.U./mg creat.)	8.3 ± 0.7	9.3 ± 0.3	4.7 ± 0.4 (**)
Urinary Kallikrein (umol PNA/min/24h)/ UV (ml/min)	33.13 ± 0.72	33.11 ± 0.72	24.84 ± 1.8 (**)

(*) p < 0.05 compared to control - (**) p < 0.01 compared to control

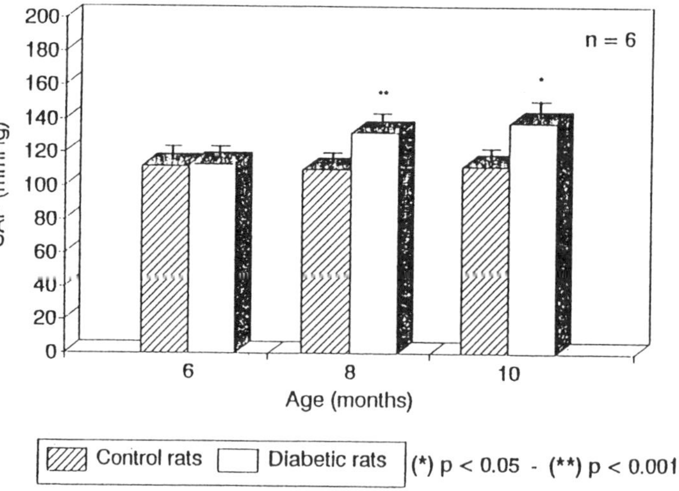

Fig. 1. Systolic arterial pressure

The diuresis of diabetic animals showed a sharp increase, reaching its highest values at 10 months of age: Urine volume (ml/24 hs) 4.75 $\pm$ 0.35 (C.R) vs 40.78 $\pm$ 6.8 (D.R), p < 0.02 (Fig. 2).

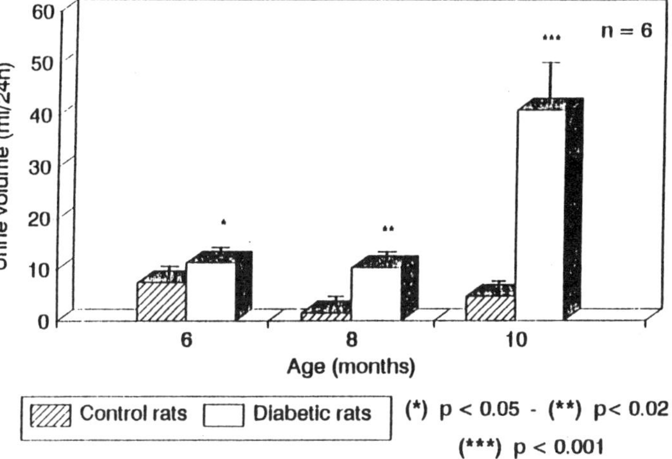

Fig. 2. Diuresis

Urinary proteins were also increased in diabetic rats although this determination offers a wide variability among not only experimental animals but also among control animals depending upon their ages: Urinary proteins (mg/24 hs) at 6 months of age 18.7 $\pm$ 1.1 (C.R) vs 21.1 $\pm$ 1.0 (D.R), no sign; at 8 months of age 12,5 $\pm$ 1.6 (C.R) vs 20.6 $\pm$ 2.4 (D.R), p < 0.05; at 10 months of age 21.9 $\pm$ 1.0 (C.R) vs 26.8 $\pm$ 8.3 (D.R), no sign (Fig. 3).

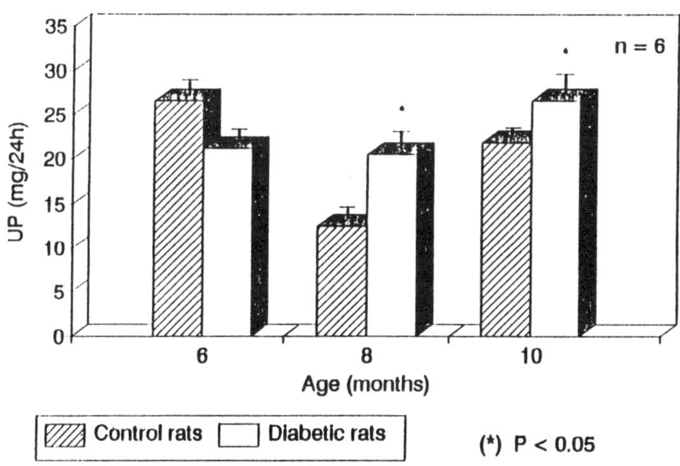

Fig. 3. Urinary Protein

Active kallikrein (UAK) expressed in relation to urinary volume (UV) showed no significant modifications at 6 months of age just when arterial blood pressure seemed to reach normal values: UAK (umol/min/24 hs) UV (ml/min) x 10^3 31.5 $\pm$ 7.0 (C.R) vs 30.8 $\pm$ 3.3 (D.R), no sign. As systolic arterial pressure rose again active kallikrein was markedly reduced: UAK (umol/min/24 hs) UV (ml/min) at 8 months of age 46.9 $\pm$ 3.0 C.R) vs 28.5 $\pm$ 2.5 (D.R), $p < 0.005$; at 10 months of age 39.2 $\pm$ 4.0 (C.R) vs 25.2 $\pm$ 3.3 (D.R), $p < 0.005$ (Fig. 4).

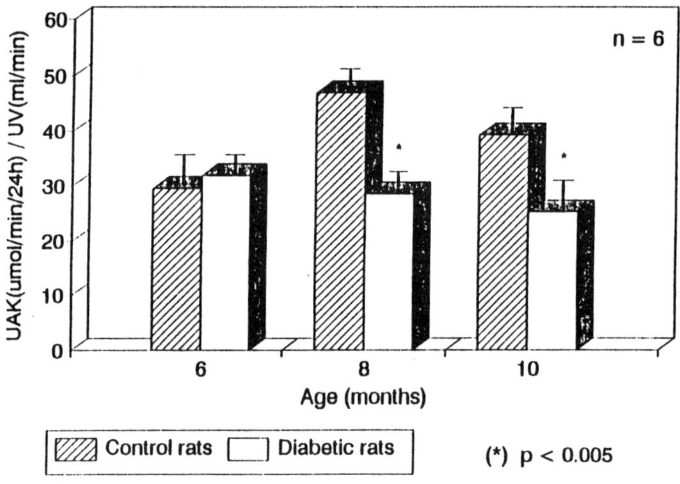

Fig. 4. Urinary Active Kallikrein

Percentage of prekallikrein (UpreK) remained increased in an experimental animals along all ages considered: UpreK (%) at 6 months of age 7.95 $\pm$ 0.99 (C.R) vs 21.37 $\pm$ 0.94 (D.R), $p < 0.001$; at 8 months of age 8.85 $\pm$ 0.75 (C.R) vs 12.23 $\pm$ 0.83 (D.R), $p < 0.02$; at 10 months of age 10.86 $\pm$ 0.26 (C.R) vs 22.20 $\pm$ 5.13 (D.R), $p < 0.05$ (Fig. 5).

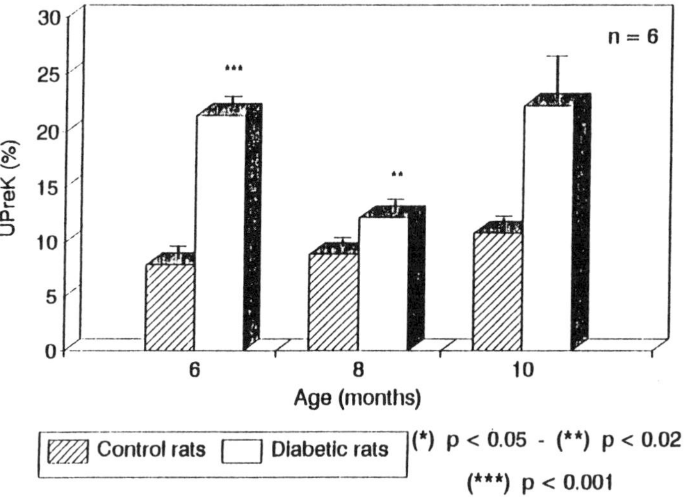

Fig. 5: Urinary Prekallikrein

Creatinine clearance (CC) was determined at 8 and 10 months of age: CC (ml/min) at 8 months of age 0.29 ± 0.03 (C.R) vs 0.34 ± 0.05 (D.R), no sign; at 10 months of age 0.46 ± 0.03 (C.R) vs 0.70 ± 0.14 (D.R), $p < 0.05$ (Fig. 6).

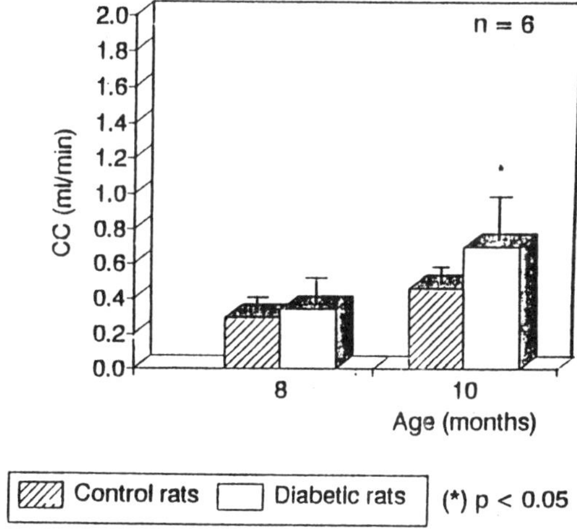

Fig. 6. Creatinine Clearance

DISCUSSION

Hemodynamics alterations in the kidneys of diabetic animals have been shown to aggravate the severity of glomerular lesion (7). Identifications of the mechanisms underlying this hyperfiltration in the diabetes may allow modifications of early hemodynamics changes and perhaps inhibit the development of later structural damage (8).

On the other hand the recognition of functional abnormalities in the early stages of diabetes may provide a theroretical basis for elucidating the pathogenesis of later clinical diabetic nephropathy and renal failure (9, 10). Glycemic test of glucose tolerance tended to be higher at the end of the study in the diabetic rats, time where the renal alteration and hypertension are installed. Early those complications the systolic pressure increased at 3 months of age and later at 8 months of age. Also diuresis and urinary proteins increased during the time of the study.

This data is very important since the increased blood glucose between others alterations produce osmotic diuresis and proteinuria. It is well known that blood pressure elevation contributes to the major causes of morbidity and mortality in the diabetic population. Several investigators have suggested that increased transcapillary escape rate of plasma proteins may indicate a generalized endothelial injury (11).

This motel of diabetes could involved microvascular passage of plasma proteins, increase vascular permeability and/or raised hydraulic pressure in the microcirculation, specially in the later stage of the diseases. The relationship between renal hemodynamic and renal kallikrein activity was observed in several publications (12, 13). The decreasing of urinary kallikrein at 3 months of age reflect the early filtration abnormalities in diabetes.

The mechanisms of kinin is to dilate the glomerular arterioles when infused into the kidney or antiluminal side of kidney (14). This suggests that early modifications in the hemodynamics renal function can contribute significantly to development hypertension on the later stages, as was observed by the decreasing of active kallikrein at 8 and 10 months of age.

REFERENCES

1. Mongensen CE, Osterby R, Gundersen HJG. Diabetology 1979; 17:71-76.

2. Mongensen CE, Steffes MW, Deckert T, Christiansen JS. Diabetology 1981; 21:81-93.

3. Weir GC, Clore ET, Zmachinski CJ, Bonner-Weir S. Diabetes 1981; 30:590-595.

4. Mayfield RK, Margolius HS, Levine JH, Wohltmahn CB, Loadholt, Colwell JAJ. Clin Endocr Metab 1984; 59:278-286.

5. Lowry OH, Rosenbrough NJ, Farr AL, Randall RJ. J Biol Chem 1951; 193:267-275.

6. Test combination creatinine. Método Jaffé. Boehringer Argentina S.A.

7. Mayfield RK, Margolius HS, Bailey GS, Miller DH, Sens DA, Squires J, Nann DH. Diabetes 1985; 34:22-28.

8. Keen H, Niseman MJ, Viberti GC. In: Biology and Pathology of the Vessel Wall. Woolf E, editor. Eastbourne NY: Praeger 1982:189-196.

9. Maver SM, Steffes MW, Brown DM. Am J Med 1981; 70:603-612.

10. Catanzaro OL, Pivetta OH, Zuccollo A, Buzzalino ND, de Matos DG, Vila SB. Adv Exp Med Biol 1989; 247A:593-597.

11. Parving HH. Dan Med Bull 1975; 22:217-233.

12. Harvey JN, Jaffa AA, Loadholt CB, Mayfield RK. Dliabetes Res 1988; 9:67-72.

13. Jaffa AA, Miller DH, Bailey GS, Chao J, Margolius HS, Mayfield RK. J Clin Invest 1987; 80:1651-1659.

14. Mayfield RK, Margolius HS. Am J Nephrol 1983; 3: 145-155.

AAS 38/II
Recent Progress on Kinins
© 1992 Birkhäuser Verlag Basel

ISOLATION OF A THIOL-DEPENDENT ACID KININOGENASE FROM RAT SPLEEN

K.Yamafuji, Y.Matsui

Nakamura Gakuen College, Fukuoka 841-01,Japan

SUMMARY: The enzyme which could produce kinin-like peptides from rat plasma at acidic condition and at coexistence of thiol compound was separated from acid extract of rat spleen. The isolation procedure of this enzyme was established. Substrate specificity was examined against fluologenic substrates and two types of collagen. The purified enzyme was proved to have kinin-forming activity and also collagenlytic activity,

INTRODUCTION

In the circumstances such as injury or inflammation, the intracellular enzymes which are active at weakly acidic condition may have the role in releasing mediators or degrading structural materials. We have been working on the acidic enzymes from spleen of bovine (1,2) and rat (3,4). The acid extract of rat spleen has SH-independent kininogenase, SH-dependent kininase and multiple forms of SH-dependent kininogenases in the decreasing order of molecular weight. The order was reverse in the case of bovine. In this paper, our report will be restricted to one of the SH-dependent kininogenases. Z-Phe-Arg-NMec is the best substrate of this enzyme. Enzyme has affinity to the double hydrophobic residue prior to arginine. Bz-Arg-NMec or Arg-NMec could hardly be creaved. We found this acid kininogenase had collagenolytic activity. It is not likely identical with cathepsin L (5) or collagenolytic cathepsin (6). The precursor of kinin-like peptide was found to be T-kininogen and not HMW-kininogen (4,7,8) in rat plasma. As a physiological role of released kinin-like peptide, the effect on glucose transport and matabolism at rat jejunum was investigated.

MATERIALS AND METHODS

Some spleens were collected from used Wister rats and others were purchased as deep frozen spleens from Kyudoh K.K. Heated plasma was prepared as described previously (3,9). Bovine tendon type I insoluble collagen was obtained from SIGMA, porcine cartilage type II soluble collagen was from WAKO. Z-Phe-Arg-NMec, Bz-Arg-NMec, and other peptidyl-NMec were the products of Peptide Research Foundation. Sephadex G-100,DEAE-Sephadex A-50 and Butyl-Sepharose 4B are obtained from Pharmacia Fine Chemicals. Reagents for PAGE are from Bio Rad.

Enzyme preparation. <u>Ammonium sulfate fractionation</u> and <u>Gel filtration on Sephadex G-100</u>. 280 pieces (206g) of spleen were homogenized in 1mM EDTA and extracted with sulfuric acid at pH 3.6 and fractionated by ammonium sulfate to obtain precipite at 40~70% saturation as described previously (4). Thus obtained 330mg of protein was applied on halves on Sephadex G-100. The corresponding fractions collected from two chromatograms were combined and subjected to following steps.

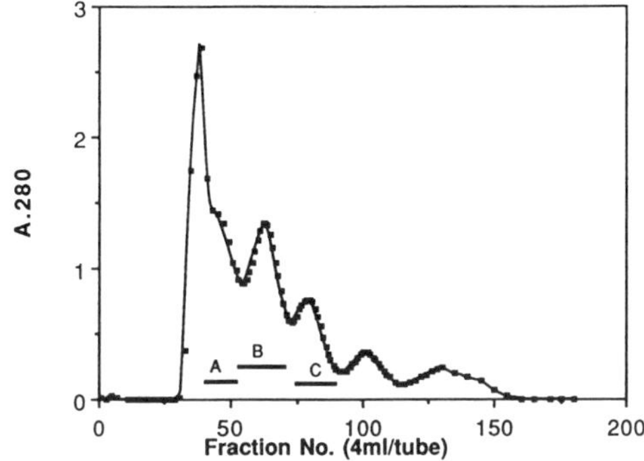

Figure 1. Gel filtration on Sephadex G-100; Column size: 3x90cm, Flow rate: 15ml/hr, Eluting solution: 0.9%NaCl,1mM EDTA, Sample: 330mg of 40~70%SAS, dialyzed against eluting solution

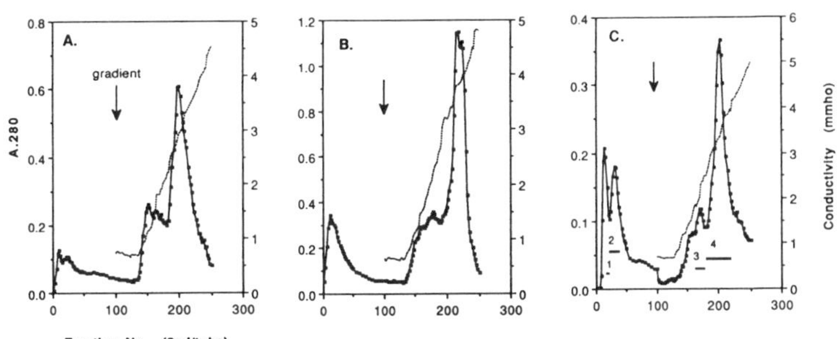

Figure 2. DEAE-Sephadex A-50 column chromatography; Column size: 1.5x45cm, Flow rate: 8ml/hr, Elution buffer: 0.01MPhosphate, 1mM EDTA, pH7.5 with NaCl gradient from 0.02M to 0.5M, Sample: G-100 fractions (A 58mg, B 115mg, C 54mg) concentrated and dialysed against starting buffer

<u>DEAE-Sephadex A-50</u> The precipitate of 80% ammonium sulfate saturation of each combined fractions were dialyzed against 0.01M, pH7.5 phosphate buffer containing 1mM EDTA. The resulting solution was applied on DEAE-Sephadex column. The same system was used in case of

rechromatography. The fractions eluted at the concentration of NaCl from 0.25M to 0.37M were collected, concentrated through AMICON DIAFLO YM3 membrane and equilibrated with 0.05M, pH6.8 phosphate buffer containing 1mM EDTA and 1.7M ammonium sulfate.

<u>Butyl-Sepharose 4B</u> Then sample was applied to Butyl-Sepharose 4B column. After eluting with this starting buffer, gradient of ammonium sulfate concentratiom from 1.7M to 0.0M was performed. The peak fractions were collected, concentrated and dialyzed, then applied to DEAE-Sephadex A-50 once more.

Enzyme assay. The enzyme activity of each fraction was examined by the following method. The hydrolysis of metylcoumarylamide substrate was analyzed as described in previous paper by fluorometric assay (10) using HITACH F-2000 fluorescene spectrophotometer. Kinin formation was estimated from the contraction of isolated rat uterus using Natsume isotonic transduser. Cleavage of collagen (6) was estimated by determining the increase of terminal amino group by means of o-phthaldialdehyde (11) or also determining hydroxyproline after acid hydrolysis by the colorimetry using chloramine T, perchloric acid and p-dimetylbenzaldehyde (12). The incubation procedure is as follows. 0.2ml of 10mg/ml suspension of bovine tendon collagen (type I) or of 3mg/ml solution of porcine cartilage collagen (type II) was incubated with 0.09mg of enzyme in 0.3ml and 0.1ml of 0.2M, pH 4.7, formate buffer at 37°C. After 3hours, 25µl was subjected to free amino groupe analysis and 500µl was hydrolyzed with conc.HCl at 110°C for 16hrs, neutralyzed and diluted to 25ml. 2ml from this resulting solution was used for hydroxyproline determination.

Effect on glucose transport and metabolism. Glucose transport and lactate formation was measured according to the method described by Kellet and Barker (13) with a little modification. Dessected jejumum (20cm) was suspended in measured volume (around 10ml) of Krebs-Henseleit buffer containing 5mM glucose (serosal solution) and luminal solution 25ml was circulated with pump at the speed of 25ml/min. Both of the solutions were oxygenated. 50µl alliquotes were taken from luminal and serosal solution at 5min interval for each assay. The amount of glucose and lactate was determined by Glucose C-test (WAKO) and Lactate test (BMY) respectively.

RESULTS　　AND　　DISCUSSION

The fractions from Sephadex G-100 were devided into three peaks, A,B, and C as shown in Fig.1, where A contain SH-independent kininogenase, B contain SH-independent kininogenase and SH-dependent kininase and C contain SH-dependent kininogenase. The proteins consisting each peak were purified by DEAE-Sephadex A-50 as shown in Fig.2, A,B,C. SH-dependent kininogenases were mainly found in the fraction notified as C-3 and C-4 in the figure. The peaks from A,B,C were all purified further, and investigated the ability of kinin formation or hydrolysis of synthetic substrates. Among them, the chromatogrum of C-4, largest fraction containing SH-dependent kininogenase activity, on Butyl-sepharose 4B was shown in Fig.3.a. This enzyme could not be recovered from Phenyl- or Octyl-sepharose 4B. The fractions designated by solid bar was collected and subjected to rechromatography on DEAE-Sephadex A-50 as shown in Fig.3.b. The comparison of the specific activity of acid kininogenase and trypsin in kinin formation was shown in Table 1. There shown much high substantial activity of this enzyme. The moleculer weight of this purified enzyme of C-4 was estimated by SDS-PAGE as 31kD, which is larger than 28kD we usualy found. In small peak of C-3, 28kD was found with higher activity. These two protein sometimes exist together and 28kD increased by standing in ice box. Thus we posturate that the autodegradation to make 28kD. Now we are trying to make antibody of 31kD to identify or differentiate two enzymes. Enzyme activities of C-4-I-I, a purified SH dependent acid kininogenase, and C-1 were summarized in Table 2. C-1 fraction which could hydrolyze Bz-Arg-NMec has potent collagenolytic activity and possibly be collagenolytic cathepsin. C-1 liberate much higher amount of free amino group from tendon than C-4, but the difference is not so dramatic as for cartilage. Hydroxyproline liberation from tendon were 68% of total content for C-1 and 45% for C-4. This means C-1 digest collagen into smaller peptides and C-4 to rather large soluble peptide. As the enzyme was found to be contained in macrophage or lynphocyte (3), this enzyme might be expected to have synergistic effect on osteoporosis, releasing a mediator and hydrolyzing collagen. As to the physiological role of peptide formed, we started to investigate the effects on the transport and metaborism of glucose. The effect of kinin on the small intestine was said to be varied by the composition of fatty acid in the diet on which the rat was grown (16). We used female wister rats which were fed CE-2 of Clea Japan. CE-2 contain 49% of linoleic acid and 3.8% of

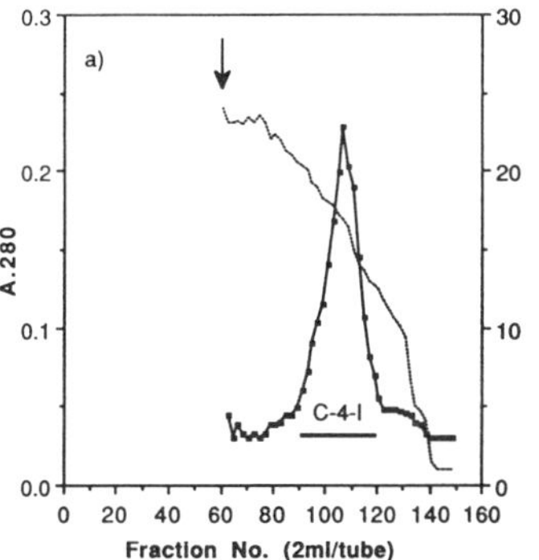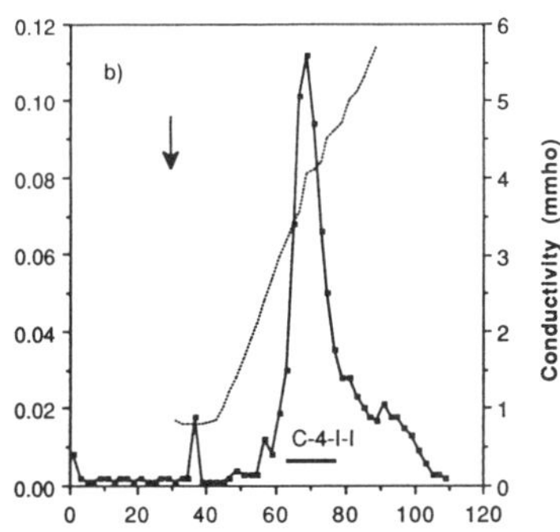

Figure 3 a) Affinity chromatography on butyl-Sepharose 4B; Column size: 1x25cm, Flow rate: 10ml/hr. Elution buffer: 1mM EDTA, pH6.8 with Ammonium sulfate gradient from 1.7M to 0.0M, Sample: C-4 , b) Rechromatography on DEAE-Sephadex A-50; Column size: 1x25cm, Flow rate: 8ml/hr, Sample: C-4 Butyl Sepharose 90~120 fraction

Table 1. Kinin liberation from rat plasma or T-kininogen by spleen kininogenase

Substrate		Enzyme	Librated kinin (µg BK eq)	Specific activity (µg BK eq/mg E)
Rat heated	1ml	Trypsin	11.9	0.95 (14)
plasma		Pancreatic Kallikrein	0.02	0.02
		Spleen kininogenase	10.0	125
T-kininogen*	1mg	Trypsin	14.1	0.014 (15)
	1U	Spleen kininogenase	14.1	288
HMW-kininogen	1U	Spleen kininogenase	0.36	7.2

* Gift from Drs. K. Enjyoji and H. Kato

Table 2. Enzyme activity of C-4-I-I and C-1 fraction

	BK eq from plasma	Bz-Arg NMec	Z-Phe-Arg NMec		Tendon collagen		Cartilage collagen	
	(µg/Unit E)	(AMC µmole/Unit E)			nmole	S.G.	nmole	S.G.
C-1	0.47	8.5	6.3	NH2	157	873	51	938
(Fig.2)				Hpro	255	1422		
C-4-I-I	14.2	ND	195	NH2	35	193	37	689
(Fig.3)				Hpro	167	927		

S.A.: nmole/mg Substrate mg Enzyme; Unit E: A280 x ml of enzyme fraction

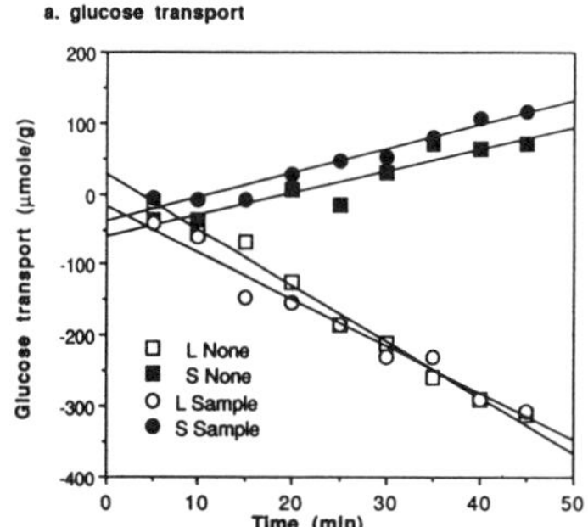

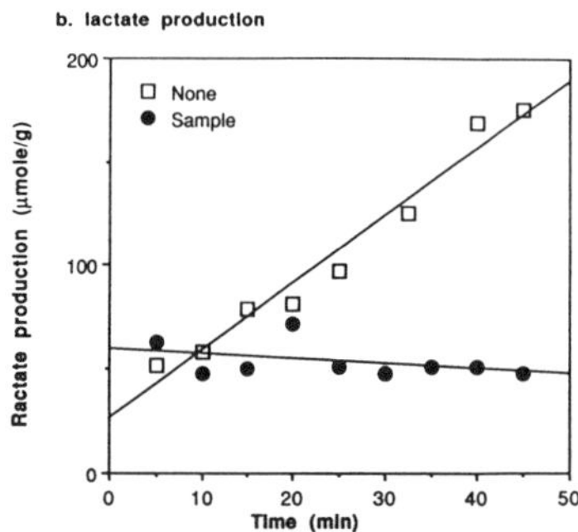

Figure 4. Time course of glucose transport and lactate production in rat jejunum; Sample: Product from SH-dependent reaction, 0.2µg BK eq., Enzyme: Fraction C-4-I (Fig.3), Substrate: TKNG rich fraction

linoleinic acid. The amounts of glucose and lactate in serosal or luminal solution was plotted as shown in Fig.4 for anexample. And some of the preliminary result were shown in Table 3. Bradykinin may not have possitive effect on transport because the diet contain adeqnate unsaturated fatty acid. Though the condition incruding the rate of oxygen bubling shold be reexamined carefully, and also the diet controle shoud be designed, so far, kinins were shown to have some effect on rat jejunum. The peptide released by acid kininogenase was shown to inhibit lactate formation as can be seen in Figure 4.

Table 3. The effects on glucose transport and metabolism at rat jejunum

Diet	Addition		Glucose		Lactate
		absorption(L)	TMtransport*(S)	utilisation	production
CE-2	None(n=4)	488±47	218±33	273±20	203±48
	BK 100nM	345	187	158	53
	Sample	397	205	192	-14

Rates are expressed in μmole/h per g dry weight.
* Transmural transport

CONCLUSION

One of the SH dependent kininogenase was separated and shown to have collagenolytic activity. The relationship among the multiple forms of SH-dependent kininogenase and also the relationship of these enzymes with known cathepsins should be elusidated by means of immunological techniques in near future.

REFERENCES

1. Yamafuji,K. and Takeishi,M.,Substrate specificities of acid kininogenase. Adv Exp Med Biol 1979; 120A(KININS-II,Pt.A),335-349 .

2. Yamafuji, K. and Watanabe,M.,Studies on the kinin formation by bovine spleen acid kininogenases. Adv Exp Med Biol 1983; 156A (KININS-III,Pt.A), 409-418 .

3. Watanabe,M. and Yamafuji,K.,Intracellular and intercellular distri-butions of acid kininogenases in spleen. Adv Exp Med Biol 1989; 198A (KININS-IV,Pt.A), 19-28 .

4. Yamafuji,K. and Matsui(Matsuki),Y., Kinin formation from T-kininogen by spleen acid kininogenases. Adv Exp Med Biol 1989; 247B (KININS-V,Pt.B) 97-102.

5. Turk,V. and Kregar,I., Cathepsin B, Cathepsin H, and Cathepsin L. Methods of Enzymatic Analysis. third Ed. Hans Ulrich Bergmeyer et al, editors. Weinheim(Germany): VCH., 1988;195-210.

6. Etherington,D.J., The nature of the collagenolytic cathepsin of rat liver and its distribution in other rat tissues. Biochem J 1972; 127,685-692.

7. Enjyoji,K. et al, Purification and characterization of two kinds od low molecular weight kininogens from rat(non-inflamed) plasma. J Biol Chem 1988;263,965-972.

8. Enjyoji,K. et al, Purification and characterization of rat T-kininogens isolated from plasma of adjuvant-treated rats. J Biol Chem 1988; 263,973-979.

9.Oh-ishi,S. et al, Bromelain, A thiolprotease from pinapple stem, depletes high molecular weight kininogen by activation of hageman factor(factor 12). Thrombo Res 1979; 14,665-672.

10.Barret,A.J., Fluorimetric assays for Catepsin B and Cathepsin H with Methylcoumarylamide Substrates. Biochem J 1980; 187,909-912.

11. Torres,A.R., Alvarez,V.L. and Sandberg,L.B., The use of O-phthal-dialdehyde in the detection of proteins and peptides. Biochem Biophys Acta 1976; 434,209-214.

12.Woessner,J.F.Jr., The determination of hydroxyproline in tissue and protein samples containing small proportions of this imino acid. Arch Biochem Biophys 1961; 93,440-447.

13. Kellet,G.L. and Baker E.D., The effect of vanadate on glucose transport and metabolism. Biochem Biophys Acta 1989; 979,311-315.

14. Okamoto H. and Greenbaum,L.M., Isolation and structure of T-kinin. Biochem Biophys Res Comm 1983;112.701-708.

15.Moreau,T.,et al, Relationship between the cystein-proteinase-inhibitory function of rat T kininogen and the release of immunoreactive kinin upon trypsin treatment. Eur J Biochem 1986;159,341-346.

16.Kellet,G.L. and Baker,E.D., The stimulation of glucose absorption and matabolism in rat jejunum by bradykinin: dependence on the composition of commercial diets. Biochem Biophys Acta 1989;992, 128-130.

CHLORIDE CONDUCTANCE CHANGES IN CULTURED COLONIC EPITHELIUM INDUCED BY KININS

A.W. Cuthbert, L.J. MacVinish and R. Henderson

Department of Pharmacology, University of Cambridge,
Tennis Court Road, Cambridge CB2 1QJ, UK

The first descriptions of kinin effects on electrogenic chloride secretion in epithelia were made almost a decade ago (1,2). During this time it has been shown that many epithelia secrete anions electrogenically in response to kinins (3). The response in many epithelial tissues is dependent in part on the generation of eicosanoids (4,5) although there is not a mandatory requirement for this (6). Much kinin stimulated eicosanoid generation takes place not in the epithelium, but in the underlying connective tissue (7). However, once it was known that cultured epithelial monolayers responded to kinins (8) it became clear that eicosanoid formation can take place in epithelial cells or that kinins can activate alternative mechanisms to induce secretion. This paper describes some recent results obtained in two human colonic cell lines derived from a human adenocarcinoma, namely HCA-7 and HCA-7 Colony 29. The parent cell line was described first by Kirkland (9) and Colony 29 was derived from the parent line by cloning after transformation with sodium butyrate.

In many respects these two lines are similar in sensitivity to agonists, each having both apical and basolateral kinin receptors (10,11), those on the apical surface being apparently more sensitive. In each cell line kinins cause an increase in intracellular calcium (Ca_i), which precedes but does not outlast the change in chloride secretion (11). Kinin responses in HCA-7 epithelia are unaffected by piroxicam, a cyclooxygenase inhibitor (10), while Colony 29 responses are partially inhibited by the same compound. Thus it appears that eicosanoid formation may be responsible, in part, for the chloride secretory response to kinins in Colony 29 cells. The kinin antagonist, Hoe 140, inhibits kinin effects (only tested in Colony 29 cells) and curiously the mechanism appears to be competitive when secretory responses are measured as short circuit current, but are non-competitive when Ca_i increases are used to monitor the response. The kinin receptors are therefore of the B_2 type.

Recently we have investigated these epithelial cell types using patch clamp and $^{125}I^-$ efflux techniques (12). The reasons to do this were to further define the membrane entities involved in the transepithelial transport of Cl^- and to understand more fully the mechanisms involved. Conventional inside-out patch and cell attached patch methods have been employed. The aim was to uncover the nature of ion channels present in the apical membrane of epithelial cells. However, all types of ion channels present are not necessarily detected using the patch clamp technique. For example, their conductance may be too small to be resolved by the technique or the frequency of opening and closing may be outside the bandwidth for recording. Further inside-out patches may show run-down, i.e. diffusion of cytoplasmic materials needed for the functioning of the channels in the patch may be lost. One way to detect the activation of all types of chloride channel (and exchangers) is to measure the efflux of $^{125}I^-$ from preloaded cells. All chloride channels appear to be able to conduct I^- as well as Cl^- so the rate constant for $^{125}I^-$ efflux gives a measure of chloride permeability.

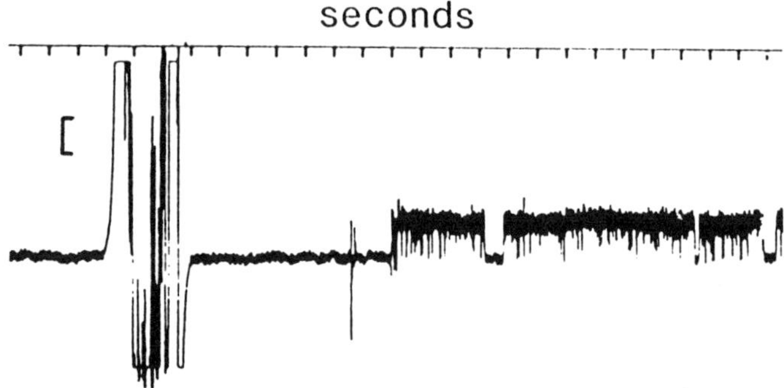

Figure 1. Inside-out membrane patch from an HCA-7 cell containing a chloride channel. When cAMP (100 µM) was added to the bath (causing interference) the quiescent channel was reactivated after a diffusive delay. Holding potential was +40 mV. Calibration 1 pA. Taken from (12).

Recently we have described outwardly-rectifying chloride channels in the apical membranes of HCA-7 cells. Their conductance is $g_{in} \approx 26$ pS, $g_{out} \approx 40$ pS with a selectivity for Cl^- over K^+ of ≈ 7.5 (12). The chloride channels are not unlike those found in other epithelia such as *Necturus* enterocytes (13), human pancreas (14), dog trachea (15) and HT_{29} and T84 cells (16,17). The Cl^- channels in HCA-7 cells were sensitive to cAMP but not to Ca^{2+}. An example of the response to the nucleotide is given in Fig. 1.

Activity of single chloride channels often disappeared after prolonged observation of a patch and activity could not be restored by repeated depolarisation. It was in quiescent patches such as these that the effect of cAMP was best demonstrated. Addition of cAMP to the bath containing a quiescent patch gave, after a diffusive delay, reactivation of the chloride channel activity. The demonstration of apical chloride channels however does not mean they are relevant to the chloride secretory response caused by kinins.

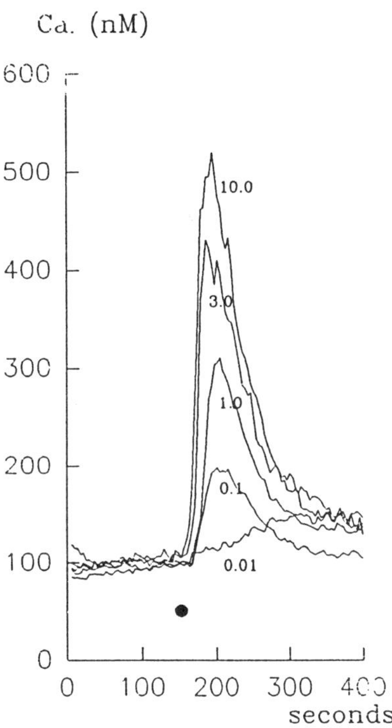

Figure 2. Ca_i increase in Colony 29 monolayers following lysylbradykinin (applied at ●) measured using Fura-2 fluorescence. Concentrations of the kinin (in μM) are indicated. Each response is from a separate monolayer and the data are superimposed.

First, kinins cause a rapid increase in Ca_i in these cells (Fig. 2) (11), yet these channels are insensitive to Ca^{2+}, at least up to 1 mM. It is possible that eicosanoid generation in Colony 29 cells following kinin gives rise to activation of adenylate cyclase as shown for rat colon epithelium (5) although this has not been tested directly here. Certainly these cells are able to generate cAMP in response to appropriate stimuli (18). A second reason for rejecting the possibility that outward rectifying chloride channels are part of the kinin secretory mechanism relates to relation between the membrane potential and the open state probability, P_o. This is illustrated in Fig. 3 showing that P_o increases as the membrane is depolarised. At the normal membrane potentials in intact cells (around -30 mV) the open state probability is low. Furthermore it is likely that the increase in Ca_i, which is consequent on kinin action, activates Ca^{2+} sensitive basolateral K^+ channels which further hyperpolarises the cell so that P_o is further reduced, although the electrical gradient for chloride exit across the apical membrane is increased.

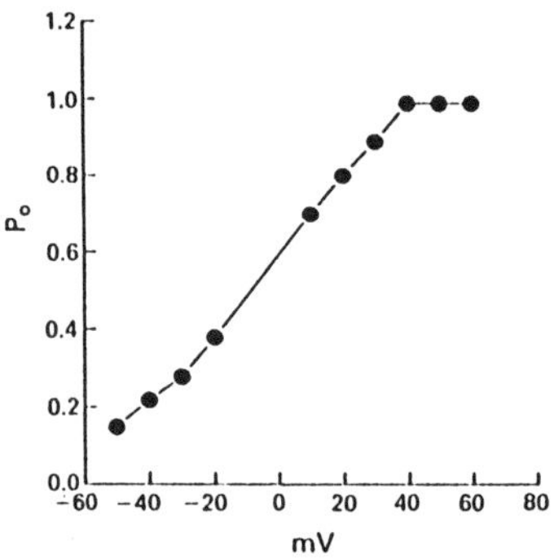

Figure 3. Open state probability (P_o) versus holding potent (V_h) for an outward rectifying chloride channel from an HCA-7 cell. Taken from (12).

However, it can be shown that kinins do activate channels in the apical surface of Colony 29 cells and, furthermore, this must involve the generation of intracellular messengers. This is shown using the cell attached patch clamp method as illustrated in Fig. 4. In this configuration records are obtained from channels situated below the patch pipette, while kinin is ejected from a second pipette by a pressure pulse and diffuses to the membrane. Any activity caused by kinin cannot be due to direct action since the peptide cannot reach the membrane patch and must result from the generation of intracellular messengers, which diffuse through the cell to reach the cytoplasmic face of the patch. In the experiment illustrated the membrane is held at 0 mV so the channel activity which appears is not due to voltage activation. The record shows more than one type of channel is involved and preliminary evidence indicates that some are non-selective cation channels. How any of these kinin activated channels are involved in chloride ion secretion is not yet clear. Further, it must be emphasised that kinins may activate a chloride conductance which cannot be resolved by patching. We have investigated the increase in chloride conductance following kinin by measuring the rate constant for $^{125}I^-$ efflux from Colony 29 monolayers.

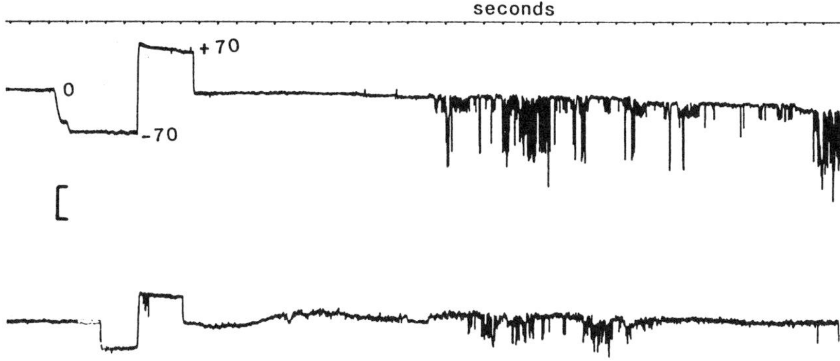

Figure 4. Whole cell patch recording from a Colony 29 cell. The patch was held at 0 mV, clamping at either +70 mV or -70 mV caused no channel activity to appear. Lysylbradykinin was pressure ejected onto the cell and led to an almost immediate burst of channel activity. Note channels of various sizes are seen. On a second application predominantly smaller channels were activated. Calibration 1 pA.

Two experiments using this approach are given in Fig. 5. In the first of these anion efflux was stimulated with the calcium ionophore, A23187. The result shows that an agent which increases Ca_i increases anion efflux. If Ba^{2+} is added to block calcium-sensitive K-channels the response is attenuated. This indicates that part of the anion efflux response results from membrane hyperpolarisation, increasing the gradient for efflux. The residual efflux increase in the presence of Ba^{2+} may be indicative of a Ca^{2+} sensitive conductance, located in the apical membrane of the cells. Kinins can also stimulate anion efflux as shown in the second experiment. Part of this response must be due to increase in Ca_i since the response was attenuated by the intracellular Ca^{2+} chelator, BAPTA.

To summarise the data suggest that the apical membrane of HCA-7 and HCA-7 Colony 29 cells have conductances which are sensitive to both cAMP and Ca^{2+}. Two separate chloride conductances have also been found in T84 cells (19) but the current-voltage relationship was linear for the cAMP stimulated conductance, whereas here the cAMP sensitive Cl⁻ channel was outwardly rectifying. However, the experiments with T84 cells used the whole cell patch clamp technique and has the advantage that all Cl⁻ conductances are measured, as with the [125]I⁻ efflux method, avoiding problems with 'undetectable' channels. As well as affecting apical membrane Cl⁻ conductance kinins, through the elevation of Ca^{2+}, influence transport via an effect on basolateral Ca^{2+}

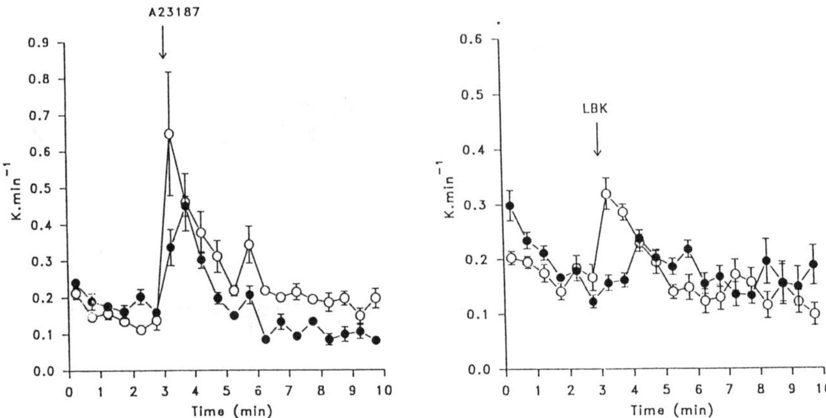

Figure 5. Rate constants for $^{125}I^-$ efflux from Colony 29 monolayers. Each point gives the mean value ± standard errors for 6 measurements. All monolayers in a given experiment were from the same batch of cultures. In one experiment A23187, 1 µM, was used to stimulate anion efflux. This agent was used alone (open symbols) or in the presence of Ba^{2+}, 1 mM (closed symbols). The latter attenuated the response to the ionophore. In a second experiment lysylbradykinin (LBK, 0.1 µM) was used to stimulate efflux in the absence (open symbols) or the presence of intracellular BAPTA (closed symbols). Chelation of intracellular Ca^{2+} by BAPTA attenuated the response to LBK. Monolayers were preincubated with BAPTA-AM, 5 µM, resulting in free BAPTA being trapped in the cells.

conductances are measured, as with the $^{125}I^-$ efflux method, avoiding problems with 'undetectable' channels. As well as affecting apical membrane Cl^- conductance kinins, through the elevation of Ca^{2+}, influence transport via an effect on basolateral Ca^{2+} sensitive K^+ channels. Two modes of stimulation of Cl^- secretion by bradykinin via apical cAMP sensitive channels and basolateral Ca^{2+} sensitive K^+ channels have been proposed for cultured canine tracheal epithelium (20). The ways kinins stimulate Cl^- secretion in simple epithelia is clearly more complex than for many other secretagogues which have only basolateral receptors linked to a single G-protein mechanism. It seems likely that even in simple epithelia more complex mechanisms may yet be revealed. For example, in other systems kinins activate the Na K 2 Cl cotransporter (21), a mechanism which here would facilitate Cl^- entry through the basolateral face. Considering that kinins also activate release of autacoids, particularly prostanoids, from submucosal elements (7) and that prostaglandins are potent releasers of neuropeptides from intramural nerves (22) the effect of kinins produced *in vivo* on epithelial function must be even more complex than on simple epithelia *in vitro*. The advent of potent kinin antagonists will help delineate the overall functional responsibility of kinin peptides.

REFERENCES

1. Cuthbert AW, Margolius H.S. Kinins stimulate net chloride secretion by the rat colon. Br J Pharmacol 1982; 75:587-598.
2. Manning D, Snyder SH, Kachur JF, Miller RJ, Field M. Bradykinin receptor mediated Cl⁻ secretion in the intestine. Nature 1982; 299:256-259.
3. Cuthbert A.W, MacVinish LJ. Diversity of kinin effects on transporting epithelia. In 'Kinins V', part A. Keishe A, Moriya H, Fujii S, editors. Plenum Press 1989: 105-111.
4. Cuthbert AW, Halushka PV, Margolius HS, Spayne JA. Role of calcium ions in kinin-induced chloride secretion. Br J Pharmacol 1984; 82:587-595.
5. Cuthbert AW, Halushka PV, Margolius HS, Spayne JA. Mediators of the secretory response to kinins. Br J Pharmacol 1984; 82:597-607.
6. Cuthbert AW, Halushka PV, Kessel D, Margolius HS, Wise WC. Kinin effects on chloride secretion do not require eicosanoid synthesis. Br J Pharmacol 1984; 83:549-554.
7. Warhurst G, Lees M, Higgs NB, Turnberg LA. Site and mechanisms of action of kinins on rat ileal mucosa. Am J Physiol 1987; 252:G293-G300.
8. Cuthbert AW, Kirkland SC, MacVinish LJ. Kinin effects on ion transport in monolayers of HCA-7 cells - a line from a human colonic adenocarcinoma. Br J Pharmacol 1985; 86:3-5.
9. Kirkland SC. Dome formation by a human colonic adenocarcinoma cell line (HCA-7). Cancer Res 1985; 45:3790-3795.
10. Cuthbert AW, Egléme C, Greenwood H, Hickman ME, Kirkland SC. MacVinish, L.J. Calcium- and cyclic AMP-dependent chloride secretion in human colonic epithelia. Br J Pharmacol 1987; 91:503-515.
11. Pickles RJ, Cuthbert AW. Relationship of anion secretory activity to intracellular Ca^{2+}.in response to lysylbradykinin and histamine in a cultured human colonic epithelium. Eur J Pharmacol 1991; 199:77-91.
12. Henderson RM, Ashford MLJ, MacVinish LJ, Cuthbert AW. Chloride channels and anion fluxes in a human colonic epithelium (HCA-7). Br J Pharmacol 1992: In Press.
13. Giraldez F, Murray KJ, Sepulveda FV, Sheppard DN. Characterisation of a phosphorylation activated Cl⁻ selective channel in isolated necturus enterocytes. J Physiol 1989; 416:517-537.
14. Gray MA, Greenwell JR, Argent BE. Secretin-regulated chloride channel on the apical plasma membrane of pancreatic duct cell. J Memb Biol 1988; 105:131-142.
15. Welsh M. Single apical membrane anion channels in primary cultures of canine tracheal epithelium Pflügers Arch 1986; 407:S116-S122.
16. Hayslett JP, Gogelein H, Kunzelmann K, Greger R. Characteristics of apical chloride channels in human colon cells (HT₂₉). Pflügers Arch 1987; 410:487-494.
17. Halm DR, Rochkemmer GR, Schoumacher RA, Frizzell RA. Apical membrane chloride channels in a colonic cell line activated by secretory agonists. Am J Physiol 1988; 254:C505-C511.
18. Cuthbert AW. Transepithelial ion transport in cultured colonic epithelial cell monolayers. In 'Advances in Cell Physiology and Cell Culture'. Jones C, editor. Kluwer Academic Publications, 1990: pp 49-64.
19. Cliff WH, Frizzell RA. Separate Cl⁻ conductances activated by cAMP and Ca^{2+}.in Cl⁻-secreting epithelial cells. Proc Natl Acad Sci USA 1990; 87:4956-4960.
20. Smith JJ, McCann JD, Welsh MJ. Bradykinin stimulates airway epithelial chloride secretion via two second messenger pathways. Am J Physiol 1990; 258:L369-L377.

21.   O'Neill C, Klein JD. Bradykinin effects on the Na-K-2 Cl cotransporter. This
       symposium.
22.   Bern MJ, Sturbeaum CW, Karayaicin SS, Berschneider HM, Wachsman JT,
       Powell DW. Immune system control of rat and rabbit colonic electrolyte transport.
       Role of prostaglandins and the enteric nervous system. J Clin Invest 1989;
       83:1810-1820.

CELL MEMBRANE POTENTIAL OSCILLATIONS INDUCED BY KININS IN FIBROBLASTS EXPRESSING THE HA-RAS ONCOGENE

F. Lang, E. Wöll, S. Waldegger, F. Friedrich, M. Ritter, G. Pinggera, K. Kloiber, I. Bichler, H. Heitzenberger, K. Maly, H. Grunicke

Institutes for Physiology and Biochemistry, University of Innsbruck, Austria

SUMMARY: In NIH-3T3 fibroblasts expressing the ras oncogene (+ras) bradykinin (BK) elicits sustained oscillations (1/min) of cell membrane potential (PD) due to oscillations of intracellular calcium activity with subsequent activation of calcium sensitive K+ channels. In NIH-3T3 fibroblasts not expressing the oncogene (-ras), BK leads to a single transient hyperpolarization of the cell membrane, not followed by oscillations. The oscillations of cell membrane potential require the presence of extracellular calcium and are abolished by K+ channel blocker barium (1 mmol/l), as well as by calcium channel blockers cadmium (1 mmol/l), lanthanum (0.1 mmol/l) and nifedipine (10 μmol/l). However, the oscillations are not modified by 1 μmol/l nifedipine, or by other calcium channel blockers, such as verapamil (10 μmol/l) or diltiazem (10 μmol/l). Cell proliferation is inhibited by nifedipine (10 μmol/l) but not by verapamil or diltiazem, indicating that the oscillations of intracellular calcium are a prerequisite for the growth factor independent proliferation of ras oncogene expressing cells.

INTRODUCTION

The products of ras oncogenes are GTP binding proteins resistant to inactivation by GTPase activating protein (1). They are thought to be involved in the cellular signal transduction of growth factors and expression of ras oncogenes has been shown to be followed by growth factor independent cell proliferation (2).

Very little is known about the celluar events following activation of the ras proteins (1). The present study has been performed to elucidate the possible involvement of ion transport at the cell membrane. Specifically, the possibility was tested, whether the expression of ras oncogenes modifies the regulation of ion transport at the cell membrane by bradykinin.

MATERIALS AND METHODS

Experiments were performed on NIH-3T3 fibroblasts transfected with a transforming Ha-ras MMTV-LTR construct expressing the oncogene, which is pointmutated at position 12, upon a 24h treatment with 1 μmol/l dexamethasone (+ras) (3). As controls served transfected cells not treated with dexamethasone (-ras). It has previously been shown that the response to bradykinin was similar in -ras cells and in nontransfected cells treated with dexamethasone (4).

The cells were grown on cover glasses in Dulbecco's modified Eagle's medium (DMEM) at 37 °C, 5 % CO_2 and 95 % air supplemented with 10 % fetal calf serum (FCS) (3). Prior to the experiments the cells were incubated in low serum medium (0.5 % FCS) for 48 - 72 h. Cover glasses with incompletely confluent cell layers were mounted into a perfusion chamber (volume: 0.1 ml, perfusion rate 12 ml/min). The control perfusate was composed of (in mmol/l) 114 NaCl, 5.4 KCl, 0.8 $MgCl_2$, 1.2 $CaCl_2$, 0.8 Na_2HPO_4, 0.2 NaH_2PO_4, 20 $NaHCO_3$, 5.5 glucose and continuously bubbled with 95 % O_2 and 5 % CO_2 (pH 7.4). The experiments were performed at 37 °C. Chemicals were from Sigma, Munich, FRG. Measurements of the potential difference across the cell membrane (PD) were made using conventional microelectrodes (tip diameter < 0.5 μm, input resistance 100 - 200 MΩ, tip potential < 5 mV), back filled with 1 mol/l KCl, versus an Ag/AgCl electrode connected with the bath via a 3 mol/l KCl-agar bridge. Impalements were made under an inverted phase-contrast microscope (Invertoscop ID Zeiss, Oberkochen, FRG), using a piezostepper (PM 20 N, Frankenberger, Germering, FRG) mounted on a Leitz micromanipulator (Leitz, Wetzlar, FRG).

Patch-clamp experiments were carried out according to the method of Sakmann and Neher (5) as described previously in detail (6,7). Single channel current events were measured by means of a L/M-EPC-7 amplifier (LIST-Electronics, Darmstadt, FRG), stored on a VHS-video-tape recorder (ELIN-6101, Vienna, Austria) via pulse code modulation (SONY PCM-501ES). The experiments were performed under cell-attached and excised-patch configuration. Outward current from the cytoplasm to the pipette is given as positive. The potential of the pipette (Vp) is given in reference to the bath.

Determinations of intracellular calcium have been made utilizing fura 2 fluorescence. As described previously in detail (4) the cells were incubated for 45 min with 2.5 μm fura 2-AM (Molecular Probes, Junction City, OR, USA, and Calbiochem, Geneva, CH). Fluorescence measurements were made under an inverted phase-contrast microscope (IM-35, Zeiss, FRG) equipped for epifluorescence and photometry (Hamamatsu, Herrsching, FRG) (8). Light from a xenon arc lamp (XBO75, Osram, Berlin, FRG) was directed through a grey-filter (nominal transmission 3.16 %, Oriel, Darmstadt, FRG), alternatively through a 340 nm or a 380 nm interference filter (halfwidth 10nm, Oriel, Darmstadt, FRG), respectively, and a diaphragm and was deflected by a dichroic mirror (FT425, Zeiss, FRG) into the objective (Plan-Neofluar 63 x oil immersion, Zeiss, FRG). The emitted fluorescence was directed through a 420 nm cut-off filter to a photomultiplier tube (R4829, Hamamatsu, Herrsching, FRG). To reduce the region from which fluorescence was collected, a pinhole was placed in the image plane of the phototube (limitation to a circular area of 60 μm diameter).

The fluorescence values are expressed as the ratios obtained at the two different excitation wavelengths (340 nm/380 nm). For calculation of intracellular calcium activity ([Ca]i), the following equation was utilized (9):

$$[Ca2+]i = Kd\ Sf2\ (R - Rmin)/\ Sb2\ (Rmax - R)$$

where R, Rmin and Rmax are the fluorescence ratios corrected for autofluorescence at experimental conditions, at maximal and at minimal calcium binding. Kd is the dissociation constant for fura 2 (= 225), Sf2 and Sb2 are the proportionality coefficients for the fluorescence at 380 nm excitation of free and calcium bound dye, respectively.

For isolation of inositolphosphates fibroblasts were seeded onto 35-mm culture dishes (6-well plates) at a density of 105 cells per dish and grown in inositol-free DMEM containing 10 % FCS in the presence of 10 μCi myo-[2-3H]inositol per ml for 48 hours. Subsequently the cells were exposed to inositol-free DMEM containing 0.5 % FCS in the presence of 10 μCi myo-[2-3H]inositol per ml for 24 hours. Cell density at this time was approximately 3.5 x 105 cells per dish. At 15 min before the experiment the cells were incubated in 1 ml Hepes buffer [140 mmol/l NaCl, 5 mmol/l KCl, 1 mmol/l CaCl2, 0.5 mmol/l MgCl2, 5.5 mmol/l glucose, 10 mmol/l HEPES, pH 7.4] and stimulated with 1 μmol/l bradykinin where indicated. The incubation was terminated by aspiration of the buffer and addition of 1 ml of ice-cold 15 % trichloroacetic acid per dish. After 10 min on ice, the trichloroacetic acid extract was collected. The trichloroacetic acid present in the extract was removed by three sequential washes with 8 ml diethylether, and the water soluble inositolphosphates were separated by HPLC (Beckman, System Gold) as described previously (10, 11). Elution times of inositolphosphates were calibrated using [3H]-standards of inositolphosphates. Fractions of 0.5 ml were collected and counted for [3H]-radioactivity using a liquid scintillation counter (Beckman LS3801).

Applicable data are expressed as arithmetic means $\pm$ SEM. Statistical analysis was made by t-test, where appropriate. Significant difference was assumed at p < 0.05.

RESULTS AND DISCUSSION

As shown in Fig. 1, in cells not expressing the ras oncogene (-ras) bradykinin leads to a single, transient hyperpolarization of the cell membrane. In contrast, in cells expressing the ras oncogene (+ras) bradykinin leads to a sustained oscillation of the cell membrane potential throughout the presence of the hormone. The oscillations require 1 nmol/l bradykinin and the full length of the peptide.

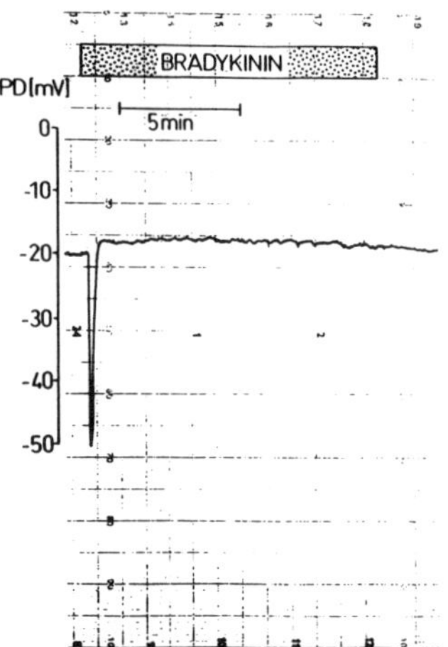

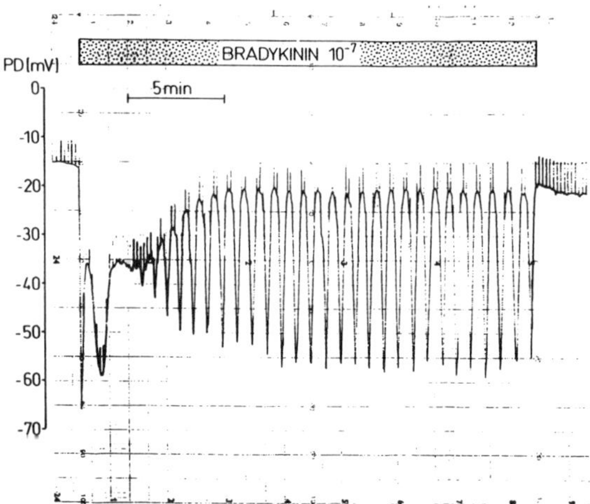

Figure 1. Original tracings showing the effect of 0.1 μmol/l bradykinin on the potential difference across the cell membrane (PD) in NIH fibroblasts expressing (right tracing) or not expressing (left tracing) the ras oncogene.

The amplitude of the cell membrane potential oscillations is strongly dependent on extracellular potassium concentration (Fig.2), suggesting that the oscillations are due to intermittent activation of K+ channels.

Patch clamp experiments reveal the existence of inwardly rectifying K+ channels (Fig. 3), which are closed (Po = 0.01 ± 0.02) at 0.1 μmol/l but activated (Po = 0.21 ± 0.04) at 1 μmol/l intracellular calcium activity.

According to fluorescence measurements, bradykinin elicits a single, transient increase of intracellular calcium activity in both, +ras and -ras. Oscillations of intracellular calcium activity are observed in +ras but not in -ras, when extracellular sodium is replaced by choline (Fig. 4). This maneuver presumably impairs the Na+/Ca++ exchanger and thus amplifies intracellular calcium oscillations.

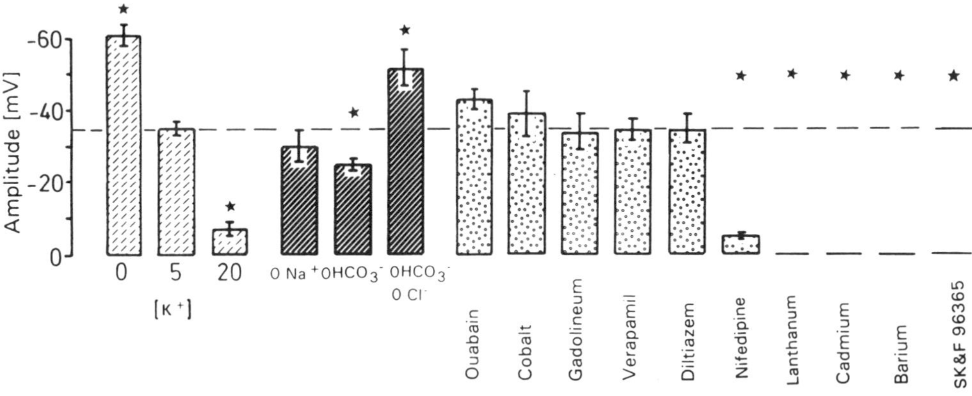

Figure 2. Effect of various experimental maneuvers on the amplitude of the bradykinin induced cell membrane potential oscillations in ras oncogene expressing cells (arithmetic means ± SEM, asterix indicates significant difference from control).

Taken together, the data suggest that the oscillations of cell membrane potential are due to oscillations of intracellular calcium activity with subsequent activation of calcium sensitive K+ channels.

The oscillations of cell membrane potential are slowed upon reduction of extracellular calcium activity from 1.2 to 0.2 mmol/l and are abolished following complete removal of extracellular calcium. Thus, the oscillations obviously depend on the entry of calcium from the extracellular space. The oscillations thus reflect either oscillating Ca++ channel activity at the cell membrane or pulsatile release of intracellular calcium triggered by continuous entry of calcium through receptor operated Ca++ channels.

As shown in Fig. 2, the oscillations of cell membrane potential are not dependent on the presence of extracellular sodium, bicarbonate or chloride. They are not inhibited by 0.1 mmol/l ouabain, 0.1 mmol/l dimethylamiloride, 1 mmol/l furosemide, 0.1 mmol/l hydrochlorothiazide, 0.1 mmol/l cobalt, 0.1 mmol/l zinc, 0.1 mmol/l gadolineum, 10 μmol/l verapamil and 10 μmol/l diltiazem. They are, however, virtually abolished by 10 μmol/l nifedipine, 0.1 mmol/l lanthanum, 1 mmol/l cadmium and 25 μmol/l SK&F 96365, a putative inhibitor of receptor operated calcium channels (12).

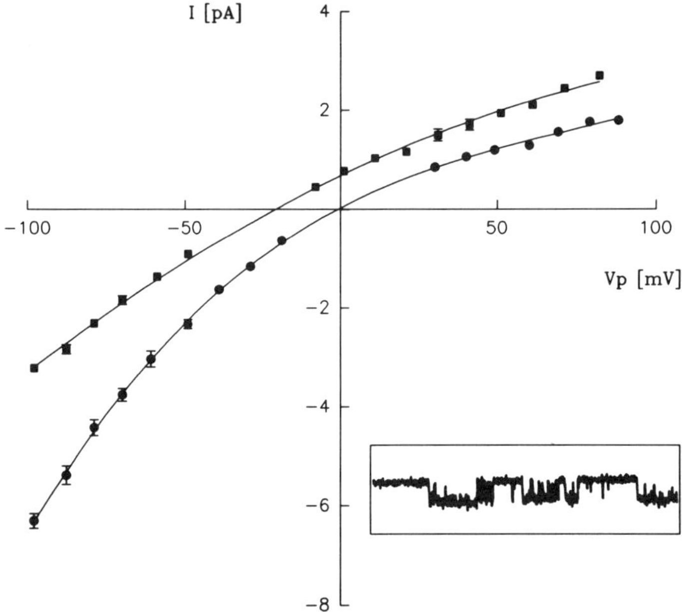

Figure 3. Current voltage relation of calcium sensitive K+ channels in ras oncogene expressing cells. The single channel current (I) is plotted versus the potential difference (Vp) across excised inside out cell membrane patches. Circles refer to 150 mmol/l K+ in pipette and bath, squares to 50 mmol/l K+ in pipette and 150 mmol/l K+ in bath (arithmetic means ± SEM, insert original tracing).

The oscillations are further inhibited by 0.2 mmol/l TMB-8, a putative inhibitor of intracellular calcium release (13) and by 10 μmol/l phorbolester TPA. Thus, circumstantial evidence suggests that the oscillations require intracellular calcium release and are inhibited by activation of protein kinase C.

The cellular concentration of both, 1,4,5 inositoltrisphosphate (1,4,5 InsP3) and 1,3,4,5 inositoltetrakisphosphate (1,3,4,5 InsP4) is significantly greater in +ras as compared to -ras, by factors of 1.8 $\pm$ 0.2 and 3.0 $\pm$ 0.2, respectively. Bradykinin leads to a transient increase of 1,4,5 InsP3 and 1,3,4,5 InsP4 in both, -ras and +ras. Following 10 min of continued exposure to bradykinin, 1,4,5 InsP3 is no more significantly different between +ras and -ras but 1,3,4,5 InsP4 remains significantly greater in +ras as in -ras. Thus, the oscillations could well be secondary to enhanced intracellular concentrations of 1,3,4,5 InsP4 in +ras.
In media depleted of growth factors (0.5 % fetal calf serum), -ras are unable to grow, whereas +ras still proliferate under those conditions. Nifedipine (10 μmol/l) abolishes the growth of +ras without significantly modifying the cell number of -ras cells.

In conclusion, in ras oncogene expressing NIH fibroblasts but not in normal fibroblasts, bradykinin elicits sustained oscillations of intracellular calcium leading to intermittent activation of calcium sensitive K+ channels and subsequent oscillations of cell membrane potential. These oscillations appear to be a prerequisite for the growth factor independent proliferation of these cells.

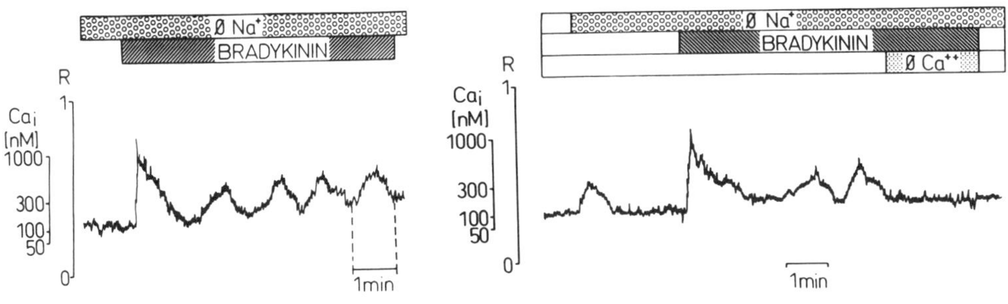

Figure 4. Bradykinin induced oscillations of intracellular calcium activity in ras oncogene expressing cells as evident from fura 2 fluorescence (original tracings).

REFERENCES

1. McCormick F. ras GTPase activating protein: signal transmitter and signal terminator. Cell 1989; 56: 5-8.

2. Barbacid M. ras genes. Annual Review of Biochemistry 1987; 56: 779-827.

3. Jaggi R, Salmons B, Muellener D, Groner B. The v-mos and H- ras oncogene expression represses glucocorticoid hormone-dependent transcription from the mouse mammary tumor virus LTR. EMBO Journal 1986; 5: 2609-16.

4. Lang F, Friedrich F, Kahn E, Wöll E, Hammerer M, Waldegger S et al. Bradykinin-induced oscillations of cell membrane potential in cells expressing the Ha-ras oncogene. Journal of Biological Chemistry 1991; 266: 4938-42.

5. Sakmann B, Neher E. Single channel recording. Plenum, New York 1983.

6. Friedrich F, Paulmichl M, Kolb HA, Lang F. Inward rectifier K channels in renal epitheloid cells (MDCK) activated by serotonin. Journal of Membrane Biology 1988; 106: 149-55.

7. Friedrich F, Weiss H, Paulmichl M, Lang F. Activation of potassium channels in renal epitheloid cells (MDCK) by extracellular ATP. American Journal of Physiology 1989; 256: C1016-21.

8. Almers W, Neher E. The Ca signal from fura-2 loaded mast cells depends strongly on the method of dye loading. Federation of European Biochemical Societies 1985; 192:13-18.

9. Grynkiewicz G, Poenie M, Tsien RY. A new generation of Ca2+ indicators with greatly improved fluorescence properties. Journal of Biological Chemistry 1985; 260: 3440-50.

10. Heslop JP, Irvine RF, Tashjian AH, Berridge MJ. Inositol tetrakis and pentakisphosphates in GH4 cells. Journal of Experimental Biology 1985; 119: 395-401.

11. Oberhuber H, Maly K, Berall F, Hoflacher J, Kiani A, Grunicke HH. Mechanism of desensitization of the Ca2+-mobilizing system to bombesin by Ha-ras. Journal of Biological Chemistry 1991; 266: 1437-42.

12. Merritt JE, Armstrong WP, Benham CD, Hallam TJ, Jacob R, Jaxa-Chamiec A, et al. SK&F 96365, a novel inhibitor of receptor-mediated calcium entry. Biochemical Journal 1990; 271: 515-22.

13. Carr FE, Galloway RJ, Reid AH, Kaseem LL, Dhillon G, Fein HG, et al. Thyrotropin-releasing hormone regulation of thyrotropin a-subunit gene expression involves intracellular calcium and protein kinase C. Biochemistry 1991; 30: 3721-3728.

REGULATION OF BRADYKININ-INDUCED CHLORIDE SECRETION IN A HUMAN EPITHELIAL CELL LINE

D. H. Miller, A. W. Baird, S. Bennet, M. Halushka
M. Sasaguri, H. Schomer, and H. S. Margolius

Department of Cell and Molecular Pharmacology and Experimental Therapeutics
Medical University of South Carolina, Charleston, SC, USA

SUMMARY: The chloride secretory response to bradykinin in T84 cells is regulated. The efflux rate of ^{125}I from these cells can be used to measure this response, and to demonstrate that the sensitivity to bradykinin varies with time in culture. The response in NuT84 cells is greater than that in T84, and can be blocked by the B2 receptor antagonist HOE-140.

INTRODUCTION

Bradykinin has been shown to induce an active secretion of chloride in rat colonic tissue (1, 2), canine airway epithelial cells (3), and the human colonic epithelial cell line T84 (4). This effect involves an increase in chloride channel conductance, a circumstance known to include activation of B2 receptors with, ultimately, increases in intracellular calcium and cAMP (5). Various other responses to bradykinin have been shown to be regulated (6-9), and these changes can result from alterations in receptor number (8, 9) or in signaling pathways (7). Recently, the sensitivity of T84 cells to bradykinin-induced chloride secretion has also been shown to change (4), though the mechanisms responsible for this adaptation have not been defined. A fast and simple gauge of chloride conductance in T84 cells involves measuring the rate of efflux of ^{125}I from the cells (10), and we have begun to use this method to study changes in responsiveness to bradykinin.

MATERIALS AND METHODS

T84 cells were maintained in 6-well plastic culture dishes (9.6 cm2/well) as previously

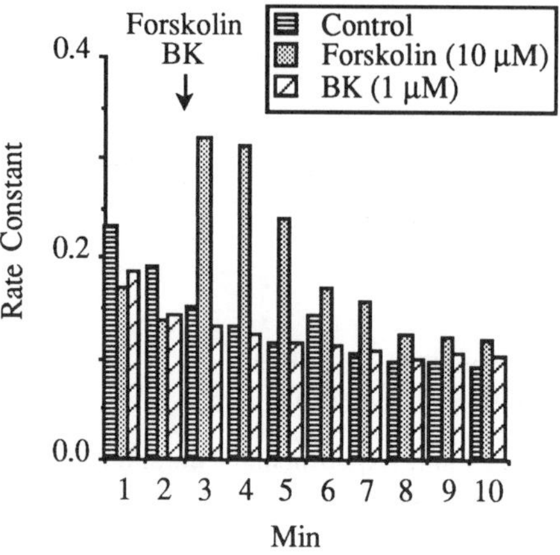

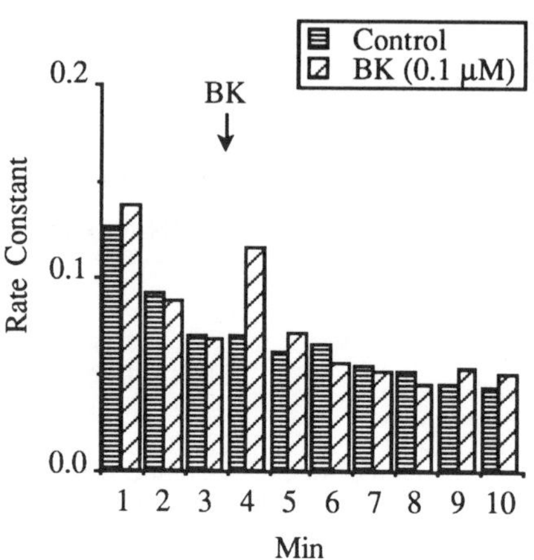

Fig. 1: Forskolin-stimulated 125-I efflux from T84 cells two months after plating. There is no response to bradykinin.

Fig. 2: Bradykinin-stimulated 125-I efflux in T84 cells 10 days after plating.

described (4). They were grown in a 1:1 mixture of Dulbecco's modified Eagle's medium and Ham's F-12 (DME/F12), supplemented with 5% fetal bovine serum, 100 units/ml penicillin G, and 100 µg/ml streptomycin. At least 24 hours before an experiment, the medium was changed to a serum-free medium containing 2 µg/ml insulin, 0.2 µg/ml glucagon, 2 µg/ml transferrin, 1 ng/ml epidermal growth factor, 50 nM hydrocortisone, 0.5 nM triiodothyronine, 25 nM sodium selenite, and 57 µM ascorbic acid (11). The cultures were kept at 37 °C in a 95% air-5% CO_2 atmosphere.

NuT84 cells were also produced as described (4). These are T84 cells that have been grown as subcutaneous explants in nude mice, and subsequently recovered and grown again in culture. This procedure results in increased kallikrein content of the cells, and increased responsiveness to bradykinin.

The ^{125}I-efflux assay was as described by Venglarik (10). T84 or NuT84 cells in 6-well plates were incubated in 95% air-5% CO_2 at 37 °C for one hour in Krebs-Henseleit solution ([in mM] 118 NaCl, 4.7 KCl, 2.5 $CaCl_2$, 1.2 $MgSO_4$, 1.2 KH_2PO_4, 25 $NaHCO_3$, 11.1 glucose) containing 2.5 µCi/ml Na[125]I. After the incubation period, the wells were quickly washed four times with 1 ml Krebs-Henseleit solution, then incubated further in 1 ml of the same solution. Every one minute thereafter, for a total of ten minutes, the solution was collected for counting,

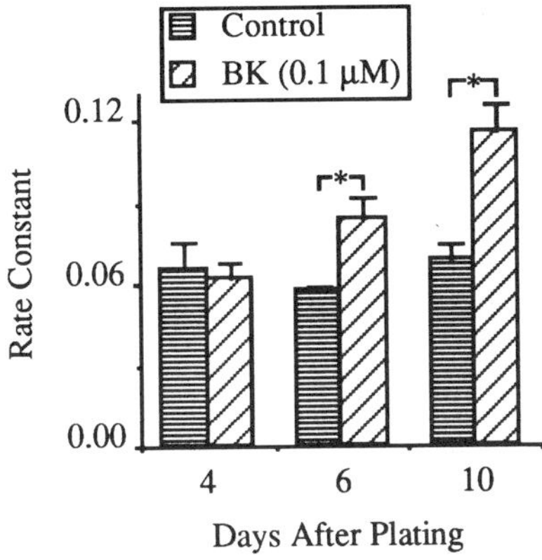

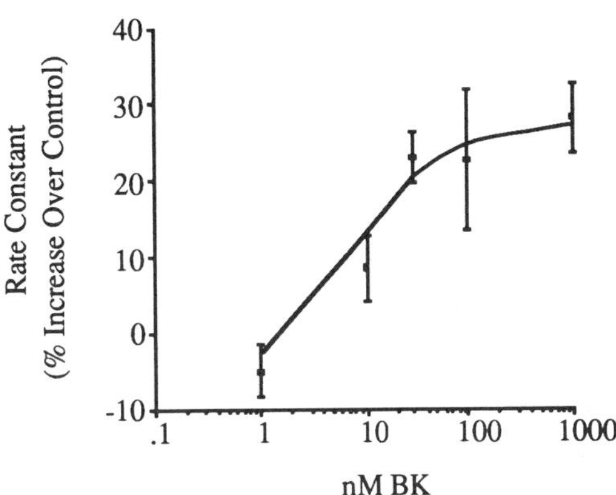

Fig. 3: Development of 125-I efflux responsiveness to bradykinin in T84 cells. Rate constants were determined in triplicate for the one minute period following the addition of bradykinin. P=0.026 at 4 days, and 0.016 at 10 days.

Fig. 4: Bradykinin dose-response relationship of 125-I efflux from T84 cells near confluence. Rate constants were determined as in Fig. 3. n=6 for each point.

and replaced with fresh solution. The rate of efflux of ^{125}I from the cells is taken as an indication of chloride channel conductance. The rate constant is calculated as $r = [\ln(R_1) - \ln(R_2)]/(t_1 - t_2)$, where R is the percent of counts remaining in the cells at time t.

Statistical significance for the data in Fig. 3 was determined by analysis of variance (ANOVA).

RESULTS

When T84 cells were grown in the same wells for two months, then loaded with ^{125}I and challenged with bradykinin, no change in the rate of ^{125}I-efflux was seen (Fig. 1). That the cells were competent to respond to a chloride secretagogue, however, was seen in the response to forskolin, an activator of adenylyl cyclase. A prompt increase in the rate of ^{125}I-efflux was seen, indicative of an increase in chloride channel conductance.

To test whether a bradykinin response might be temporally regulated, six 6-well plates were seeded with T84 cells at a density of 5×10^4 cells/cm^2, and ^{125}I-efflux experiments were carried out on separate days using two of the plates. At four days after plating, no response to bradykinin was seen, but six and 10 days after plating, as the cells had reached confluence (as judged by microscopic observation) a response was evident (Fig. 2). Note that the response is short-lived, and is no longer apparent in the second minute after bradykinin addition.

Fig. 3 shows the rate constants for the ^{125}I-efflux obtained in the minute after bradykinin addition for each day on which this experiment was carried out. It has been a consistent observation that prior to confluence, no response to bradykinin occurs. Furthermore, in cells kept in culture for periods of time well past confluence, as in Fig. 1, there is also no response. We have not further defined the duration of bradykinin responsiveness, but it is clear that the phenomenon is transient.

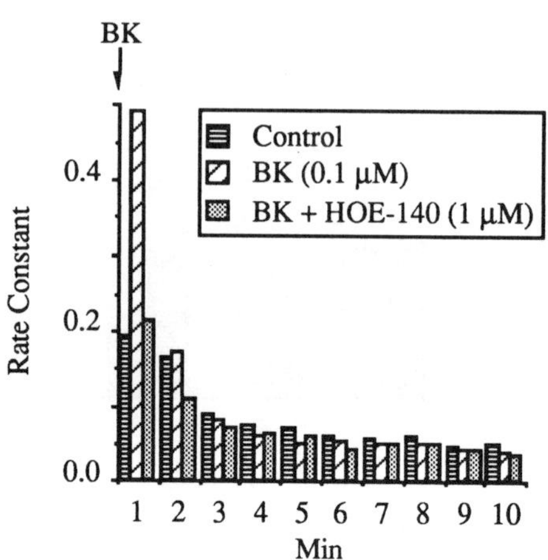

Fig. 5: Bradykinin-stimulated 125-I efflux from NuT84 cells (duplicate samples).

It was possible to construct a dose-response curve to bradykinin for the ^{125}I-efflux by testing cultures just reaching confluent growth. Fig. 4 shows an EC_{50} of 10 nM for this response, when measured in the minute immediately after adding bradykinin. At a dose of 1 μM, the rate constant in these experiments was increased by up to 30 per cent over the control.

The increase in short-circuit current (a measure of chloride secretion) brought about in NuT84 cells by bradykinin is 30-40-fold greater than in T84 (4). The ^{125}I-efflux response to bradykinin in NuT84 cells nine days after plating is seen in Fig. 5. The bradykinin (0.1 μM) was added at the start of the efflux period instead of after the third minute, as in the previous Figs. Nevertheless, such a robust response was never seen in T84 when the bradykinin was added at this time.

The effect in the NuT84 cells is probably a B2 receptor-mediated phenomenon. When the B2 antagonist HOE-140 was added to the incubation medium 15 min prior to starting the efflux collections, the bradykinin effect was completely blocked (Fig. 5).

DISCUSSION

The regulation of bradykinin receptors is complex. In cultured human foreskin fibroblasts, downregulation of receptor number occurs in response to bradykinin exposure and to treatment with dexamethasone (8). In contrast, interleukin-1 treatment of human synovial cells results in an upregulation of bradykinin receptor number and an increase in bradykinin-stimulated PGE_2 production (9). Interleukin-1 also increased bradykinin-stimulated PGE_2 production in 3T3 cells, but in this case the increased responsiveness did not involve changes in receptor number, but probably involved induction of the receptor-coupling G-protein, as well as other intracellular signaling pathways (7).

We have not yet determined the basis for the changes in T84 cell responsiveness. A decrease in thromboxane A_2 receptor number with an increase in cell density has been reported for rat aortic vascular smooth muscle cells (12), a growth-associated phenomenon that may relate to the results of Fig. 3. The responsiveness in the NuT84 cells (Fig. 5) may also be growth-related, but in view of our previous results (4), is likely to also derive from the particular environment provided in the mouse. The fact that the chloride secretory response to bradykinin is regulated in this epithelial cell line suggests a physiological purpose, and we are continuing to investigate the factors controlling bradykinin actions.

ACKNOWLEDGMENTS

This work was supported by NIH Grants HL44671 and HL17705.

REFERENCES

1. Cuthbert AW, Margolius HS. Kinins stimulate net chloride secretion by the rat colon. Br J Pharmacol 1982; 75:587-598.

2. Manning DC, Snyder SH, Kachur JF, Miller RJ, Field M. Bradykinin receptor-mediated chloride secretion in intestinal function. Nature 1982; 299:256-259.

3. Leikauf GD, Ueki IF, Nadel JA, Widdicombe JH. Bradykinin stimulates Cl secretion and prostaglandin E_2 release by canine tracheal epithelium. Am J Physiol 1985; 248:F48-F55.

4. Baird AW, Miller DH, Schwartz DA, Margolius HS. Enhancement of kallikrein production and kinin sensitivity in T84 cells by growth in the nude mouse. Am J Physiol 1991; 261:C822-C827.

5. Cuthbert AW, Halushka PV, Margolius HS, Spayne JA. Mediators of the secretory response to kinins. Br J Pharmacol 1984; 82:597-607.

6. Roscher AA, Manganiello VC, Jelsema CL, Moss J. Autoregulation of bradykinin receptors and bradykinin-induced prostacyclin formation in human fibroblasts. J Clin Invest 1984; 74:552-558.

7.   Burch RM, Connor JR, Axelrod J. Interleukin 1 amplifies receptor-mediated activation of phospholipase A_2 in 3T3 fibroblasts. Proc Nat Acad Sci, USA 1988; 85:6306-6309.

8.   Roscher AA, Klier C, Dengler R, Faussner A, Müller-Esterl W. Regulation of bradykinin action at the receptor level. J Cardiovascular Pharmacol 1990; 15(Suppl. 6):S39-S43.

9.   Bathon M, Manning DC, Goldman DW, Towns MC, Proud D. Characterization of kinin receptors on human synovial cells and upregulation of receptor number by interleukin-1. J Pharmacol Exp Therap 1992; 260:384-392.

10. Venglarik CJ, Bridges RJ, Frizzell RA. A simple assay for agonist-regulated Cl and K conductances in salt-secreting epithelial cells. Am J Physiol 1990; 259:C358-C364.

11. Murakami H, Masui H. Hormonal control of human colon carcinoma cell growth in serum-free medium. Proc Nat Acad Sci, USA 1980; 77:3464-3468.

12. Masuda A, Halushka PV. Thromboxane A_2 receptors are influenced by cell density in cultured rat aortic smooth muscle cells. Life Sci 1991; 48:2391-2395.

BRADYKININ SIGNAL TRANSDUCTION IN FIBROBLASTS

Ronald M. Burch

Nova Pharmaceutical Corporation, 6200 Freeport Centre, Baltimore MD 21224 USA

SUMMARY: Signal transduction induced by G protein-linked bradykinin B2 receptors in fibroblasts is mediated through primary activation of phospholipase C and phospholipase A_2

INTRODUCTION

Binding of bradykinin to B2 receptors can lead to activation of several second-messenger systems, the systems activated depending upon the tissue. In nearly all tissues, bradykinin induces release of arachidonic acid and its metabolism, leading to a variety of products, termed eicosanoids. Depending upon the tissue these may include prostaglandins, leukotrienes, hydroxyeicosatetraenoic acids, and platelet activating factor (1). These metabolites are of great importance in mediating bradykinin's effects, because inhibition of their synthesis completely blocks bradykinin-induced physiological effects, or markedly attenuates the responses induced by low concentrations of the peptide. Activation of bradykinin receptors also stimulates phosphatidylinositol-specific phospholipase C in most tissues. The released inositol phosphates mediate release of calcium from intracellular stores and contribute to the calcium currents generated by "receptor-operated calcium channels." The other metabolite produced by phospholipases C is diacylglycerol, which activates protein kinases C. In murine 3T3 fibroblasts, we have found that activation of phospholipases leads to generation of biologically active lipids, in particular prostaglandin E_2 (PGE_2), and to generation of inositol phosphates and diacylglycerol.

MATERIALS AND METHODS

SV-T_2 BALB/c 3T3 fibroblasts and BALB/c 3T3 fibroblasts were obtained from the American type culture collection. Cells were cultured in Dulbecco's modified Eagle's medium containing 10% calf serum. PGE_2 was quantitated using a radioimmunoassay and inositol phosphates were measured as the radioactive products recovered from cells prelabeled with [3H]inositol (2), or quantitated as mass of 1,4,5-inositol trisphosphate using a radioreceptor assay (3).

RESULTS AND DISCUSSION

Figure 1 shows the time course for formation of PGE_2 and IP_3 following stimulation by bradykinin in $SV-T_2$ cells. PGE_2 synthesis is maximal by 5 minutes, whereas IP_3 formation is delayed and more prolonged. Similar results were obtained when measuring release of labeled IP_3 or using a radioreceptor assay to quantitate IP_3

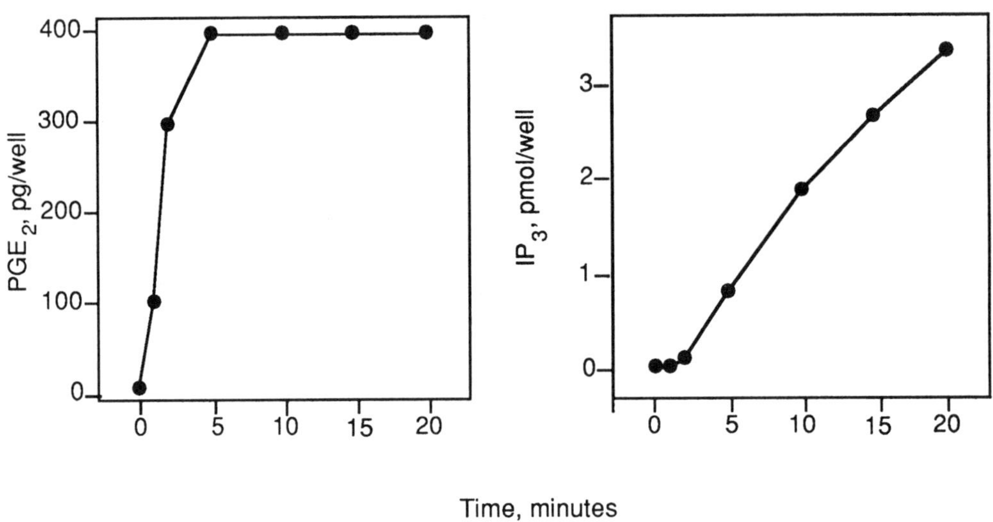

Figure 1. Time course for synthesis of PGE_2 and IP_3 after addition of 1 μM bradykinin to $SV-T_2$ 3T3 fibroblasts. Results are means of 6 determinations.

We have shown in these cells that stimulation of PGE_2 synthesis is the result of activation of phospholipase A_2, whereas IP_3 formation is the result of activation of phosphatidylinositol-specific phospholipase C (2). Both of these enzymes are coupled to the receptor by G proteins. Activation of the two phospholipases is independent. Dexamethasone and indomethacin completely inhibit bradykinin-stimulated PGE_2 synthesis while not affecting IP_3 formation at all.

Pretreatment of cells with phorbol esters greatly augments PGE_2 synthesis while inhibiting IP_3 formation. Neomycin inhibits IP_3 formation while not affecting PGE_2 synthesis (2).

Even though the pathways leading to PGE_2 and IP_3 are independent early on (5 minutes), at later times the two pathways do interact. As noted above, pretreatment with phorbol esters enhances PGE_2 synthesis. Phorbol esters activate protein kinase C. The endogenous stimulator of protein kinase C is diacylglycerol. Diacylglycerol is produced upon activation of phospholipase C. If 3T3 cells are stimulated with an agonist, such as thrombin or bradykinin to stimulate the production of diacylglycerol, then another agonist added which also stimulates diacylglycerol synthesis, the two agonists synergistically stimulate PGE_2 synthesis (Table 1). While we assume for the purpose of this report that diacylglycerol and phorbol esters increase PGE_2 release as a consequence of activation of protein kinase C, other studies have suggested that other mechanisms may contribute, as well (4,5).

Table 1. Interaction between bradykinin and thrombin

Treatment	Diacylglycerol % increase above basal	PGE_2 ng/well above basal
Bradykinin, 1 μM	50	0.4
Thrombin, 2U/ml	150	1.05
Bradykinin + Thrombin	240	2.2
Bradykinin then Thrombin	400	3.0
Thrombin then Bradykinin	760	5.1

cAMP production may also be elicited by bradykinin in 3T3 fibroblasts. This is a secondary effect of the peptide. Bradykinin stimulates PGE_2 synthesis, which in turn binds to its own receptor and stimulates cAMP synthesis (7). The use of a related 3T3 cell line has yielded the suggestion that cAMP-dependent protein kinase may also be important in PGE_2 synthesis. BALB/c 3T3 is the parent line for SV-T_2. However, if BALB/c 3T3 cells are stimulated with bradykinin, no PGE_2 synthesis occurs (8). This cell line expresses bradykinin receptors as revealed using radioligand binding studies. The receptors are coupled to transduction pathways, since bradykinin is mitogenic in BALB/c 3T3 cells. Further, if one examines arachidonate release, it is found to occur in response to bradykinin stimulation. However, the release of arachidonate is not reflected in enhanced PGE_2 synthesis. If the cells are pretreated with cAMP analogs, or synthetic activators of cAMP-dependent protein kinase, or agonists of receptors that stimulate adenylate cyclase, then bradykinin stimulation leads to synthesis of PGE_2. Apparently, fatty acid cyclooxygenase is dependent upon cAMP to be expressed (8).

In 3T3 fibroblasts PGE_2 also increases intracellular free calcium activity. This is achieved by inducing influx of extracellular calcium (9).

Studies in murine fibroblasts have shown that bradykinin initiates its biological effects by activation of phospholipases. Phosphatidylinositol-specific phospholipase C catalyzes the synthesis of inositol phosphates which release calcium from intracellular stores (Figure 2), and diacylglycerol which

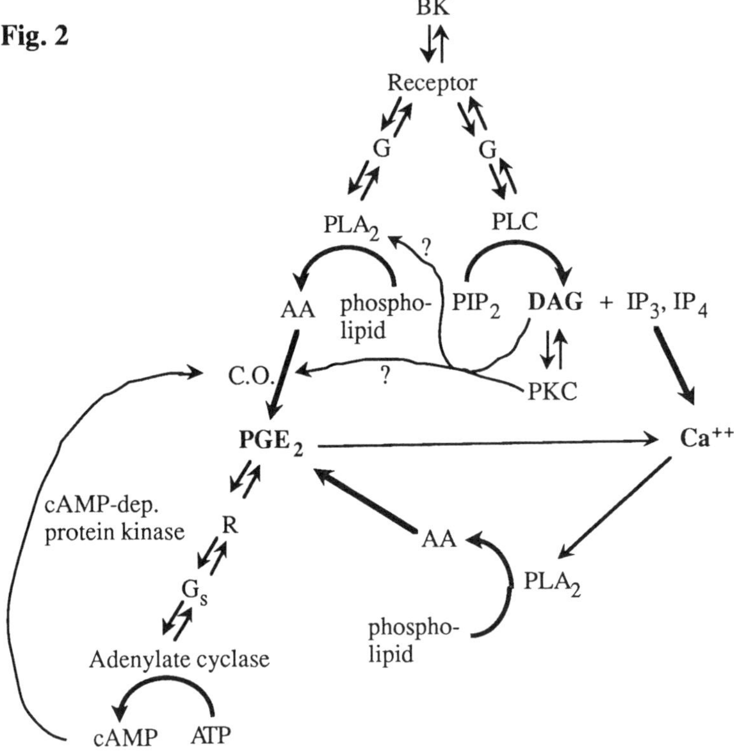

activates protein kinase C to increase PGE_2 synthesis. In these cells, protein kinase C is also known to feed back to inhibit inositol phosphate synthesis. Phospholipase A_2 releases arachidonic acid, which is converted to PGE_2 in these cells. PGE_2 binds to its own receptor and increases cAMP synthesis, and increases intracellular free calcium independent of inositol phosphates. The pathways leading to activation of phospholipase C and phospholipase A_2 are, at least for 5 minutes, pharmacologically distinct. However, interaction between the pathways becomes apparent downstream as the biologically active metabolites interact. Also drawn in Figure 2, but not directly investigated by us, is the calcium-sensitive phospholipase A_2 which has been found in many cell types and which is implicated in release of arachidonic acid for eicosanoid synthesis (10). In murine fibroblasts this enzyme may contribute to the prolonged arachidonic acid release and PGE_2 synthesis observed after stimulation of the cells with the cytokines interleukin 1 and tumor necrosis factor (11,12).

REFERENCES

1.   Burch, RM, Farmer, SG, Steranka, LR. Bradykinin receptor antagonists. Med Res Rev 1990; 10:237.

2.   Burch, RM, Axelrod, J. Dissociation of bradykinin-stimulated arachidonic acid release from inositol phosphate formation in Swiss 3T3 fibroblasts. Evidence for a G protein-coupled phospholipase A_2. Proc Natl Acad Sci USA 1987; 84:6374.

3.   Bredt, DS, Mourey, RJ, Snyder, SH. A simple, sensitive, and specific radioreceptor assay for inositol 1,4,5-trisphosphate in biological tissues. Biochem Biophys Res Commun. 1989; 159:976.

4.   Burch, RM, Ma, AL, Axelrod, J. Phorbol esters and diglycerides amplify bradykinin-stimulated prostaglandin synthesis in Swiss 3T3 fibroblasts. Possible independence form protein kinase C. J Biol Chem 1988; 263:4764.

5.   Burch, RM. Diacylglycerol stimulates phospholipase A_2 from Swiss 3T3 fibroblasts. FEBS Lett 1988; 234:283.

6.   Burch, RM. Diacylglycerol in the synergy of bradykinin and thrombin stimulation of prostaglandin synthesis. Eur J Pharmacol 1989; 168:39.

7.   Burch, RM, White, M, Connor, JR. Interleukin 1 stimulates prostaglandin synthesis and cyclic AMP production in Swiss 3T3 fibroblasts: interactions between two second messenger systems. J Cell Physiol 1989; 139:29.

8.   Burch, RM, Connor, JR. Amplification of interleukin 1-stimulated prostaglandin synthesis in fibroblasts cy cyclic nucleotides. J Cell Physiol. 1992; in press.

9.   Yamashita, T, Takai, Y. Inhibition of prostaglandin E1-induced elevation of cytoplasmic free calcium ion by protein kinase C-activating phorbol esters and diacylglycerol in Swiss 3T3 fibroblasts. J Biol Chem 1987; 262:5536.

10.   Clark, JD, Lin, L-L, Kriz, RW, Ramesha, CS, Sultzman, LA, Lin, AY, Milona, N, Knopf, JL. A novel arachidonic acid-selective cytosolic PLA$_2$ contains a homology to PKC and GAP. Cell 1991; 65:1043.

11.   Burch, RM, Connor, JR, Axelrod, J. Interleukin 1 amplifies receptor-mediated activation of phospholipase A$_2$ in 3T3 fibroblasts. Proc Natl Acad Sci USA 1988; 85:6306.

12.   Burch, RM, Tiffany, CW. Tumor necrosis factor causes amplification of arachidonic acid metabolism in response to interleukin 1, bradykinin, and other agonists. J Cell Physiol 1989; 141:85.

DESENSITIZATION OF BRADYKININ-INDUCED ACTIVATION OF PERIPHERAL NOCICEPTORS

A. Dray, I.A. Patel, M.N. Perkins, A. Rueff and L. Urban

Sandoz Institute for Medical Research, 5 Gower Place, London WC1E 6BN, UK

SUMMARY: Bradykinin-induced activation of peripheral nociceptors has been studied in an isolated spinal cord/tail preparation from the neonatal rat. Prolonged administration of bradykinin consistently produced a selective desensitization which could be prevented by concanavalin A but not by succinyl concanavalin A or phenylarsine oxide. These data indicate that mannose-containing glycoproteins occur in or close to the bradykinin receptor site. In addition the desensitization observed under the present conditions, did not involve the internalization of bradykinin receptors.

INTRODUCTION

Bradykinin is a pain producing and pro-inflammatory nonapeptide which activates a sub-population of polymodal nociceptors. Studies of nociceptor activation by bradykinin have been made in vivo [1,2] but these experiments provide little quantitative information about the events and factors on which the effects of bradykinin depend. This is mainly due to the physical and biochemical restrictions imposed on studies of fine sensory nerve terminals in situ.

A common feature of the action of bradykinin on many cell systems, including nociceptors, is rapid desensitization [3,4,5,6,7] which occurs with repeated or prolonged exposure to bradykinin. Judging from studies on other sytems, desensitization may involve several mechanisms including dislocation of receptor from second messenger or translocation and internalization of membrane receptor protein [5,6,8]. In order to study this phenomenon in nociception we have used an in vitro preparation of the spinal cord with functionally connected tail, maintained in vitro. This preparation allows the composition of the superfusate in contact with peripheral fibres to be altered. This is advantageous for evaluating the mechanisms of nociceptor activation.

We have investigated desensitization to bradykinin which acts via a B_2 receptor and the subsequent activation of second messenger systems in this preparation [9,10]. We have used concanavalin A, a plant lectin, previously shown to prevent desensitization of other nerve membrane receptors [11,12].

METHODS

The intact spinal cord and the functionally connected tail were removed from 1-2 day old rats following decapitation. The skin was carefully removed from the tail. This procedure exposed cutaneous fibres and their endings to allow activation by bradykinin. The efficacy of bradykinin and other noxious stimuli suggested that nociceptors were preserved in our viable preparations. The preparation was placed in a chamber such that the cord and tail could be separately superfused (2-4ml/min) with a physiological salt solution (composition mM: NaCl 138.6, KCl 3.35, $CaCl_2$ 1.26, $MgCl_2$ 1.16, $NaHCO_3$ 21.0, $NaHPO_4$ 0.58, glucose 10; at $24^{\circ}C$ and gassed with 95% O_2/5% CO_2). Peripheral nociceptive fibres were activated by superfusion of the tail with bradykinin, capsaicin and by superfusate heated to $48^{\circ}C$ (noxious heat). Each stimulus was applied for 10 sec with an intervening period of 15 minutes between stimuli. Bradykinin applications were separated by at least 40-60min to avoid tachyphylaxis.

The activation of peripheral fibres was assessed by measuring the depolarization produced in a spinal ventral root (L_3-L_5). The ventral root potential was recorded (dc with respect to the spinal cord which was earthed) using a low impedence glass pipette which was placed in an electrolyte-filled well containing the selected ventral root. The signals were amplified using conventional means (Neurolog System) and displayed simultaneously on an oscilloscope and on a rectilinear chart recorder.

RESULTS

Brief administration of bradykinin in the tail superfusate at submaximal concentrations (10s, 200-350nM; maximal concentration 1μM) produced a ventral root response due to the activation of capsaicin sensitive nociceptors [9]. These responses were reproducible if bradykinin applications were separated by periods of 30-60min to avoid tachypylaxis. Responses were also evoked by other noxious stimuli, incuding capsaicin (10s, 300-700nM) and heat ($48^{\circ}C$). Selective tachyphylaxis to bradykinin could be produced by prolonged exposure (5min, 1µM) such that subsequent brief applications of bradykinin were ineffective, whereas responses to heat and capsaicin were unchanged (Figure 1).

Exposure of the tail to concanavalin A (1µM) at a concentration shown to prevent desensitization of other receptors [11] completely prevented the bradykinin-induced desensitization (n=6) (Figure 1). This effect of concanavalin A was prevented by co-administration of α-methyl mannoside (10mM) which is bound to mannose sugar recognition sites on concanavalin A. Under these circumstances the bradykinin-induced desensitization was produced once again. Similar exposure of the tail to succinyl concanavalin A (1µM) did not prevent bradykinin-induced desensitization. Finally pretreatment with phenylarsine oxide (100µM) did not affect bradykinin-induced desensitization.

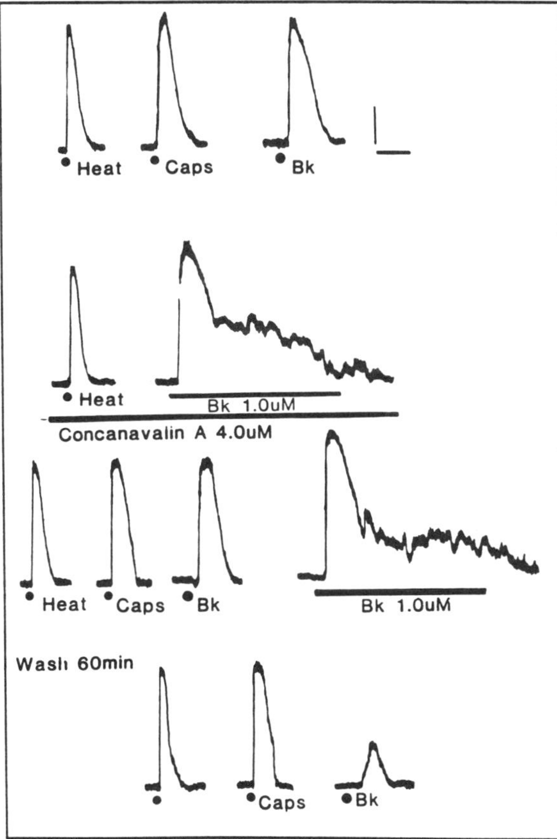

Figure 1. Concanavalin A prevents bradykinin desensitization.

The top traces show control responses to heat (48°C), capsaicin (700nM) and bradykinin (350nM). The second row of traces show a response to a prolonged administration of bradykinin (5min, 1µM) in the presence of concanavalin A (1µM, indicated by the bar below the trace). Following this, the subsequent responses to heat, capsaicin and bradykinin (3rd row) were unchanged. The repeated, prolonged administration of bradykinin, in the absence of concanavalin A, evoked a prolonged response which was not sustained. Following this however the response to further application of bradykinin was significantly attenuated without changes in the responses evoked by heat or capsaicin. The calibration bars are 0.2mV and 60s.

DISCUSSION

The present experiments have demonstrated that bradykinin-induced activation of peripheral nocicepors undergoes a rapid desensitization. This phenomenon was consistently and selectively prevented by the lectin, concanavalin A which has been shown previously to prevent desensitization of bradykinin receptors in fibroblasts [5,6] and NG-108-15 cells [7]. In addition concanavalin A has been shown to prevent desensitization in a number of other ligand-receptor interactions including glutamate [11], β-adrenergic receptors[8].

The effect of concanavalin A appeared to depend on an interaction with mannose sugar residues, as previously indicated [12], since its action was prevented by α-methyl mannoside. In addition cross-linking of membrane glycoproteins by the four identical polypeptide subunits of concanavalin A , would appear to be necessary for this effect since cross linking would not occur with the dimeric analogue, succinyl concanavalin A which did not prevent desensitization to bradykinin. Finally bradykinin desensitization was unaffected by phenylarsine oxide which has been suggested to interact with membrane sulphydryl groups to stabilize membrane structure and thereby prevent sequestration of receptor protein prior to internalization [5,13]. Receptor internalization has been proposed as a mechanism to account for desensitization of several receptors including insulin, epidermal growth factor, β-adrenergic receptor and bradykinin receptors in human fibroblasts [5,12,13].

It would seem unlikely that the activity of membrane proteases and the rapid breakdown of bradykinin could explain bradykinin desensitization. Our previous unpublished studies have indicated that the effects of bradykinin in this preparation, were unchanged in the presence of a number of kininase inhibitors. The most likely explanation for the present observations would be a transformation of bradykinin-receptors from high to lower affinity state, as suggested from studies on other tissue [4,7].

In summary, the present study has shown that bradykinin-receptor desensitization can be prevented by concanavalin A, indicating the presence of mannose containing glycoproteins in, or close to, the bradykinin receptor site. In addition receptor desensitization, under the present conditions, did not involve the internalization of bradykinin receptors.

REFERENCES

1. Beck PW, Handwerker HO. Bradykinin and serotonin effects on various types of cutaneous nerve fibres. Pfluegers Arch., 1974; 347: 209-222.

2. Franz M, Mense S. Muscle receptors with Group IV afferent fibres responding to applications of bradykinin. 1975; Brain Res. 92: 369-383.

3. Burgess GM, Mullaney I, McNeil M, Dunn PM, Rang HP. Second messengers involved in the mechanism of action of bradykinin in sensory neurones in culture. J. Neurosci.,1989; 9: 3314-3325.

4. Roberts RA, Gullick WJ. Bradykinin receptors undergo ligand-induced desensitization. Biochem. 1990; 29: 1975-1979.

5. Roscher AA, Klier C, Faussner A. Bradykinin receptor desensitization and down-regulation. 1991; (This symposium).

6. Roscher AA, Manganiello V, Jeselma CL, Moss J. Autoregulation of bradykinin receptors and bradykinin-induced prostacyclin formation in human fibroblasts 1984; J.Clin Invest. 74; 552-558.

7. Wolsing DH, Rosenbaum JS, Bradykinin stimulated inositol phosphate production in NG108-15 cells in mediated by a small population of binding sites which rapidly desensitize. J. Pharm Exp. Ther., 1991; 257: 621-633.

8. Sibley DR, Lefkowitz RJ. Molecular mechanisms of receptor desensitization using the β-adrenergic receptor-coupled adenylate cyclase sytem as a model. Nature 1985; 317: 124-129.

9. Dray A, Bettaney J, Forster P, Perkins MN. Bradykinin-induced stimulation of afferent fibres is mediated through protein kinase C. Neurosci. Lett., 1988; 91: 301-307.

10. Dray A, Bettaney J, Forster P, Perkins MN. Activation of a bradykinin receptor in peripheral nerve and spinal cord in the neonatal rat in vitro. Br. J. Pharmacol. 1988; 95: 1008-1010.

11. Huettner JE. Glutamate receptor channels in rat DRG neurons: activation by kainate and quisqualate and blockade of desensitization by con A. Neuron 1990; 5: 255-266.

12. Lin SS Levitan IB Concanavalin A: a tool to investigate neuronal plasticity. TINS 1991; 14: 273-277.

13. Hartel C, Coulter SJ, Perkins JP. A comparison of catecholamine-induced ineternalization of β–adrenergic receptors and receptor-mediated endocytosis of epidermal growth factor in human astrocytoma cells. Inhibition by phenylarsine oxide. J. Biol Chem. 1985; 260: 12547-12553.

AAS 38/II
Recent Progress on Kinins
© 1992 Birkhäuser Verlag Basel

EFFECTS OF BRADYKININ ON ION CONDUCTANCES IN NG108-15 NEUROBLASTOMA x GLIOMA HYBRID CELLS RECORDED WITH PATCH-CLAMP ELECTRODES

[1]J.Robbins,[2]I.McFadzean & [1]D.A.Brown

[1]Department of Pharmacology, University College London, Gower Street, London, WC1E 6BT, U.K. and [2]Department of Pharmacology, Kings College London, Manresa Road, London, SW3 6LX, U.K.

SUMMARY: Under whole-cell recording, bradykinin (BK) produced an initial outward membrane current followed by an inward current in voltage-clamped NG108-15 cells. The initial outward current was associated with a rise in intracellular Ca^{2+} and was accompanied by the opening of Ca^{2+}-dependent K^+-channels recorded with a cell-attached patch electrode. This current was inhibited by intracellular Mg^{2+}. The inward current was associated with inhibition of the voltage-dependent K^+-current $I_{K(M)}$. These effects accord with those previously observed in microelectrode-impaled cells, with the difference that BK produced much more pronounced and long-lasting desensitization in the patch-clamped cells.

INTRODUCTION

NG108-15 mouse neuroblastoma x rat glioma cells are particularly convenient neural cells for correlating the biochemical effects of bradykinin (BK) with their effects on neural ionic conductances. Thus, they express a high density of BK receptors, which couple avidly to the phosphoinositide pathway (14). Further, when differentiated, these cells express a variety of neural ionic currents conferring excitable properties (1).

In previous experiments on microelectrode-impaled cells, it has been established that activation of BK receptors induces two principal ionic conductance changes: an initial outward (hyperpolarizing) current, caused by the formation of IP_3, release of internal Ca^{2+} and subsequent activation of Ca^{2+}-dependent K^+ channels; and a later inward (depolarizing) current, caused primarily by the inhibition of a voltage-dependent K+-current, the M-current $I_{K(M)}$ (2,5,6). It was suggested that this latter effect might result from formation of diacylglycerol and activation of protein kinase C (5).

In the present experiments we have examined to what extent these previously-recorded effects of BK are maintained in NG108-15 cells following intracellular dialysis with patch-clamp electrodes.

Fig. 1

Examples of BK (10μM, bath applied at arrows)-induced intracellular Ca²⁺ rises in NG108-15 cells. Top trace is from a cell loaded with Indo-1/AM (5μM, 45 mins) and not voltage clamped. The lower trace is from a cell loaded with Indo-1 tetrapotassium salt (100μM) from a patch pipette and voltage clamped at resting membrane potential (-63 mV).

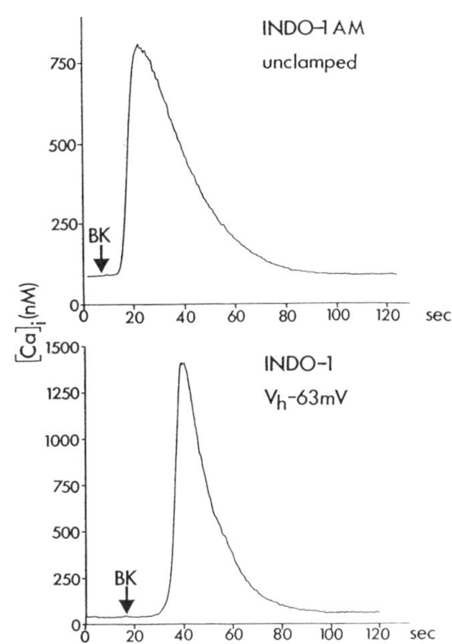

Fig. 2

Single $I_{K(Ca)}$ channels recorded in cell attached mode (asymmetrical [K⁺]) activated by pressure-applied ionomycin (50μM) (A) and bradykinin (10μM) (B). Traces on the right show an expanded section of the traces on the left. Pipette potential -60mV for both cells.

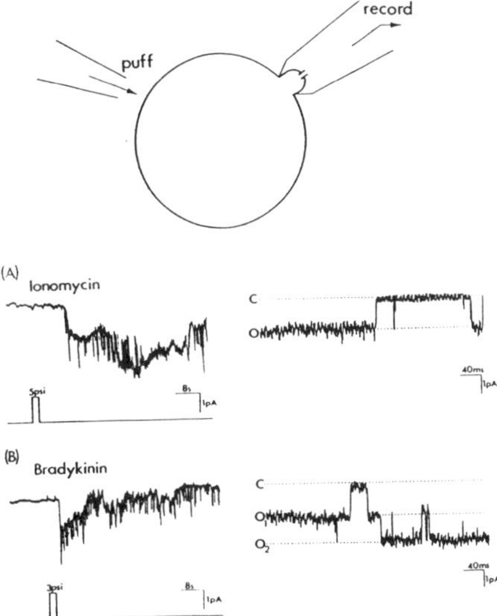

METHODS

NG108-15 cells were cultured and differentiated as described by Docherty (3). Cells were superfused with bicarbonate-buffered Krebs solution at 35°C and patch-clamped with electrodes containing 90 mM $KOOCH_3$, 20 mM KCl, 40 mM HEPES, 3 mM $MgCl_2$ and 3 mM EGTA. For Ca^{2+}-current recording, electrodes were filled with a CsCl solution (7). Current recordings were made using a switching voltage-clamp amplifier (see (12) for details). In some experiments, intracellular $[Ca^{2+}]$ was measured using 100 μM Indo-1 without EGTA in the pipette, or using Indo-1/AM ester (12).

RESULTS

1. Intracellular Ca^{2+}

In unclamped, unpatched cells, application of 10 μM BK produced a brisk rise in intracellular $[Ca^{2+}]$ after a few seconds delay (Fig.1a), in agreement with previous reports (8,9). This response was preserved when cells were voltage-clamped with a patch-electrode (Fig.1b). Hence, the essential elements of the Ca-releasing pathway were well maintained following dialysis with the patch electrode. This experiment also shows that the rise in intracellular $[Ca^{2+}]$ was not secondary to membrane depolarization and opening of Ca^{2+} channels (cf.ref.8).

2. Outward current

Notwithstanding the brisk rise in intracellular $[Ca^{2+}]$ seen with Indo-1, in initial experiments on patch-clamped cells we could only rarely (3/22 cells) detect any substantial Ca^{2+}-activated K^+-current comparable to that previously recorded in microelectrode-impaled cells (5). For the latter, microelectrodes filled with K citrate were used. Accordingly, when the normal anion in the patch pipette was replaced with K citrate, an outward K^+-current was detected in 7/10 cells tested. Likewise, intracellular iontophoretic injections of inositol trisphosphate only generated outward currents in cells patched with K citrate-filled electrodes. The reason for this appears to be that citrate reduces the intracellular free $[Mg^{2+}]$ concentration from about 1 mM to 0.07 mM in our pipette solution: thus, simply reducing intracellular $[Mg^{2+}]$ to 0.1 mM restored the outward current, even in acetate-filled pipettes (11).

In agreement with previous observations (2,5), the outward current induced by BK or by IP_3 injections was frequently blocked by apamin. However, in some cells the current appeared insensitive to apamin, and instead was blocked by charybdotoxin (Fig.2), whilst in others the current was partly blocked by both peptides. Hence, the current seems to be carried by two pharmacologically-distinct populations of Ca^{2+}-activated K^+-channels.

Also in confirmation of previous observations (6), single K^+-channels within cell-attached patch-pipettes of about 40 pS conductance could be activated by extra-patch application of BK (Fig.3B). Identical channels were also activated when cell Ca^{2+} was increased by external application of ionomycin (Fig.3A). This confirms that (a) K^+-channel activation by BK involves a cytoplasmic messenger, and (b) the final messenger is Ca^{2+}.

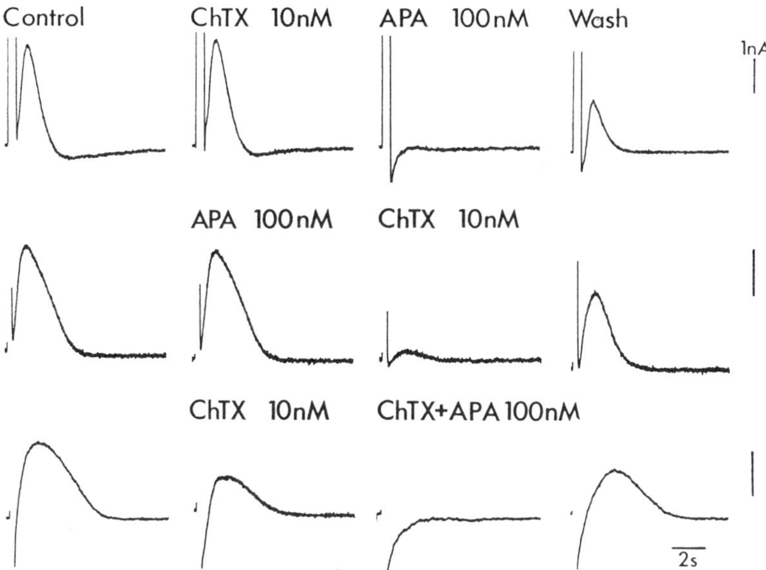

Fig. 3 IP_3-activated K^+ currents from NG108-15 cells. Examples of the relative proportions of current sensitive to charybdotoxin (ChTX) and apamin (APA). Top traces show a cell sensitive to apamin whereas the middle traces show a cell sensitive to only ChTX. The lower traces show the most frequently observed situation where both apamin and ChTX are needed to block the current. IP_3 ($100\mu M$) iontophoretic injections (10-20 nA, 100-300 ms), holding potential -30 mV for all the cells.

3. Inward Current

Also in agreement with previous experiments on microelectrode-impaled cells, BK consistently produced an inward current accompanied by a decreased input conductance (Fig.4). This conductance decrease reflected a reduction in the time- and voltage-dependent K$^+$-current, $I_{K(M)}$, as evidenced by the inhibition of the time-dependent deactivation relaxations induced by hyperpolarizing steps in Fig.4A. In NG108-15 cells, $I_{K(M)}$ is activated from about -70 mV upwards (12). As shown in Fig.5, this induces a very substantial outward rectification to the steady-state current-voltage (I/V) curve. BK reduced this outward rectification, but did not change the conductance negative to -70 mV, where $I_{K(M)}$ is deactivated (Fig.5a). This is seen more clearly where external [K$^+$] is raised to 24 mM (Fig.5b): the initial activation of $I_{K(M)}$ then induces inward rectification, which is also reduced

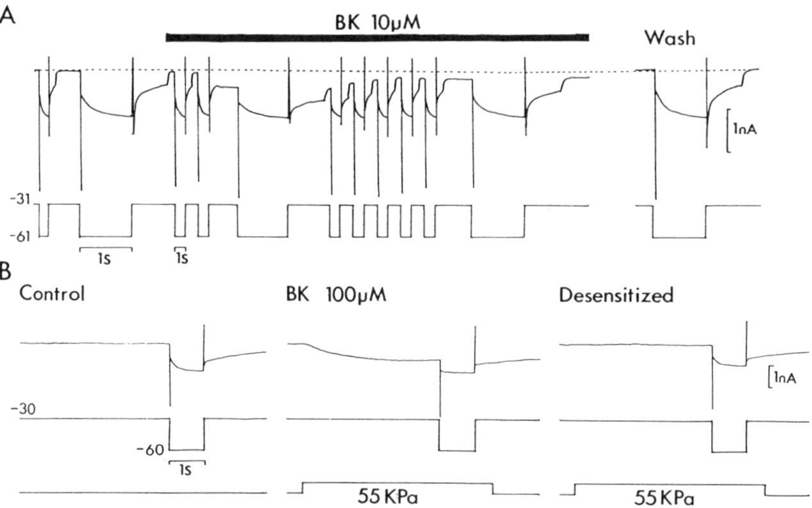

Fig. 4 Inhibition of $I_{K(M)}$ by bradykinin. **A**: continuous recording of clamp current (upper trace) and membrane voltage (lower trace). The cell was held at -31 mV and commanded to -61 mV for 1s every 30s; the recorder was accelerated x100 or x500 for each step-command. Bradykinin (BK, 10µM) was added to the superfusing fluid for the period shown by the bar. The last record ("wash") was obtained 4 min after reperfusion with normal Kreb's solution. **B**: responses to pressure-application of bradykinin from a micropipette filled with 100µM bradykinin. Note that the second application (last trace) made 5 min after the first application (middle trace) was ineffective.

Fig. 5 Currents recorded in response to voltage ramps applied before (C), and during (BK) superfusion with $5\mu M$ bradykinin, (a) in normal Krebs' solution containing 3mM [K$^+$] and then (b) after raising to 24mM. Arrows denote the calculated K$^+$ equilibrium potentials (E_K). Dashed lines show zero holding current (I_0). The voltage ramp was applied from a holding potential of 0mV to -120 mV, at a rate of 2.5 mV.s^{-1}.

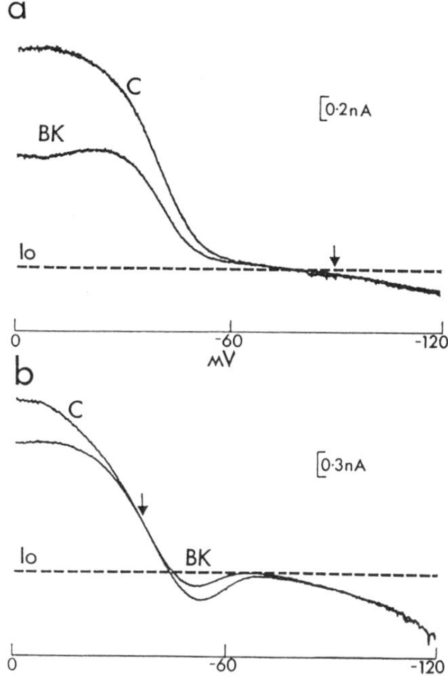

Fig. 6 Inhibition of I_{Ca} by BK is not PTX sensitive. Cell pretreated with PTX ($1\mu g/ml$, 24 hr). (A) pressure application of BK inhibits I_{Ca}. (B) Bath applications of noradrenaline (NA) and acetylcholine (ACh) had no effects on this same cell as their responses are pertussis sensitive (B). Cells were recorded with CsCl filled electrodes and tetraethylamonium-based Krebs solution. The holding potential was -90 mV and command steps every 30 s to 0 mV.

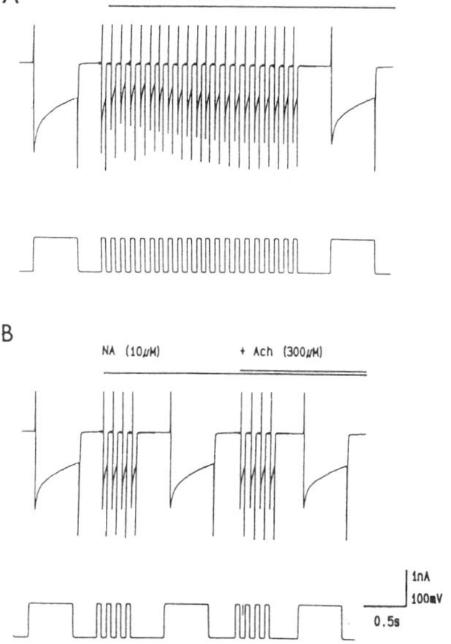

by BK. Thus, in confirmation of earlier conclusions (2), the inward currentinduced by BK in NG108-15 cells can be ascribed entirely to inhibition of the voltage-gated current $I_{K(M)}$.

Unlike the outward current, this response was not sensitive to the concentration of Mg^{2+} in the pipette solution, so could be recorded using either acetate or citrate in the pipette (11). Thus, with acetate, only the inward current response was observed (as in Fig.4), so that outward and inward current responses could be dissociated under these conditions.

By comparison with previous (and concurrent) experiments with microelectrode-impaled cells, two differences in the $I_{K(M)}$-inhibitory action of BK were noticeable in patch-clamped cells. Firstly, the magnitude of the inhibition was rather less, rarely exceeding 50 %. Secondly, the response showed very pronounced desensitization either during continuous application of BK (Fig.4A) or with repeated brief pressure-applications (Fig.4B). Moreover, no recovery from desensitization could be detected after quite prolonged washing (up to 30 min or so). Addition of ATP or GTP to the pipette solution did not hasten recovery from desensitization.

<u>4. Ca-current inhibition</u>

We previously noted that the inward current produced by BK in microelectrode-impaled cells was accompanied by a partial inhibition of the inward Ca-current I_{Ca} (2). This we originally suggested to arise from the increased intracellular $[Ca^{2+}]$, but more recent experiments (13) have suggested the two phenomena to be independent. In the present experiments, we have also detected an inhibition of I_{Ca} (Fig.6), which persisted under conditions where intracellular Ca2+ was buffered with 20 mM BAPTA and hence is unlikely to be secondary to a rise in intracellular Ca^{2+}.

<u>5. G-proteins</u>

Neither inhibition of $I_{K(M)}$ nor inhibition of I_{Ca} was prevented by Pertussis toxin (PTX). Thus, for inhibition of $I_{K(M)}$ by pressure-applied BK (100 μM, 2-8 psi), values were (mean $\pm$ s.e.m.): +PTX (1 μM, 24 hr), 57.2 $\pm$ 4.7 % (n = 9); -PTX, 65.0 $\pm$ 8.6 % (n = 8). For inhibition of I_{Ca}, corresponding values were: +PTX, 34.2 $\pm$ 5.1 % (n = 5); - PTX, 32.4 $\pm$ 7.7 % (n = 5). This accords with the PTX-resistant inhibition of $I_{K(M)}$ by acetylcholine (10), but contrasts with the PTX-sensitive inhibition of I_{Ca} by noradrenaline (7).

It also accords with the PTX-resistant stimulation of GTPase in these cells by BK (4). Hence, it is possible that inhibition of both currents might be mediated by the same G-protein.

DISCUSSION

The present experiments confirm the two principal actions of BK on resting membrane currents in NG108-15 cells previously observed in microelectrode-impaled cells - namely, initial activation of a Ca^{2+}-dependent K^+-current $I_{K(Ca)}$, followed by inhibition of the voltage-dependent K^+-current $I_{K(M)}$.

Activation of $I_{K(Ca)}$ undoubtedly results from the formation of IP_3 and consequent rise in intracellular Ca^{2+}, for reasons stated previously (6). In the present experiments we have confirmed both the parallel rise in intracellular Ca^{2+}, and the ability of either iontophoretically-injected intracellular IP_3 or Ca^{2+} (11) or Ca^{2+}-loading with ionomycin to activate the outward current. The current appears to be carried by at least two pharmacologically-distinct classes of K^+-channel, one sensitive to apamin and one to charybdotoxin, the proportional contributions of which seem to vary considerably from one cell to another. In cell-attached patch recordings we confirm the contribution of one class of channels with a conductance of about 40 pS (cf.ref.5) but the pharmacological identity of this channel has not yet been determined. We also noted that the current appears to be suppressed when internal Mg^{2+} exceeds 0.5 mM or so (11). This may be an important determinant of the extent to which the current (and the consequent hyperpolarization) is expressed in intact cells. Our estimates of resting $[Mg^{2+}]$ (0.14 mM: ref.11) suggest that BK-induced $I_{K(Ca)}$ should normally be expressed, but might be inhibited by rises in intracellular $[Mg^{2+}]$.

The mechanism responsible for inhibition of $I_{K(M)}$ is less clear. It is unlikely to result directly from the rise in intracellular $[Ca^{2+}]$ since it persists when intracellular Ca^{2+} is heavily buffered with 20 mM BAPTA (J.Robbins, unpublished observations). We originally suggested that it might result from formation of DAG and activation of PKC since application of phorbol dibutyrate (PDBu) or oleoylacetylglycerol (OAG) also inhibited $I_{K(M)}$ and occluded the effect of BK (5). However, in our experiments with patch-electrodes PDBu did not inhibit $I_{K(M)}$ under conditions where BK was effective: while this does not exclude a contribution by PKC to the inhibition produced in intact cells, it implies that activation of PKC is unlikely to be an obligatory step in the pathway for $I_{K(M)}$-inhibition by BK. On the other hand, the absence of such a step might explain why BK was less effective in our patch-clamped cells than in microelectrode-impaled cells.

The most striking difference between the present tests on patch-clamped cells and our previous experiments on microelectrode-impaled cells was the remarkably intense and persistent desensitization to BK. This suggests that recovery from desensitization requires some intracellular substance which might have been dialysed out by the patch electrode. This substance is not ATP or GTP, but we have not yet tested other cytoplasmic constituents. It is noticeable that no equivalent desensitization to the comparable effects of acetylcholine in patch-clamped cells occurs (10). Likewise, inhibition of I_{Ca} in patch-clamped NG108-15 cells by the peptide agonists enkephalin and somatostatin shows much more pronounced desensitization than that produced by small ligands such as noradrenaline (7). This suggests that some property inherent to peptide receptors is responsible for desensitization. Further experiments to elucidate this would clearly be useful.

REFERENCES

1. Brown,D.A. & Higashida,H. (1988). Voltage- and calcium-activated potassium currents in mouse neuroblastoma x rat glioma hybrid cells. *J.Physiol.* **357**, 149-165.

2. Brown,D.A. & Higashida,H. (1988). Membrane current responses of NG108-15 mouse neuroblastoma x glioma hybrid cells to bradykinin. *J.Physiol.* **397**, 167-184.

3. Docherty,R.J. (1988). Gadolinium selectively blocks a component of calcium current in rodent neuroblastoma x glioma hybrid (NG108-15) cells. *J.Physiol.*, **398**, 33-47.

4. Grandt,R., Greiner,C., Zubin,P. & Jakobs,K.H. (1986). Bradykinin stimulates GTP hydrolysis in NG108-15 membranes by a high-affinity, pertussis toxin-insensitive GTPase. *FEBS Lett.*, **196**, 279-283.

5. Higashida,H. & Brown,D.A. (1986). Two polyphosphoinositide metabolites control two K^+ currents in a neuronal cell. *Nature*, **323**, 333-335.

6. Higashida,H. & Brown,D.A. (1988). Ca^{2+}-dependent K^+ channels in neuroblastoma hybrid cells activated by intracellular inositol trisphosphate and extracellular bradykinin. *FEBS Lett.*, **238**, 395-400.

7. McFazdean,I. & Docherty,R.J. (1989). Noradrenaline and enkephalin-induced inhibition of voltage-sensitive calcium currents in NG108-15 hybrid cells. *Eur.J.Neurosci.*, **1**, 141-147.

8. Osugi,T., Uchida,S., Imaizumi,T. & Yoshida,H. (1986). Bradykinin-induced intracellular Ca^{2+} elevation in neuroblastoma x glioma hybrid NG108-15 cells: relationship to the action of inositol phospholipid metabolites. *Brain Res.*, **379**, 84-89.

9. Reiser,G. & Hamprecht,B. (1985). Bradykinin causes a transient rise of intracellular Ca^{2+} activity in cultured neural cells. *Pflueg.Arch.*, **405**, 260-264.

10.Robbins,J., Caulfield,M.P., Higashida,H. & Brown,D.A. (1991). Genotypic m3-muscarinic receptors preferentially inhibit M-currents in DNA-transfected NG108-15 neuroblastoma x glioma hybrid cells. *Eur.J.Neurosci.*, **3**, 820-824.

11.Robbins,J., Cloues,R. & Brown,D.A. (1992). Intracellular Mg^{2+} inhibits the IP_3-activated $I_{K(Ca)}$ in NG108-15 cells. *Pflueg.Arch.*(in press).

12.Robbins,J., Trouslard,J., Marsh,S.J. & Brown,D.A. (1992). Kinetic and pharmacological properties of the M-current in rodent neuroblastoma x glioma hybrid cells. *J.Physiol.*(in press).

13.Shimahara,T., Icard-Liepkins,C., Ohmori,H. & Shigemoto,T. (1990). Mobilization of intracellular Ca^{2+} and suppression of inward currents in a neuronal hybrid cell line triggered by bradykinin. *Brain Res.*, **524**, 219-224.

14.Yano,K., Higashida,H., Inoue,R. & Nozawa,Y. (1984). Bradykinin-induced rapid breakdown of phosphatidylinositol 4,5-bisphosphate in neuroblastoma x glioma hybrid NG108-15 cells. *J.biol.Chem.*, **259**, 10201-10207.

AAS 38/II
Recent Progress on Kinins
© 1992 Birkhäuser Verlag Basel

CHARACTERIZATION OF RECEPTOR-MEDIATED ACTION OF T-KININ AND [D-ILE[1]]-T-KININ , INDICATING THE EXISTENCE OF A SUBTYPE OF BRADYKININ B_2 RECEPTORS

XiaoXing Gao, John M. Stewart*, Raymond J. Vavrek* and
Lowell M. Greenbaum

Department of Pharmacology/Toxicology, Medical College of Georgia,
Augusta, Ga 30912, USA and *Department of Biochemistry, University of Colorado,
Denver, Co 80262, USA

INTRODUCTION

The receptors of kinins are classified into two types, the B_1 receptor which has high affinity for des-Arg^9-bradykinin, the product of carboxypeptidase action on bradykinin, and the B_2 receptor which is more sensitive to bradykinin itself (1). Recently, it was proposed that there are B_3 receptors in the guinea-pig trachea because the effects of kinins on the guinea-pig trachea contraction was completely insensitive to both B_1 and B_2 receptor antagonists (2).

As an endogenous peptide, T-kinin (Ile-Ser-bradykinin) generated from T-kininogen (3,4) by the action of T-kininogenase found in the rat submandibular gland (5) has very similar pharmacological properties to those of bradykinin. The purpose of this study is to characterize the type of receptors for T-kinin existing in the rat uterus.

MATERIALS AND METHODS

Animals and Agents used.
Female Sprague-Dawley rats weighing 200-250 g were injected with diethylestilbesterol (200 µg) subcutaneously 20 hours before the experiments.

T-kinin, bradykinin, [Des-Arg^9]-bradykinin were purchased from Peninsula Lab., Inc., Belmont, Ca. [D-Arg^0, Hyp^3, D-Phe^7] bradykinin was kindly supplied by Dr. Regoli, Univ. of Sherbrooke, Canada. [D-Ile1]-T-kinin was synthesized by Drs. Stewart and Vavrek. ^{3}H-bradykinin was purchased from Dupont-NEN, Boston, MA.

Bioassay of T-kinin on isolated tissues.
The method used was described by Freer et al (6). Under ether anesthesia the rat uterus was removed. The isolated intact tissue was trimmed of fascia and suspended in a tissue bath and bathed in de Jalon's solution (NaCl, 0.15 M; KCl, 5.6 mM; CaCl$_2$, 0.4 mM; MgCl$_2$, 25 µM; NaHCO$_3$, 6 mM; Glucose, 3 mM) continuously bubbled with 97% oxygen and 3% carbon dioxide at 24°C. The rat uterus was placed under 1 g of tension until a stable baseline was obtained (approx. 1 hr). Changes in tension after addition of kinins and their agonists or antagonists were recorded using a polygraph (Grass model 79D) with force-displacement transducers (Grass model FT03C). In the assays of antagonist activities, the antagonist was preincubated in the tissue bath for 20 sec before the addition of T-kinin, bradykinin or agonists. In the studies of the effects of indomethacin on T-kinin- and bradykinin-induced contractions of the rat uterus, the tissue was incubated with indomethacin for 60 min before it was exposed to kinins.

Binding assay of T-kinin on rat uterus. The method used was modified from Manning et al. (7). The saturation analysis of [^{3}H]-bradykinin binding to the receptors in rat myometrial plasma membrane was accomplished by incubating the partially purified receptor preparation with [^{3}H]-bradykinin (NEN, 78.4 Ci/mmol) in a total volume of 1 ml. Specific binding was calculated by subtracting the non-specific binding measured in the presence of 1 µM of unlabeled bradykinin from the total binding. In the experiments of displacement of kinins on [^{3}H]-bradykinin binding, 100 µl of kinin-containing solutions was incubated with [^{3}H]-bradykinin and receptor preparation.

Data analysis. Values were expressed as mean ± standard error. The Student's unpaired t tests were used for testing the difference between means of different groups. A level of probability <0.05 was considered to represent a statistically significant difference. ED50 and IC50 values were obtained using nonlinear least squares regression of curves (Michaelis-Menten equation). Ki values were calculated from IC50.

RESULTS AND DISCUSSION

T-kinin is similar to bradykinin in terms of its pharmacological properties. It was reported by several investigators that T-kinin was active in the regulation of blood pressure. Peripheral administration of T-kinin reduces blood pressure of the rat (8); however, T-kinin exhibits hypertensive activity following intraventricular injection (9). The studies on isolated vascular smooth muscles by Rhaleb et al (10) showed that T-kinin caused relaxation of dog carotid and renal arteries and contraction of rabbit jugular vein, but was less potent in these effects than bradykinin. In contrast, T-kinin showed higher potency than bradykinin in increasing the vascular permeability of rat and guinea pig skin (11) and in changing short-circuit current across the rat colon (12).

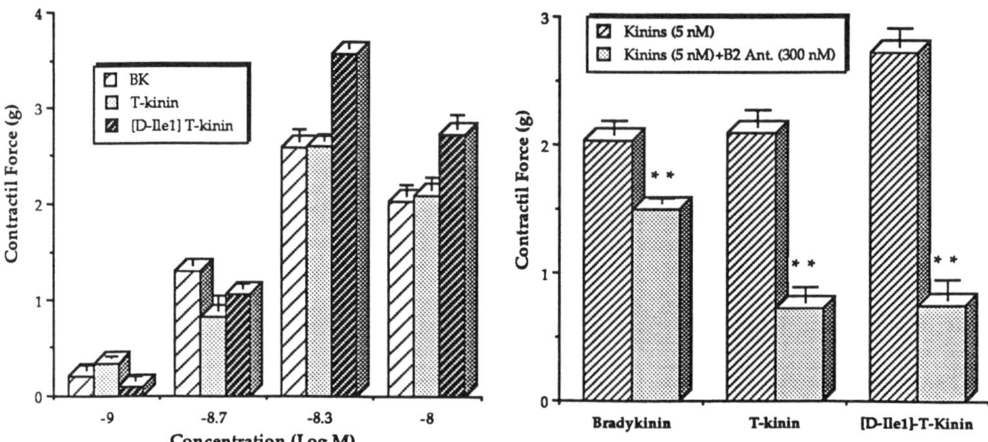

Fig. 1. Response of the rat uterus to T-kinin (n=4), bradykinin (n=4), and [D-Ile^1]-T-kinin (n=3).

Fig. 2. Effect of [D-Arg^0, Hyp^3, D-Phe^7]-bradykinin, a B$_2$ antagonist, on response of rat uterus to T-kinin. The antagonist was added to the tissue bath 20 sec prior to the addition of the kinins. n=4; **p<0.01

Our current results showed that on the contraction of isolated intact rat uterus, the potency of T-kinin (ED50: 2.3±0.24 nM) and bradykinin (ED50: 2.04±0.22 nM) were very similar; however, the D-configuration of T-kinin, [D-Ile1]-T-kinin was much more potent (ED50: >10 μM) than T-kinin and bradykinin in contracting rat uterus smooth muscle (Fig 1). Following the treatment with a bradykinin B_2 antagonist, [D-Arg^0, Hyp^3, D-Phe^7] bradykinin, responses of the rat uterus to these three peptides were inhibited significantly to different degrees (Fig 2). T-kinin and [D-Ile^1]-T-kinin were more sensitive to this B_2 antagonist when compared with bradykinin. On the other hand, [Des-Arg^9]-bradykinin, a bradykinin B_1 receptor agonist, did not show any activity on rat uterus smooth muscle; the addition of [Des-Arg^9, Leu^8]-bradykinin prior to the application of bradykinin, T-kinin and [D-Ile^1]-T-kinin did not interfere with the actions of these three bradykinin receptor agonists (data not shown).

The results from the studies on the inhibition of [^{3}H]-bradykinin binding to partially purified rat myometrium receptors demonstrated that T-kinin and its D-analogue, [D-Ile^1]-T-kinin were able to displace [^{3}H]-bradykinin binding (Table 1). Along with the evidence of the absence of their actions in the bioassays, the high Ki values of [Des-Arg^9-bradykinin and [Des-Arg^9, Leu^8]-bradykinin (Table 1) suggest that they do not bind to receptors to which [3H]-bradykinin binds in rat uterus smooth muscle (i.e., B_2 receptors). The data further confirm the finding that bradykinin B_1 receptors are not present in rat uterus smooth muscle (1). Therefore, the actions of T-kinin and its D analogue on rat uterus smooth muscle were through bradykinin B_2 receptors. [D-Ile^1]-T-kinin had a higher affinity for the receptors than T-kinin This property may account for the higher potency of this T-kinin D analogue on rat uterus smooth muscle contraction. It is of interest that studies on kinins-induced vascular permeability in rats showed that [D-Ile^1]-T-kinin had little activity when compared with bradykinin and T-kinin (11). This implies that the smooth muscle in rat uterus and in blood vessels involved in capillary permeability have different subclasses of kinin B_2 receptors.

It should be noted that the affinity of the B_2 antagonist, [D-Arg^0, Hyp^3, D-Phe^7] bradykinin, for bradykinin B_2 receptor was lower than bradykinin (Table 1). This may explain why this B_2 antagonist was less potent against the action of bradykinin on rat uterus contraction.

Table 1. Inhibition Constants of Kinins and their analogues on [^{3}H]-bradykinin Binding

Kinins	Ki (nM)
Bradykinin	1.38
[D-Ile1]-T-kinin	4.07
[D-Arg^0, Hyp^3, D-Phe^7] bradykinin	7.69
T-kinin	13.24
[Des-Arg^9]-bradykinin	> 1250
[Des-Arg^9, Leu^8]-bradykinin	> 1250

The phenomenon that T-kinin and [D-Ile^1]-T-kinin had lower affinities for the B$_2$ receptors, but similar or higher potencies on rat uterus contraction, respectively, is still a mystery. Nevertheless, when the tissue was incubated with indomethacin, the activity of T-kinin on rat uterus contraction was significantly lower than that of bradykinin. This suggests that prostaglandins are a major component of T-kinin's action. Thus, T-kinin and bradykinin probably differ with respect to their intracellular signal transduction mechanisms which triggers

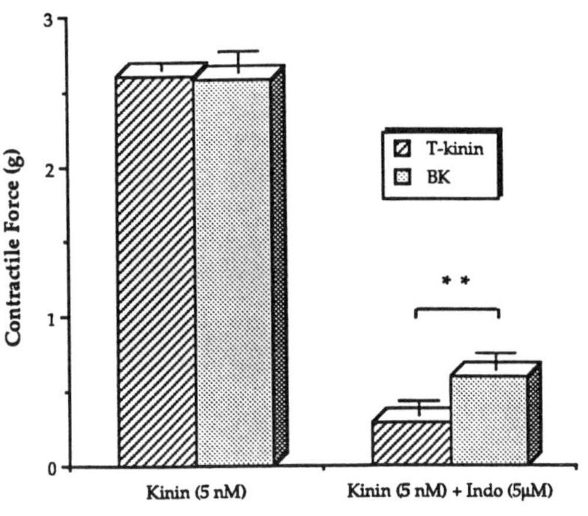

Fig. 3. Response of the rat uterus to T-kinin and bradykinin in the presence of indomethacin. The isolated tissue was incubated with indomethacin (5 μM) for 60 min before the application of 5 nM of T-kinin or bradykinin. The mean percentage of inhibition between the two groups had significant difference. **p<0.01; n=4

synthesis or release of prostaglandins. There is increasing evidence that bradykinin may, through the same receptor, stimulate different G proteins ; one for activation of phospholipase A$_2$, the other for hydrolysis of phosphoinositol which results in mobilization of intracellular calcium followed by smooth muscle contraction (13). However, additional investigations are needed to support this hypothesis.

In conclusion, the studies carried out using both intact rat uterus and rat uterus membrane receptor preparations to characterize T-kinin receptor interations indicated that T-kinin and its D analogue, [D-Ile^1]-T-kinin, functioned through bradykinin B_2 receptors in rat uterus smooth muscle. The D-configuration at Ile^1 of T-kinin increased the potency of T-kinin on rat uterus contraction due to the improvement of T-kinin's affinity for the receptors. Comparing these findings to published data indicates that the receptors in the rat uterus are not the same as those previously reported in smooth muscle of the vasculature, i.e. there exists subclasses of kinin B_2 receptors. While T-kinin had similar potency as bradykinin in causing the contraction of the isolated rat uterus, [D-Ile^1]-T-kinin had more potency than bradykinin. The receptor binding assay showed that both T-kinin and its D-analogue had lower affinities for the B_2 receptors than bradykinin. The evidence that T-kinin-induced rat uterus contraction is more sensitive to indomethacin than that of bradykinin may suggest that T-kinin and bradykinin may differ in their intracellular signal transductions which results in different rates of synthesis and release of prostaglandins.

ACKNOWLEDGEMENTS

This work was supported by NIH Grant HL-32183.

REFERENCES

1. Regoli D and Barabé J, Pharmacology of bradykinin and related kinins. Pharmacological Reviews 1980; 32: 1-46.

2. Farmer SG, Burch RM, Meeker SN, and Wilkins DE, Evidence for a pulmonary B_3 bradykinin receptor. Mol Pharmacol 1989; 36: 1-8.

3. Okamoto H and Greenbaum,LM, Isolation and structure of T-kinin. Biochem Biophys Res Commun 1983; 112(2): 701-708.

4. Okamoto H and Greenbaum LM, Kininogen substrates for trypsin and cathepsin D in human, rabbit and rat plasmas. Life Sciences 1983; 32: 2007-2013.

5. Barlas A, Gao X and Greenbaum LM, Isolation of a thiol-activated T-kininogenase from the rat submandibular gland. FEBS 1987; 218(2): 266-270.

6. Freer T, Chang J and Greenbaum LM, Studies on leukokinins — III, pharmacological activities of leukokinins M and PMN. Biochem Pharmacol 1972; 21: 3107-3110.

7. Manning DC, Vavrek R, Stewart JM and Snyder SH, Two bradykinin binding sites with picomolar affinities. J Pharmacol Exp Ther 1986; 237: 504-512.

8. Greenbaum LM and Okamoto H, T-kinin and T-kininogen, in: Methods in Enzymology 1988; 163: 272 - 281, Academic Press N.Y.

9. Lindsey CJ, Nakaie CR and Martins DT, Central nervous system kinin receptors and the hypertensive response mediated by bradykinin. Br J Pharmacol 1989; 97(3): 763-768.

10. Rhaleb NE, Drapeau G, Dion S, Jukic D, Rouissi N and Regoli D, Structure-activity studies on bradykinin and related peptides: agonists. Br J Pharmacol 1990; 99(3): 445-448.

11. Sugio K and Greenbaum LM, Increase in vasular permeability of rat and guinea-pig skin by T-kinin. Inflammation 1988; 12: 407-412.

12. Tien X, Wallace LJ, Kachur JF, Won-kim S and Gaginella TS, Characterization of Ile, Ser-bradykinin-induced changes in short-circuit current across the rat colon. J Pharmacol Exper Therap 1990; 354: 1063-1067.

13. Burch RM, Gprotein regulation of phospholipase A_2. Molecular Neurobiology 1989; 3: 155-171.

ON THE MECHANISM OF RAT UTERUS DESENSITIZATION TO KALLIKREIN

I. F. Heneine[1]*, M. H. Feitosa[2], W. T. Beraldo[2], G. M. R. Oliveira[2], and J. L. Pesquero[1]

[1]Biophysics Laboratory, [2]Peptides Laboratory, Department of Physiology and Biophysics, Institute of Biological Sciences, Federal University of Minas Gerais, 31270 Belo Horizonte, Brazil

SUMMARY: An inactive form of kallikrein prepared by iodination with cold iodine, did not show any enzymatic or oxytocic action. However, a competitive pattern between this inactive and active kallikrein was observed in rat uterus preparation: When the inactive form was applied several times in the muscle, a single dose of active kallikrein was unable to cause contraction, but a double dose elicited a response. The rhythmic movement caused by a singular dose of active kallikrein, had its time curtailed by adding the inactive kallikrein to the bath. The inactive kallikrein did not interfere with bradykinin activity

INTRODUCTION

It is well known that repeated additions of kallikrein will induce a state of unresponsiveness of the rat uterus preparation (1). This finding was attributed to kininogen exaustion, for when several doses 100 times more concentrated of kallikrein were applied, the preparation only reacted when fresh uterine horns were suspended in the organ bath (2). An inactive form of kallikrein is capable of inducing dessensitization after 15 to 20 additions to the organ bath, without causing contraction, after which the preparation only reacted with a doubled dose of active kallikrein (3). Enzyme site occupancy by inactivated kallikrein molecules could explain these findings. To obtain more evidence, we prepared an inactive derivative of rat submandibular kallikrein with stablished iodination procedures (4, 5). This method is convenient for the inactivation of kallikrein, as the molecule has a Tyr-93 in the

---

* Corresponding Author

substrate site, and a His-41 in the catalytic site (6). Recently, the derivative was employed *in vitro* in experiments using rat uterus preparation (7).

MATERIALS AND METHODS

Kallikrein Preparation.
Rat submandibular kallikrein was purified by a combined method of gel filtration and ion exchange in DEAE cellulose (3).
Activity Concentration of Kallikrein and Preparation of Inactive Derivative.
The active concentration of kallikrein was determined as described by Sampaio et. al.,(9), and iodinated to a dodecaderivative with iodine monochloride (4, 5)
Bioassay.
Rat uterus from castrated and β–*oestradiol* injected females were used. They were suspended in a 5 ml bath with a modified Tyrode solution, at 37° C. Details and quantitative data were given before (3, 9,10). Bradykinin and native kalikrein were used to standardise the uterus response.

RESULTS

Properties of the Inactive Kallikrein Derivative.
When 12 or more atoms of iodine per mol were added to kallikrein, a complete inactivation of all enzymatic and oxytocic activity was obtained. The iodinated kallikrein was stable, and no reversal to activity was observed even when staying at 4° C for at least 1 month. However, repeated freezing and thawing inactivate progressively the native kallikrein and made iodinated kallikrein to loose its property to block native kallikrein activity.
Oxytocic Activity.
As shown in Fig. 1, after 20 additions of the iodinated kallikrein, in spite of no response of the muscle was observed, the native kallikrein caused contraction only when a double dose was applied to the organ bath. When inactive kallikrein was again added 20 times, the double dose of active kallikrein was unable to induce contraction. By applying a 4 times higher dose of native kallikrein a contraction was observed. We followed this pattern up to eight doses of active kallikrein. The response to bradykinin was unaltered after the application of the inactive kallikrein. However, potentiation of bradykinin was present after a contraction elicited by native kallikrein .

On the other hand, as shown in Fig. 2, a single dose of kallikrein (curve A), when remaining into the bath, induces a pendular motion that endures from 30 to 60 min, until contractions ceased. A second dose of kallikrein did not elicit a response, but when a double dose of this enzyme is added to the bath, the preparation restarts the rhythmic motion. But, if an 30 to 100 times dose of inactive kallikrein (curve B) is applied at the begining of the experiment, the pendular motion ceased within 10 to 15 min.

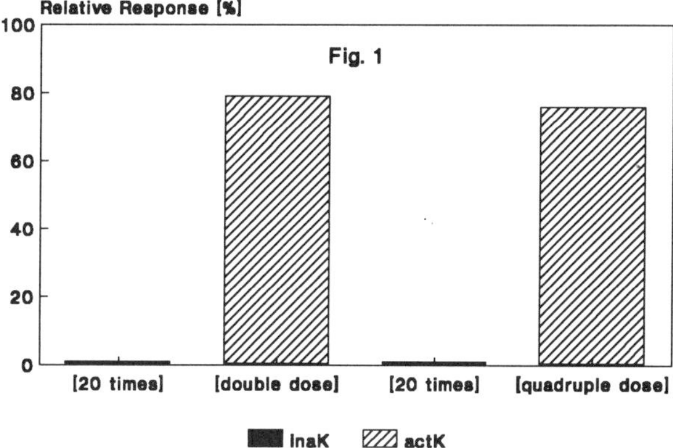

Fig. 1 - Effect of Inactive Kallikrein on the Oxytocic Response to Kallikrein on the Rat Uterus. Bars represents the response of preparation to inactive or active kallikrein. Number of 1.5×10^{-11} moles additions are in square brackets. Washing before additions were applied. **inaK**, Inactive kallikrein; **actK**, Active kallikrein

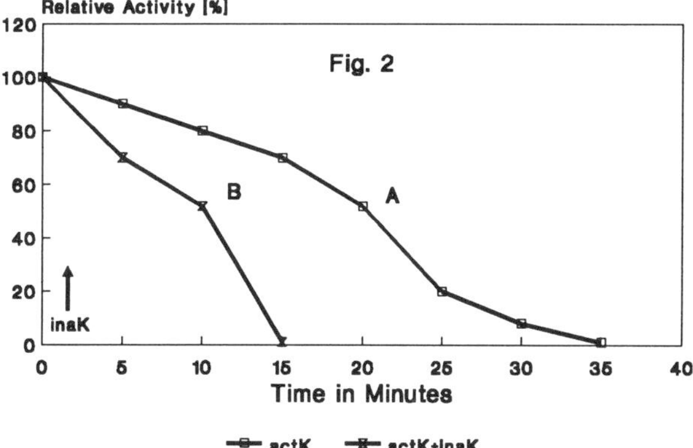

Fig. 2 - Effect of Inactive Kallikrein on the Rhythmic Contraction of Rat Uterus induced by Kallikrein. **A,** active kallikrein (1.5×10^{-11} moles) was applied and pendular motion registered for 40 min. **B,** a new uterine horn was suspended in the organ bath, active kallikrein added, and a 30 to 100 times dose of inactive kallikrein (↑)was added after first few contractions. **actK**-Active kallikrein. **inaK**- Inactive kallikrein

DISCUSSION

A possible explanation (see Fig. 3) for the results showing the inhibitory effect when inative kallikrein was applied beforehand, is the occupation of the binding sites of native kallikrein by the inactive kallikrein, without hydrolysis of bradykininogen. The site of bradykinin action was not involved, and remained free to receive the exogenous bradykinin. When a competitive dose of active kallikrein was applied, it dislocated the inactive enzyme from the tissue sites, liberating bradykinin from the substrate (bradykininogen), and a contraction ensued.

As far as the rhythmic uterine contractions is concerned, its cessation was not due to exaustion of substrate, for the pendular motion reappeared when a double dose of kallikrein was added to the bath. No clue was given on the fate of active kallikrein molecules after eliciting contraction. Nevertheless, site occupancy as inactivated molecules is suggested. This hypothesis is reinforced by the fact that inactive kallikrein, when added to the preparation induces an earlier stop of the rhythmic movement, because sites are occupied by inactive molecules. The difference of doses (20 to 100) of inactive kallikrein to block 1 dose of active kallikrein, when tested to obtain a contraction of the uterus, or to block the rhythmic uterine contraction, suggested that the affinity for receptors sites is different when native and inative kallikrein are considered.

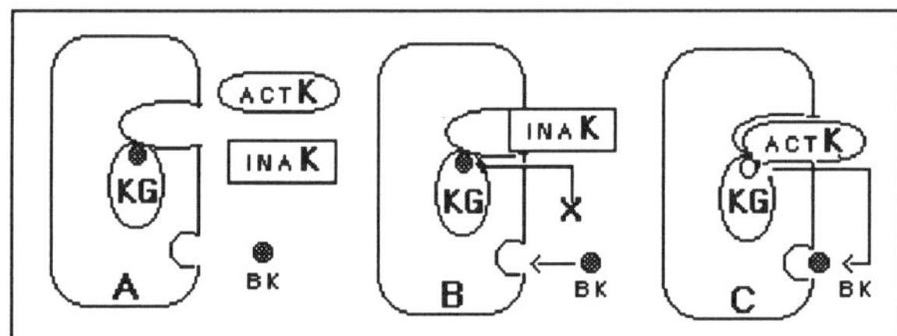

Fig. 3 - A Model Proposed to Explain the Action of Active and Inactive Kallikrein on the Rat Uterus: ACTK, active kallikrein; INAK, inactive kallikrein, **BK**, bradykinin; **KG**, kininogen.
A- Tissue receptors for kallikrein and bradykinin. Bradykinin could be endogenous, from kininogen, or exogenous. **B-** Site occupancy by inactive kallikrein. C- Site occupancy by active kallikrein.

CONCLUSIONS

Dessensitization can occur without kininogen depletion. Inactive and active kallikreins can compete each other, but site affinity of inactive molecules is lower.

ACKNOWLEDGMENTS
Supported by FAPEMIG, CNPq, PRPq-UFMG and FINEP.

REFERENCES

1. Beraldo WT, Lauar NS, Siqueira G, Heneine IF and Catanzaro OL. Peculiarities of the oxytocic action of rat urinary kallikrein. In: Chemistry and Biology of the Kallikrein-Kinin System in Health and Disease. Fogarty Int. Cent. Procc. 1974; 27:375-378.

2. Figueiredo AFS, Salgado AHI, Siqueira GTR, Veloso CR and Beraldo WT. Rat uterine contraction by kallikrein and its dependence on uterine kinnogen. Biochem. Pharmacol, 1990; 39: 763-769.

3. Feitosa MH, Pesquero JL, Oliveira GMR, Beraldo WT and Heneine IF The action of iodinated kallikrein on the rat uterus. Agents and Actions, in press.

4. Contreras MA, Bale WF and Spar IL. Iodine Monochloride (ICl) iodination techniques. Meth. Enzymol, 1983; 92: 277-292.

5. Edelhoch H. The properties of thyroglobulin. VIII-The iodination of thyroglobulin. J. Biol.Chem. 1962; 237: 2778-2787.

6. Ashley PL and MacDonald RJ. Kallikrein-Related mRNAs of the Rat Submaxillary Gland: Nucleotide Sequences of Four Distinct Types Including Tonin. Biochemistry 1985; 24: 4512-4520.

7. Feitosa MH, Pesquero JL, Oliveira GMR, Beraldo WT and Heneine IF The action of iodinated derivatives of glandular kallikrein on smooth muscle. Kinin '91 Munich International Conference. 1991, Abstract PS-1.13: p. 244.

8. Sampaio CAM, Sampaio MU and Prado ES. Active-Site Titration of Horse Urinary Kallikrein. Hoppe-Seyler's Z. Physiol. Chem. 1984, 365: 297-302.

9. Feitosa MH, Figueiredo, AFS, Beraldo, WT and Heneine, IF. Efeito da iodação nas propriedades da calicreina glandular do rato. IV FESBE, 1989, Abstract 7.42, p. 257.

10. Feitosa MH, Oliveira GMR, Pesquero JL, Beraldo WT and Heneine IF, VI FESBE, 1991, Abstract 17.16, p. 507.

Functional Aspects of Kallikreins or Proteinases, Kininogens and Kallikrein or Proteinase Inhibitors

AAS 38/II
Recent Progress on Kinins
© 1992 Birkhäuser Verlag Basel

PROLINE-SPECIFIC AMINOPEPTIDASES: POTENTIAL ROLE IN BRADYKININ DEGRADATION

Greet Vanhoof[1], Ingrid de Meester[1], Dirk Hendriks[1], Filip Goossens[1], Marc van Sande[1] Simon Scharpé[1] and Arieh Yaron[2]

[1]Laboratory of Medical Biochemistry, University of Antwerp, Universiteitsplein 1, 2610 Wilrijk, Belgium and [2]Department of Membrane Research and Biophysics, The Weizmann Institute of Science, 7100 Rehovot, Israel

SUMMARY: The N-terminus of bradykinin is shown to be sequentially degraded by the human proline-specific aminopeptidases aminopeptidase P (EC 3.4.11.9) and dipeptidyl peptidase IV (EC 3.4.14.5). Additional evidence is provided for the hypothesis that these proline-specific aminopeptidases play an essential role in the degradation of peptides containing an N-terminal Xaa-Pro sequence.

INTRODUCTION

A Xaa-Pro sequence appears at the N-terminus of a wide variety of human peptides and proteins, subsequent to proteolytic cleavage of the precursor. The proline at the penultimate position protects the resulting peptide from further undesired proteolysis by common peptidases [1,2]. Aminopeptidase P (APP; EC 3.4.11.9) and dipeptidyl peptidase IV (DPP IV;EC 3.4.14.5) are the only enzymes that recognise this sequence with a high specificity and might thus be important in the regulation of the activity of those proteins. APP catalyzes the removal of any unsubstituted, N-terminal amino acid, that is adjacant to a penultimate prolyl residue [3,4]. DPP IV removes N-terminal dipeptides from polypeptides having unsubstituted N-termini. The penultimate residue must be Pro, Hyp or Ala, with the greatest rates occuring on Pro, provided that the third residue is neither Pro nor Hyp. DPP IV has been proposed to activate substance P by removing sequentially the dipeptides Lys-Pro and Arg-Pro [5,6], and to inactivate ß-casomorphin by degrading the N-terminal sequence [7]. Apart from direct modulation of the biological activity of Xaa-Pro containing peptides, the action of APP and

DPP IV can also influence the half life of those proteins: their action might facilitate the further degradation since the sequestered residue is than susceptible to subsequent aminopeptidase attack. In proteins with penultimate Pro-Pro sequence, the removal of the N-terminal amino acid is required before DPP IV can remove the Pro-Pro sequence. Such a sequence thus imposes the concerted action of APP and DPP IV for N-terminal degradation, and comprises a double protection against undesired hydrolysis. In order to establish whether the concerted action of APP and DPP IV can remove the protective sequences, we studied the kinetic characteristics of these enzymes for the N-terminus of bradykinin.

The study of peptidases involved in the degradation of bradykinin is of clinical significance: inhibition of these peptidases can potentiate the plasma kinin levels, and modification of the cleavable bonds in bradykinin can lead to the production of peptidase-resistant analogs. The two enzymes that are considered to play a major role in the degradation of bradykinin are angiotensin converting enzyme (EC 3.4.15.1) and carboxypeptidase N (EC 3.4.17.3). Several facts strongly suggest that peptidases other than angiotensin converting enzyme and carboxypeptidase N are involved in the degradation of bradykinin *in vivo*. D-Phe[7]-containing kinin antagonists display relatively short half-lifes in vivo despite their resistance to angiotensin converting enzyme [8]. Similarly, the B2 kinin agonist [Phe[8]-ψ(CH$_2$NH)Arg[9]]bradykinin also has a relatively short duration of action despite its resistance to both angiotensin converting enzyme and carboxypeptidase N [9,10]. Significant hydrolysis of the N-terminal Xaa-Pro bond of bradykinin was found in a preparation enriched in cerebral microvasculature [11]. *Marceau et al.* [12] studied the metabolism of bradykinin in human plasma and contributed the formation of small amounts of des-Arg[1]-bradykinin to the action of a contaminant prolidase from erythrocytes. However, prolidase only cleaves dipeptides [13]. An involvement of APP in this cleavage would thus be more acceptable. Furthermore, after perfusion of bradykinin through intact rat lungs, the most abundant bradykinin fragment formed was the Pro-Pro dipeptide [14], consistent with a release of the N-terminal Arg by the action of APP, followed by removal of the Pro-Pro dipeptide by DPP IV. Whether APP can exert a function as a kininase and whether its degradation product can further be degraded by DPP IV to form the dipeptide Pro-Pro, depends largely on their kinetic behaviour. We recently showed the presence of APP in human platelets and suggested a role for platelets as scavengers for circulating peptides containing bonds susceptible for APP [15]. Now, we determined the K$_m$ of purified human platelet APP for bradykinin and of DPP IV towards des-Arg[1]-bradykinin in order to explore whether APP can be involved in the *in vivo* metabolisation of bradykinin, and whether the dipeptide Pro-Pro can subsequently be released by the action of DPP IV. In addition, because it was shown that 2-mercapto-ethanol potentiates the depressor action of bradykinin [16], and inhibits the N-terminal degradation of bradykinin in vivo [17], we investigated the effect of reducing agents on the purified APP.

MATERIALS AND METHODS

Bradykinin and des-Arg[1]-bradykinin were from Sigma Chemical Co (St. Louis, MO, USA). des-Arg[9]-bradykinin was purchased from Novabiochem (Läufelfingen, Switserland). The peptide des-Arg[1]-Pro[2,3]-bradykinin (Gly-Phe-Ser-Pro-Phe-Arg) was custom synthesized at the department of Biochemistry at the University of Leuven (Belgium). DPP IV and APP activities were measured using the substrates Gly-Pro-4-methoxy-ß-naphthylamide and Lys(2,4-dinitrophenyl)-Pro-Pro-NH-CH_2-CH_2-NH-2-aminobenzoyl respectively [18,19]. APP was purified from human platelets [20] and had a specific activity of 4672 U/g. DPP IV was purified from human lymphocytes [21] and had a specific activity of 12 285 U/g. One unit is defined as the amount of enzyme that releases one µmol of product per min under the assay conditions. HPLC analyses were performed with a M-45 solvent delivery system, a model 450 variable wavelength UV detector, and a Data Module (all from Waters, Millipore, Brussels, Belgium). Peptide products were applied onto a Waters Novapack C_{18} reversed phase column (5 mm ID x 10 cm) of 4-µm particle size.

The degradation of bradykinin by APP was studied by incubating the enzyme (10 µl) at 40° C for 4 to 7 min with bradykinin concentrations ranging from 0.015 to 0.3 mM in 0.2 M Tris-HCl, pH 8.0 with 7.0 mM trisodiumcitrate and 1.9 mM manganese sulfate (90 µl). The hydrolysis of bradykinin was terminated by the addition of 60 µl of 7% (v/v) perchloric acid, adjusted to pH 3.25 with NaOH. The sample was centrifuged for 5 min in an Eppendorf centrifuge. 50 µl of the supernatant was used for injection onto the column. The peptide products were eluted with an isocratic system of 16% acetonitrile in 60 mM phosphate buffer, pH 3.25, using a flow rate of 1 ml/min at ambient temperature. The degradation of des-Arg[1]-bradykinin by DPP IV was studied by incubating the enzyme (10 µl) at 37° C for 20 to 40 min with des-Arg[1]-bradykinin concentrations ranging from 0.04 mM to 0.48 mM in 25 mM Tris-HCl, 10 mM EDTA, pH 8.3 (90 µl). 50 µl of a 10% (v/v) perchloric acid solution was added to terminate the reaction. The solutions were cooled on ice, and centrifuged in an Eppendorf centrifuge for 5 min. 120 µl of the supernatant was collected and adjusted to pH 6 with 60 µl NaOH. 20 µl of this solution was used for injection onto the column. The products of the reactions were separated by HPLC as described above, using a flow rate of 1.2 ml/min at ambient temperature. Peaks were detected at 205 nm, sensitivity 0.02 A full scale, and identified by co-elution with the peptide standards bradykinin, des-Arg[1]-bradykinin and des-Arg[1]-Pro[2,3]-bradykinin. The influence of reducing agents on purified APP was investigated by incubating the enzyme with dithiothreitol and mercapto-ethanol in concentrations ranging respectively from 9 x 10^{-6} M to 9 x 10^{-3} M and from 9 x 10^{-5} M to 9 x 10^{-2} M during 10 min at 37° C, after which the standard assay procedure [19] was followed for determination of the remaining activity.

RESULTS

A typical chromatogram of bradykinin degradation by purified human platelet APP is shown in Fig. 1. The Michaelis-Menten constant was calculated using a Cornish-Bowden plot. Results - one representative experiment shown in Fig. 2- indicate an apparent Km of 66 µM (SD = 8 µM, n = 6).

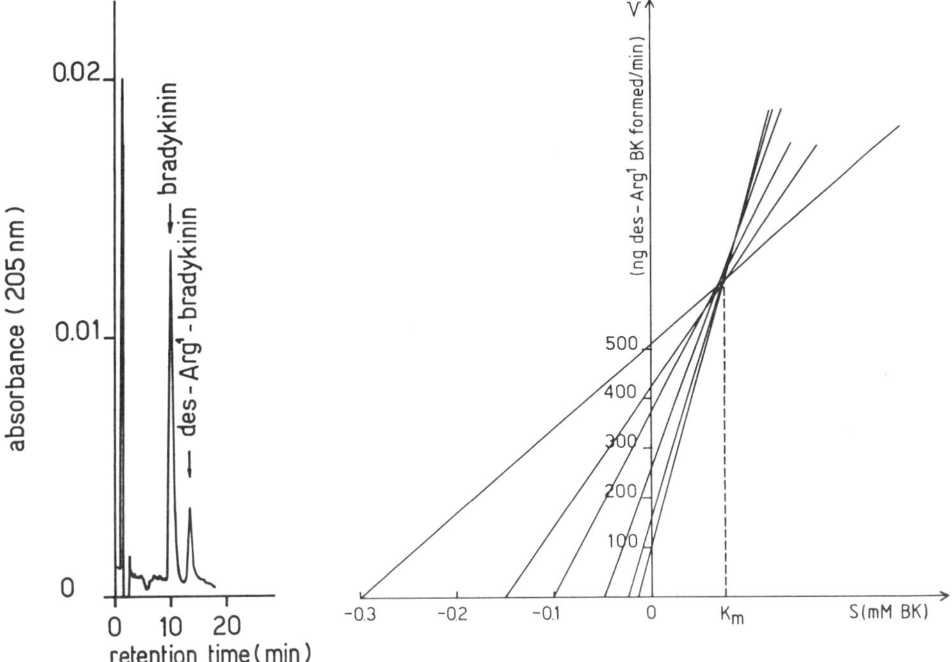

Fig. 1. Representative chromatogram demonstrating the transformation of bradykinin to des-Arg¹-bradykinin by Aminopeptidase P (left)

Fig 2. Cornish-Bowden plot of the enzymatic velocity (v) against the concentration of bradykinin (S) to determine the Michaelis-Menten constant Km (right)

The reducing agents mercapto-ethanol and dithiothreitol effectively inhibit the activity of APP at millimolar concentrations (Fig. 3). Since 2-mercapto-ethanol can potentiate the depressor action of bradykinin [16], the inhibition of APP by 2-mercapto-ethanol further supports the view that APP may play a functional role in the *in vivo* degradation of bradykinin.

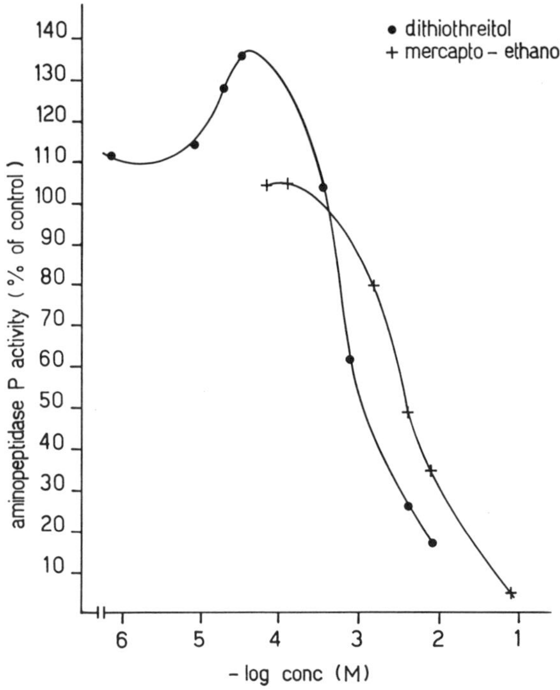

Fig. 3. Effect of dithiothreitol and mercapto-ethanol on the platelet aminopeptidase P activity

The product of bradykinin cleavage by APP, des-Arg[1]-bradykinin, was further degraded by DPP IV to des-Arg[1]-Pro[2,3]-bradykinin (Fig. 4). The Michaelis-Menten constant was calculated from a Cornish-Bowden plot. The results, shown in Fig. 5, indicate an apparent K_m of 190 μM (170 μM and 210 μM, n = 2).

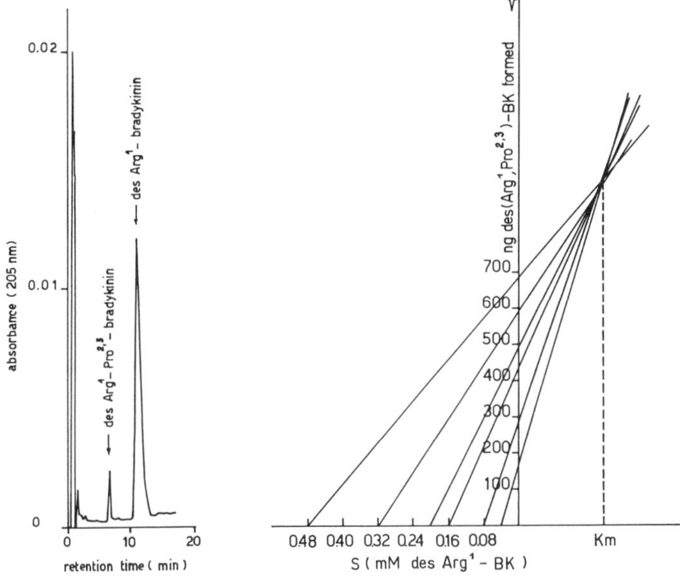

Fig. 4. Representative chromatogram demonstrating the degradation of des-Arg[1]-bradykinin to des-Arg[1]-Pro[2,3]-bradykinin by the action of dipeptidyl peptidase IV (left)
Fig. 5. Cornish-Bowden plot of the enzymatic velocity (v) against the concentration of des-Arg[1]-bradykinin (S) to determine the Michaelis-Menten constant K_m (right)

DISCUSSION

The kinetic constants of both purified human APP and DPP IV towards their respective substrates bradykinin and des-Arg[1]-bradykinin were determined for the first time. The affinity of bradykinin for APP (K_m = 66 µM) is comparable to that reported for carboxypeptidase N (K_m = 25-45 µM) [22]. The affinity of bradykinin for angiotensin converting enzyme is considerably higher (K_m = 0.4 -2 µM) [23].

The physiological significance of APP and DPP IV in bradykinin metabolism may vary considerably between different tissues and body fluids depending on the local angiotensin converting enzyme and carboxypeptidase N activity. In normal human serum, APP is probably of minor importance for bradykinin metabolism considering the abundancy of angiotensin converting enzyme and carboxypeptidase N in serum. Still, APP kininase activity may become of significant value in patients receiving converting enzyme inhibitors, or in the metabolism of bradykinin analogs containing unmodified Arg[1]-Pro[2]- N-termini. Otherwise, the N-terminal degradation of bradykinin may be important in the local control of the kinin activity. Since we showed before [15] that compared to serum, APP is present at a much higher specific activity than angiotensing converting enzyme and carboxypeptidase N in platelets, the platelet APP activity might be important for the initiation of bradykinin metabolism in e.g. inflammatory lesions. Consideration of the Arg^1-Pro^2-bond as an important cleavable site in bradykinin, may help future attempts to produce more potent bradykin analogs.

The detection of the Pro-Pro dipeptide as the most abundant metabolite of bradykinin in the rat lung [14], was the first indication of an *in vivo* degradation of biological peptides containing a penultimate proline by the concerted action of APP and DPP IV. Furthermore, the α-subunit of chorionic gonadotropin, follicle stimulating hormone, luteinizing hormone or thyroid stimulating hormone are found with and without the N-terminal Xaa-Pro sequence, while this heterogeneity does not result from differences in precursor processing [24]. Interleukin 6 (IL-6) exhibits a heterogeneity of the N-terminus by appearing with and without the N-terminal Ala or Ala-Pro dipeptide, suggesting an *in vivo* processing of the N-terminus of IL-6 by APP and DPP IV. *Yasueda et al.* [25] found that recombinant human IL-6 (N-terminal sequence Pro-Val-Pro-Pro-) overproduced in *Escherichia coli HB101*, partially retained the initiator methionine residue at the N-terminus. Using a mutant with duplicated APP genes or recombinant strains overproducing APP, they succeeded in removing the initiator methionine from Met-human IL-6 *in vivo*. These findings, together with our results on the kinetic behaviour of the human proline-specific aminopeptidases towards the N-terminus of bradykinin, suggest an essential role for these peptidases in the in vivo metabolism of peptides containing an N-terminal X-Pro sequence that include, in addition to bradykinin, substance P, ß-casomorphin, insulin-like growth factor-1, IL-1ß, IL-2, IL-6, lymphotoxin, factor XII, the fibrin α-chain, haemopexin and erythropoietin.

ACKNOWLEDGEMENTS

We would like to thank Y. Sim for her excellent technical assistance. I. De Meester is a research assistant of the NFWO, and F. Goossens and G. Vanhoof are recipients of an IWONL grant. Prof. A. Yaron is an incumbant of the Morris Belkin Professorial Chair in Cancer Research.

REFERENCES

1. Walter R, Simmons WH, Yoshimoto T. Proline-specific endo- and exopeptidases. Mol Cell Biochem 1980;30:111-127.
2. Mentlein R. Proline residues in the maturation and degradation of peptide hormones and neuropeptides. FEBS Letters 1988;234:251-256.
3. Dehm P, Nordwig A. The cleavage of prolyl peptides by kidney peptidases. Partial

purification of a "X-Prolyl-Aminopeptidase" from swine kidney microsomes. Eur J Biochem 1970;17:364-371.

4. Yaron A, Mlynar D. Aminopeptidase-P. Biochem Biophys Res Com 1968;32:658-663.

5. Conlon JM, Sheehan L. Conversion of substance P to C-terminal fragments in human plasma. Regulatory Peptides 1983;7:335-345.

6. Nausch I, Mentlein R, Heymann E. The degradation of bioactive peptides and proteins by dipeptidyl peptidase IV from human placenta. Biol Chem Hoppe-Seyler 1990;371:1113-1118.

7. Hartrodt B, Neubert K, Fisher G, Demuth U, Yoshimoto T, Barth A. Degradation of ß-casomorphin-5 by PSE and PPCE. Comparative studies of the ß-casomorphin-5 cleavage by DPP IV. Pharmazie 1982;37:72-73.

8. Togo J, Burch RM, DeHaas CJ, Connor JR, Steranka CR. D-Phe[7]-substituted peptide bradykinin antagonists are not substrates for kininase II. Peptides 1989;10:109-112.

9. Drapeau G, Rhaleb NE, Dion S, Jukic D, Regoli D. [Phe[8]ψ(CH$_2$NH)Arg[9]] bradykinin, a B2 receptor selective agonist which is not broken down by either kininase I or kininase II. Eur J Pharmacol 1988;155:193-195.

10. Drapeau G, Ward PE. Metabolism of bradykinin and bradykinin analogs. Fed Proc 1990;4:A990.

11. Bausback HH, Ward PE. Kallidin and bradykinin metabolism by isolated cerebral microvessels. Biochem Pharmacol 1988;37:2973-2978.

12. Marceau F, Fendreau M, Barabé J, St Pierre S, Regoli D. The degradation of bradykinin (BK) and of des-Arg[9]-bradykinin in plasma. Can J Physiol Pharmacol 1981;59:131-138.

13. McDonald JK, Barret AJ. In :Mammalian proteases: A glossary and bibliography. Volume 2. Exopeptidases.Academic Press, London 1986;261-268.

14. Baker CRF, Little AD, Little GH, Canizaro PC, Behal FJ. Kinin metabolism in the perfused ventilated rat lung. I: Bradykinin metabolism in a system modeling the normal, uninjured lung. Circ Shock 1991;33:37-47.

15. Scharpé SL, Vanhoof GC, De Meester IA, Hendriks DF, van Sande ME, Muylle LM, Yaron A. Exopeptidases in human platelets: an indication for proteolytic modulation of biologically active peptides. Clin Chim Acta 1990;195:125-132.

16. Ryan JW, Roblero J, Stewart JM. Inactivation of bradykinin in the pulmonary circulation. Biochem J 1968;110:795-797.

17. Ryan JW, Chen SC, Chung A, Berryer P. Aminopeptidase P inactivates bradykinin in vivo. Circukation 1987;76:IV-234.

18. Scharpé S, De Meester I, Vanhoof G, Hendriks D, van Sande M, Van Camp K, and Yaron A. Assay of dipeptidyl peptidase IV in serum by fluorometry of 4-methoxy-2-naphtylamine. Clinical Chemistry 1988;34, 2299-2301.

19. Holtzman EJ, Pillay G, Rosenthal T, Yaron A. Aminopeptidase P activity in rat organs and human serum. Anal Biochem 1987;162:476-484.

20. Vanhoof G, De Meester I, Goossens F, Hendriks D, Scharpé S, Yaron A. Kininase activity in human platelets: cleavage of the Arg[1]-Pro[2] bond of bradykinin by aminopeptidase P. Submitted.

21. De Meester I, Vanhoof G, Scharpé S, Hendriks D, Yaron A. Characterization of dipeptidyl peptidase IV (CD26) from human lymphocytes. Submitted.

22. Erdös EG, Kininases. In: Handbook of Experimental Pharmacology (Ed Erdös EG) Vol 25, Suppl I, Springer, Heidelberg 1979, p427-487.

23. Dorer FE, Kahn JR, Lentz KE, Levin M, Skeggs LT. Hydrolysis of bradykinin by angiotensin converting enzyme. Circ Res 1974;34:824-827.

24. Birken S, Fetherston J, Desmond J, Canfield R, Boime J. Biochem Biophys Res Commun 1978;85:1247-1253.

25. Yasueda H, Kikuchi Y, Kojima H, Nagase K. In-vivo processing of the initiator methioninie from recombinant methionyl human interleukin-6 synthesized in *Escherichia coli* overproducing DPP IV. Appl Microbiol Biotechnol 1991;36:211-215.

AAS 38/II
Recent Progress on Kinins
© 1992 Birkhäuser Verlag Basel

SYNTHETIC SUBSTRATES AND INHIBITORS FOR SERINE PROTEASES FROM LYMPHOCYTES, MAST CELLS, SEMEN, AND BLOOD

J. C. Powers, [≠] S. Odake,[≠] T. Ueda,[≠] D. Hudig[§], H. C. B. Graves,[†] M. Kamarei,[†] and C.-M. Kam[≠]

From [≠]School of Chemistry and Biochemistry, Georgia Institute of Technology, Atlanta, GA 30332, [§]Cell and Molecular Biology Program, School of Medicine and College of Agriculture, University of Nevada, Reno, NV 89557, and [†]Department of Urology, Stanford University Medical Center, Stanford, CA 94305

SUMMARY: The substrate specificity of several serine proteases from cytotoxic T lymphocytes, natural killer cells, mast cells, seminal fluid, and blood plasma has been determined with synthetic peptide thiobenzyl ester and *p*-nitroanilide substrates. Several new enzymatic activities have been discovered. A variety of inhibitors such as isocoumarins, trifluoromethyl ketones, and peptide chloromethyl ketones were used to study these enzymes and were found to be potent inhibitors.

INTRODUCTION

A number of serine proteases have been isolated from cytotoxic T lymphocytes (CTL) and natural killer (NK) cells, mast cells, seminal fluid, and blood plasma. These enzymes include granzymes from CTL and NK cells; chymases and tryptases from mast cells; prostate-specific antigen (PSA) protease from seminal fluid; and coagulation enzymes and kallikrein from blood plasma. These enzymes are involved in many important physiological processes such as the immune response, blood coagulation, and the inflammatory response. For example, granzymes are involved in cell-mediated killing by CTL and NK cells, which is important in defense against tumor cell proliferation and viral infection. Plasma kallikrein is involved in coagulation and

---

Abbreviations: AA = amino acid residue; ACITIC (7-NH2-CiTPrOIC) = 7-amino-4-chloro-3-(3-isothiuridopropoxy)isocoumarin; Boc = *t*-butyloxycarbonyl; CiTEtOIC = 4-chloro-3-(2-isothiureidoethoxy)isocoumarin; CiTPrOIC = 4-chloro-3-(3-isothiureidopropoxy)isocoumarin; CTL = cytotoxic T lymphocyte; Dns = 5-dimethylamino-1-naphthylenesulfonyl; Hepes = 4-(2-hydroxyethyl)-1-piperazineethane sulfonic acid; HR granzyme A = human recombinant granzyme A; IC = isocoumarin; *ly*-tryptase = lymphocyte tryptase; NA = *p*-nitroanilide; PSA = prostate-specific antigen; SBzl = thiobenzyl ester; Suc = succinyl; Z = benzyloxycarbonyl.

fibrinolysis, and glandular kallikrein may participate in the regulation of organ blood flow.

Synthetic peptide substrates have been invaluable tools for studying the active sites of serine proteases and synthetic inhibitors have been used to elucidate the enzymatic mechanism and physiological roles of these enzymes. Here we report studies on the substrate specificity of several biological important enzymes using peptide p-nitroanilides and thioesters, which has resulted in the discovery of new enzymatic activities. We also report various potent inhibitors of these enzymes which should be useful for defining their biological roles.

MATERIALS AND METHODS

Human recombinant (HR) granzyme A was a generous gift from Dr. Duke Virca at Immunex Research and Development Corporation. Murine granzyme B was kindly provided by Dr. Jürg Tschopp at the Univ. of Lausanne. Human Q31 chymase was a gift from Dr. Martin Poe at Merck. Human thrombin and porcine factor IXa were gifts from Dr. Sriram Krishnaswamy and Dr. Pete Lollar at Emory Univ. Human factor VIIa was kindly provided by Dr. George Vlasuk at Merck. PSA protease was purified by a previously described method (1). Z-Lys-SBzl and bovine trypsin were obtained from Sigma Chemical Co., St. Louis, MO. Suc-Phe-Leu-Phe-SBzl and all Boc-amino acids used in the synthesis of new peptide thiobenzyl esters were purchased from Bachem Bioscience Inc., Philadelphia, PA. All the Arg-containing peptide thioesters (2), Arg-containing peptide p-nitroanilides (3), Boc-Ala-Ala-AA-SBzl (4, 5), isocoumarins substituted with isothiureidoalkoxy groups (Kam and Powers, unpublished results), Arg-containing peptide chloromethyl ketones (6), and Arg trifluoromethyl ketones (7) have been synthesized previously.

Substrate Kinetics. The enzymatic hydrolysis of peptide thioester substrates were measured in 0.1 M Hepes, 0.01 M $CaCl_2$ (or 0.5 M NaCl), pH 7.5 buffer containing 8 % Me_2SO and at 25 °C in the presence of 4,4'-dithiodipyridine. Stock solution of substrate were prepared in Me_2SO and stored at -20 °C. The initial rates were measured at 324 nm ($\varepsilon_{324} = 19800\ M^{-1}cm^{-1}$) using a Beckman 35 or Varian DMS-90 spectrophotometer when a 10-25 μl of an enzyme stock solution was added to a cuvette containing 2.0 ml of buffer, 150 μl of 4,4'-dithiodipyridine (5 mM) and 25 μl of substrate. The same volumes of substrate and 4,4'-dithiodipyridine were added to the reference cell in order to compensate for the background hydrolysis rate of the substrates. Initial rates were measured in duplicate for each substrate concentration and were averaged in each case. Peptide p-nitroanilide hydrolysis was measured at 410 nm ($\varepsilon_{410} = 8800\ M^{-1}cm^{-1}$).

Inhibition Kinetics-Incubation Method. The inactivation reaction was initiated at 25 °C by adding a 25 μl aliquot of inhibitor in Me_2SO to 0.3 ml of buffered enzyme solution (30-600 nM) such that the final Me$_2$SO concentration was 8-9 %. Aliquots were removed at various time intervals, diluted into substrate solution (90 fold dilution) and the residual activity was measured spectrophotometrically. HR granzyme A, human thrombin, human factor VIIa, and tryptases were assayed with Z-Arg-SBzl, and porcine factor IXa was assayed with Z-Trp-Arg-SBzl by the procedure described above. First order inactivation rate constants (k_{obs}) were obtained from plots of ln v_t/v_o vs. time and had correlation coefficients greater than 0.98. Inactivation rate constants were the average of duplicate experiments.

RESULTS AND DISCUSSION

Substrate Studies. Synthetic peptide substrates such as *p*-nitroanilides and thioesters are very useful for monitoring the enzymatic activities of serine proteases. Thiobenzyl esters are very sensitive substrates since they have high k_{cat} values and the hydrolysis product benzyl thiol can be detected easily using a thiol reagent such as 4,4'-dithiodipyridine or Ellman's reagent contained in the assay mixture. The nitroanilide substrates are less reactive but more specific than the thioesters. We have used more than 15 Boc-Ala-Ala-AA-SBzl derivatives and several *p*-nitroanilides to determine the substrate specificity of various serine proteases.

PSA protease and kallikrein. PSA protease is one of the most abundant prostatic-secreted proteins in human semen and its primary structure is very similar to that of the Arg-restricted glandular kallikrein-like protease (8, 9). Previous studies indicated that PSA protease displayed only chymotrypsin-like activity but not trypsin-like activity (10). However, we found that aprotinin chromatography did not remove the low levels of trypsin-like activity in our PSA preparation. Using more sensitive thioester substrates, we have shown that the PSA protease has high chymotrypsin-like and low trypsin-like activity, and it hydrolyzes Suc-Phe-Leu-Phe-SBzl faster than Z-Trp-Arg-SBzl by 4 fold (Table 1). We also have shown that Suc-Phe-Leu-Phe-SBzl is a better substrate than the previous reported Tyr-containing *p*-nitroanilide substrates (10). Both porcine pancreatic and human plasma kallikrein also have trypsin-like activities and hydrolyze Z-Trp-Arg-SBzl very efficiently (11), but we found that these two kallikreins hydrolyzed Suc-Phe-Leu-Phe-SBzl more slowly than Z-Trp-Arg-SBzl.

Granzymes and rat NK proteases. Seven serine proteases (granzyme A, B, C, D, E, F, and G) have been found in mouse CTL granules and three serine proteases (granzyme A, B and chymase) have been isolated from human CTL granules. Among these proteases, granzyme A has trypsin-like activity, and granzyme B hydrolyzes Boc-Ala-Ala-Asp-SBzl preferentially (5). Rat NK granules show hydrolytic activities toward Z-Gly-Arg-SBzl (*ly*-tryptase activity),

Suc-Phe-Leu-Phe-SBzl (*ly*-chymase activity), Boc-Ala-Ala-Asp-SBzl (Asp-ase activity), Boc-Ala-Ala-Met-SBzl (Met-ase activity), and Boc-Ala-Ala-Ser-SBzl (Ser-ase activity) (12). HR granzyme A effectively hydrolyzes peptide thioesters and nitroanilides which contained Arg or Lys in the P_1 site (Table 2). The thioesters have higher hydrolysis rates than the nitroanilides. Among the nitroanilides, granzyme A preferred hydrophobic residues at the P_2 position, e.g. Z-Ala-Phe-Arg-NA is a better substrate than Z-Ala-Gly-Arg-NA. Granzyme B hydrolyzes Asp-containing peptide thioesters and Suc-Asp-Val-Asp-SBzl is the best substrate (Table 2). These results indicate that granzyme B preferres Val over Ala, Pro or Leu at the P_2 site, Asp over Ala at the P_3 site and Suc or Boc over a free N-terminal at the P_4 site, and that all the interactions at the S_1-S_4 subsites are important for substrate binding. Our substrate mapping results are consistent with the predictions made from molecular modeling of granzyme B (13). We also discovered that human chymase only showed significant hydrolytic activity toward Suc-Phe-Leu-Phe-SBzl among our series of peptide thioesters.

Table 1. Kinetic Constants for Hydrolysis of Peptide Thioesters by PSA Protease

Substrates	k_{cat} (s^{-1})	K_M(mM)	k_{cat}/K_M(M^{-1}s^{-1})
Z-Trp-Arg-SBzl	1.56	2.0	780
Suc-Ala-Ala-Met-SBzl	0.33	0.60	560
Suc-Phe-Leu-Phe-SBzl	0.30	0.09	3250
Boc-Ala-Ala-Tyr-SBzl			185

Table 2. Substrate Specificity of HR Granzyme A and Murine granzyme B

Substrate	[E] (nM)	[S] (µM)	Rate (nM/s)
HR Granzyme A			
Z-Lys-SBzl	2	55	9.5
Z-Arg-SBzl	2	94	56.4
Z-Ala-Gly-Arg-NA	16	109	0.04
Z-Ala-Phe-Arg-NA	16	112	0.2
Murine granzyme B			
Boc-Ala-Ala-Asp-SBzl		114	79
Boc-Ala-Val-Asp-SBzl		114	110
Boc-Ala-Pro-Asp-SBzl		114	67
Boc-Ala-Leu-Asp-SBzl		114	41
Suc-Ala-Val-Asp-SBzl		55	69
Suc-Asp-Val-Asp-SBzl		47	97
H-Asp-Val-Asp-SBzl		114	10

Inhibitor Studies. Reversible inhibitors such as trifluoromethyl ketones and irreversible inhibitors such as substituted isocoumarins and peptide chloromethyl ketones have been developed for serine proteases. The inhibition mechanism of serine proteases by these compounds has been investigated previously (14). Upon binding to serine proteases, trifluoromethyl ketones react with the γ-OH of Ser-195 to form a hemiketal structure resembling the transition state for peptide bond hydrolysis. Peptide chloromethyl ketones will alkylate the active site His-57 and form a tetrahedral adduct with Ser-195. Isocoumarins are mechanism-based inhibitors and the reaction involves the initial formation of an acyl enzyme intermediate with the unmasking of the reactive group such as 4-aminobenzyl chloride moiety in the case of ACITIC. This reactive group can then react with another active site residue such as His-57 to form an irreversibly inactivated enzyme.

Blood coagulation enzymes. Blood coagulation enzymes are serine proteases with trypsin-like specificity and they have much more complex structures and are more specific than trypsin. Isocoumarins substituted with basic groups such as guanidino or isothiureidoalkoxy group are potent irreversible inhibitors of blood coagulation enzymes (15). Several ACITIC derivatives with various substituents at the 7 and 3 positions (structures shown in Fig 1) are potent inhibitors of thrombin, factor VIIa, and factor IXa (Table 3). Substituted isocoumarins with isothiureidoethoxy groups at the 3-position are 4-16 fold better inhibitors than compounds with isothiureidopropoxy groups. This indicates that the charged isothiureidoethoxy group fits into the S_1 pocket better than the longer isothiureidopropoxy group. Isocoumarins substituted with a large hydrophobic group such as phenylcarbamoylamino at the 7-position have enhanced inhibitory activity toward these three enzymes by 1-2 fold.

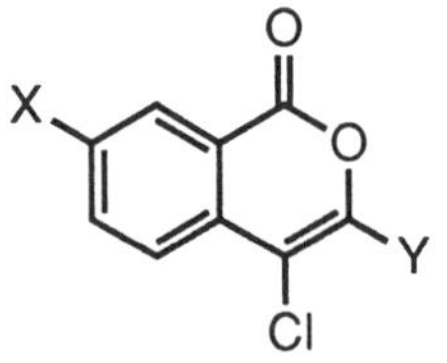

ACITIC, X = NH_2, Y = $O(CH_2)_3S\text{-}C(=NH_2^+)NH_2$

7-PhNHCONH-CiTEtOIC, X = PHNHCONH,
Y = $O(CH_2)_2S\text{-}C(=NH_2^+)NH_2$

7-PhNHCONH-CiTPrOIC, X = PHNHCONH,
Y = $O(CH_2)_3S\text{-}C(=NH_2^+)NH_2$

Fig 1. Structures of Substituted Isocoumarins

The chloromethyl ketone D-Phe-Pro-Arg-CH_2Cl is a potent and specific inhibitor of thrombin, and Dns-Glu-Gly-Arg-CH_2Cl inhibited factor Xa very effectively (6). These two compounds also inhibited factor VIIa and factor IXa (Table 3). D-Phe-Pro-Arg-CH_2Cl inhibits thrombin more effectively than the other three enzymes by 3-6 order of magnitude, and Dns-Glu-Gly-Arg-CH_2Cl inhibits factor Xa better than the other enzymes by 2-4 order of magnitude. These results indicate that peptide chloromethyl ketones are more specific than the heterocyclic isocoumarins. However, small structural changes on the isocoumarins can improve their specificities and these isocoumarins have greater potential for therapeutic use.

Table 3. Inhibition of Coagulation Enzymes by Substituted Isocoumarins and Peptide Chloromethyl Ketones

Compounds	$k_{obs}/[I]$ $(M^{-1}s^{-1})$			
	Human Thrombin	Bovine factor Xa[a]	Human Factor VIIa	Porcine Factor IXa
7-NH$_2$-CiTPrOIC (ACITIC)	760		430	80
7-PhNHCONH-CiTPrOIC	1,840		720	110
7-PhNHCONH-CiTEtOIC	22,400		3,140	1,790
D-Phe-Pro-Arg-CH$_2$Cl	11,500,000	4,500	110	20
DNS-Glu-Gly-Arg-CH$_2$Cl	630	367,000	16	180

[a]Data was obtained from reference 6.

HR Granzyme A. Substrate studies indicate that granzyme A is a trypsin-like enzyme, and we have tested this enzyme with various trypsin inhibitors such as Arg-containing peptide chloromethyl ketones and substituted isocoumarins (Table 4). Arg-containing peptide chloromethyl ketones are poor inhibitors. The better inhibitors are those containing a large hydrophobic group at the P$_2$ site such as Z-Arg-CH$_2$Cl and Phe-Phe-Arg-CH$_2$Cl. The preference for a hydrophobic group at the P$_2$ site was also shown in our substrate studies. Isocoumarins substituted with basic groups were potent inhibitors of human and murine granzyme A (5). The isothiureidoethoxyisocoumarin (7-PhNHCONH-CiTEtOIC) is a better inhibitor than the isothiureidopropoxy compound (7-PhNHCONH-CiTPrOIC) by one order of magnitude. Isocoumarins with large hydrophobic substituents on the 7-amino group inhibit granzyme A more potently than the parent compound, NH$_2$-CiTPrOIC ($k_{obs}/[I]$ = 2000 $M^{-1}s^{-1}$ for human granzyme A, 5). Isothiureidoethoxyisocoumarins inhibit granzyme A more efficiently than peptide chloromethyl ketones.

Mast Cell tryptases. Tryptases are serine proteases localized in the granule of mast cells and a few synthetic inhibitors have been reported. Arginine trifluoromethyl ketones are potent inhibitors of trypsin and coagulation enzymes (7), and we have shown that rat skin tryptase was inhibited by 1-naphthoyl-Arg-CF$_3$ and Bz-Arg-CF$_3$ with K$_I$ values of 0.9 and 1.2 μM respectively. Isocoumarins substituted with a basic isothiureidoalkoxy group such as 7-PhNHCONH-CiTEtOIC inhibited bovine trypsin, rat skin and human lung tryptases quite potently with $k_{obs}/[I]$ values of 10^4-10^5 $M^{-1}s^{-1}$. 7-PhNHCONH-CiTEtOIC formed a stable trypsin-inhibitor complex which regained less than 8 % of activity upon standing in a pH 7.5 buffer and regained 30 % of activity in the presence of 0.3 M NH_2OH after one day. The reactivation results indicate that both an acyl enzyme and irreversible inactivated enzyme are formed in the inhibition process.

Table 4. Inhibition of HR Granzyme A by Various Types of Inhibitors

Inhibitors	[I] (μM)	$k_{obs}/[I]$ ($M^{-1}s^{-1}$)
Z-Arg-CH_2Cl	450	25
H-Phe-Phe-Arg-CH_2Cl	430	24
D-Phe-Pro-Arg-CH_2Cl	420	7.8
7-PhNHCONH-CiTPrOIC	4.3	1800
7-PhNHCONH-CiTEtOIC	0.42	94050

CONCLUSION

Synthetic peptide *p*-nitroanilides and thioesters were used to study biological important serine proteases and several new enzymatic activities were discovered. Potent inhibitors with various structures have also been found for these enzymes and should be useful for studying the physiological roles of these serine proteases.

ACKNOWLEDGEMENTS

This investigation was supported by grants to Georgia Institute of Technology (HL34035, HL29307, and GM42212) and Univ. of Nevada (GM42212) from the National Institutes of Health, and a grant from the Emory/Georgia Tech Biomedical Technology Research Center.

REFERENCES

1. Graves HCB, Kamarei M, and Stamey TA. Identity of prostatic specific antigen and the semen protein p30 purified by a rapid chromatography technique. J Urol 1990; 144: 1510-1515.

2. McRae BJ, Kurachi K, Heimark RL, Fujikawa K, Davie EW, and Powers JC. Mapping the active sites of bovine thrombin, factor IXa, factor Xa, factor XIa, factor XIIa, plasma kallikrein,

and trypsin with amino acid and peptide thioester: Development of new sensitive substrates. Biochemistry 1981; 20: 7196-7206.

3. Cho K, Tanaka T, Cook RR, Kisiel W, Fujikawa K, Karachi K, and Powers JC. Active site mapping of bovine and human blood coagulation serine proteases using synthetic peptide 4-nitroanilide and thioester substrates. Biochemistry 1984; 23: 644-655.

4. Harper JW, Cook RR, Roberts CJ, McLaughlin BJ, and Powers JC. Active site mapping of the serine proteases human leukocyte elastase, cathepsin G, porcine pancreatic elastase, rat mast cell protease I and II, bovine chymotrypsin Aα, and Staphylococcus aureus protease V-8 using tripeptide thiobenzyl ester substrates. Biochemistry 1984; 23: 2995-3002.

5. Odake S, Kam CM, Narasimhan L, Poe M, Blake JT, Krahenbuhl O, Tschopp J, and Powers JC. Human and murine cytotoxic T lymphocyte serine proteases: subsite mapping with peptide thioester substrates and inhibition of enzyme activity and cytolysis by isocoumarins. Biochemistry 1991; 30: 2217-2227.

6. Kettner C, and Shaw E. Inactivation of trypsin-like enzymes with peptides of arginine chloromethylketones. Methods Enzymol 1981; 80: 826-842.

7. Ueda T, Kam CM, and Powers JC. The synthesis of arginylfluoroalkanes, their inhibition of trypsin and blood-coagulation serine proteinases and their anticoagulant activity. Biochem J 1990; 265: 539-545.

8. Lilji H. A kallikrein-like serine protease in prostatic fluid cleaves the predominant seminal vesicle protein. J Clin Invest 1985; 76: 1899-1903.

9. Watt KWK, Lee PJ, M'Timkulu T, Chan W-P, Loor R. Human prostate-specific antigen: Structural and functional similarity with serine proteases. Proc Natl Acad Sci USA 1986; 83: 3166-3170.

10. Christensson A, Laurell CB, and Lilja H. Enzymatic activity of prostate-specific antigen and its reactions with extracellar serine proteinase inhibitors. Eur J Biochem 1990; 194: 755-763.

11. Powers JC, McRae BJ, Tanaka T, Cho K, and Cook RR. Peptide thioesters and 4-nitroanilides as substrates for procine pancreatic kallikrein. Biochem J 1984; 220: 569-573.

12. Hudig D, Allison NJ, Pickett TM, Winkler U, Kam CM, and Powers JC. The function of lymphocyte proteases. Inhibition and restoration of granule-mediated lysis with isocoumarin serine protease inhibitors. J Immunol 1991; 147: 1360-1368.

13. Murphy MEP, Moult J, Bleackley RC, Gershenfeld H, Weissman IL., and James MNG. Comparative molecular model building of two serine proteinases from cytotoxic T lymphocytes. Proteins: Structure, Function, and Genetics 1988; 4: 190-204.

14. Powers JC, and Harper JW. Inhibitors of serine proteinases. In: Proteinase Inhibitors. Barrett AJ, Salvensen G, editors. Amsterdam, New York, Oxford: Elsevier, 1986: 55-152.

15. Kam CM, Fujikawa K, and Powers JC. Mechanism based isocoumarin inhibitors for trypsin and blood coagulation serine proteases: New anticoagulants. Biochemistry 1988; 27: 2547-2557.

AAS 38/II
Recent Progress on Kinins
© 1992 Birkhäuser Verlag Basel

ABSORPTION STUDIES WITH
PORCINE PANCREATIC KALLIKREIN IN MAN

W. Miska, R. Geiger[+] and W.-B. Schill

Dept. of Dermatology and Andrology University Giessen,
Gaffkystr. 14, D-6300 Giessen, Germany.
[+]MEDOR GmbH, D-8036 Herrsching, Germany

SUMMARY
Porcine pancreatic kallikrein (PPK), the main component of
Padutin[R] (Bayropharm, FRG), is used since 1974 for the
treatment of some forms of idiopathic infertility in man.
During kallikrein therapy the number of spermatozoa increases, and qualitative and quantitative sperm motility is
improved.
In order to investigate the intestinal absorption of PPK in
man a clinical study with 7 healthy volunteers was performed. 4500 KE (corresp. to 2.8 mg PPK) and 600 KE
(corresp. to 0.38 mg PPK) of kallikrein respectively was
orally adminstered in one dosis. Serum and urine samples
were collected several times within 24 hours. Seminal plasma
was collected 4-5 days before and 8 hours after treatment
with kallikrein. Absorbed PPK was determined using a highly
sensitive bioluminescence-enhanced enzyme immunoassay (1)
and a newly developed light measuring equipment (MTP reader)
(3). The limit of detection was 1 pg/ml in serum corresponding to 6 amol PPK per assay.
For both groups (600 KE and 4500 KE) absorption of PPK in
serum was found. Maximum absorption was observed between 4
and 12 h and between 2 and 6h, respectively, after oral
application of kallikrein. Renal excretion plays no important role in the elimination of PPK from serum.
In gel filtration experiments with blood samples of volunteers in which absorbed PPK was detected, one peak of
immunochemically active material corresponding to a molecular mass of 82 kDa was found.
According to our results, kallikrein is absorbed in unaltered form by the intestine. The absorbed amount of PPK is
sufficient to exert a possible effect in enzymatically
active form on the target cells in the male gonads before it
is inhibited probably by α_1-proteinase inhibitor.

INTRODUCTION

Porcine pancreatic kallikrein (PPK), the main component of Padutin[R] (Bayropharm, FRG), is used since 1974 for the treatment of some forms of idiopathic infertility in man. In several clinical trials (1) it has been shown, that orally administered PPK can be useful mainly in infertility cases with asthenozoospermia and/or oligozoospermia. During kallikrein therapy the number of spermatozoa increases, and qualitative and quantitative sperm motility is improved (2). Absorption studies with PPK have been performed only in animal species like dog and rat (3). The main reason therefore was due to the small amounts of kallikrein, which are applicated to volunteers and which could not be detected by conventional measuring systems. A recently developed ultra-sensitive detection system on the basis of enzyme-enhanced bioluminescence (4-8) enabled the quantification of the small concentrations of absorbed PPK.
In order to investigate the intestinal absorption of PPK in man a clinical study with healthy volunteers was performed (16). The aim of the study was to quantify the intestinal absorption, the renal excretion and a possible transsudation of PPK into seminal plasma. Moreover parameters like absorption rate and mean absorption maximum should also be determined.

VOLUNTEERS AND METHODS

Study Design
Padutin[R] was orally adminstered in one dose. Four volunteers obtained 4500 KE (corresp. to 2.8 mg PPK) and three 600 KE (corresp. to 0.38 mg PPK). Serum and urine samples were collected several times within 24 hours. Seminal plasma was collected 4-5 days before and 8 hours after treatment with

kallikrein. Absorbed PPK was determined using a highly sensitive bioluminescence-enhanced enzyme immunoassay (4,5) and a newly developed light measuring equipment (MTP reader) (10).

Bioluminescence-enhanced Enzyme Immunoassay for PPK
Microtiter plates were coated with rabbit anti-porcine pancreatic kallikrein-IgG (10 μg/ml corbonate buffer, pH 9.6; 0.2 ml per well) at 4 °C overnight. The plates were then washed (5 times) with washing buffer. Porcine pancreatic kallikrein standard samples and test samples were diluted with dilution buffer. 0.2 ml of these samples were added to the wells and the plates were incubated at 4 °C for 24 h. After incubation, the plates were washed (5 times) with washing buffer, 0.2 ml of rabbit anti-porcine pancreatic kallikrein-IgG biotin conjugate solution was added to each well and incubated for 2 h at 37 °C. Then the plates were washed (5 times), 0.2 ml of extravidin-alkaline phosphatase conjugate (1:100) were added to the wells and incubated for 1 h at 37 °C. The plates were washed (5 times), 0.2 ml of D-luciferin-O-phosphate substrate solution were added to the wells and incubated for 10 min at 25°C. 0.1 ml of this solution was transferred to black microtiter plates containing 0.1 ml detection solution per well and emitted light was integrated for 5 min in a MTP-reader.

Gel filtration experiments
1 ml of serum from the absorption maximum was applicated to a Sephacryl S-200 column (1x110 cm) and eluted at 4°C with PBS buffer, pH 7.4 and a pump speed of 2 ml*h^{-1}. UV absorption was measured at 278 nm. Fractions were collected each 30 min and PPK was determined by bioluminescence-enhanced enzyme immunoassay. Calibration of the column was done by elution of standard proteins in the range of 13.7-92.5 kDa.

RESULTS

All seven volunteers showed detectable absorption of PPK
into serum (Tab. 1). Maximum concentrations of 1-2.25 ng/ml
of PPK in the low dose group (600 KE administered) and 2.7-7
ng/ml in the high dose group (4500 KE administered) were
found after 4-12 h and 2-6 h respectively.
Minimum absorption rates ranged from 0.05 % (volunt. I) to
1.89 % (volunt. C) with a mean value of 0.74 % (± 0.22 %)
(Tab. 1). The extremly low absorption rate of volunteer I
possibly indicates a difference between the sensitivity to
Padutin[R] of responders and non-responders.

Table 1: Minimum absorption and absorption rates of PPK

Volunt.	max. PPK-concentr. [ng/ml]	Minimum absorption [μg/person]	Minimum absorp. rate [%]
I	0,5	1,27	0,05
II	5,0	17,1	0,61
III	7,0	21,8	0,78
IV	2,7	7,58	0,27
A	1,0	2,85	0,75
B	1,0	3,08	0,81
C	2,25	7,18	1,89

Renal excretion of PPK was only observed in the high dose
group (Tab. 2). The values ranged from 4.45 ng/person to
11.7 ng/person corresponding to an excretion of 0.02-0.92 %
of total absorbed PPK. Therefore excretion of absorbed PPK
by the kidney plays only a secondary role for the
elimination of PPK from blood.
In seminal plasma no PPK could be detected definitly
(detection limit 10 pg/ml).

In gel filtration experiments with blood samples of volunteers in which absorbed PPK was detected, one peak of immunochemically active material corresponding to a molecular mass of 82 kDa was found.

Table 2: Excretion of PPK by the kidney.

Volunt.	PPK in urine [ng/person]	percentage of absorbed PPK [%]
I	11,7	0,92
II	4,45	0,03
III	5,03	0,02
IV	7,72	0,10

DISCUSSION

With the help of the newly developed bioluminescence-enhanced enzyme immunoassay for PPK intestinal absorption of this protein in man could be demonstrated. The new detection system is more sensitive than radio immunoassays (5). By the combination of a signal system with high specific activity (4) and a measuring system with high sensitivity (MTP-Reader) (10) limits of detection in the subattomolar range are reachable.

Absorption rates could not be estimated exactly because no data concerning the distribution of PPK in other body compartments are available. The indicated absorption rates are lower than the real one and represent only lower limits (Tab. 1). In animals (rat, dog) intestinal absorption of PPK was also quantified below one percent of the applicated kallikrein (3,11) and a great variety of the absorption profiles was observed.

Renal excretion of PPK could only be measured in the high dose group (Tab. 2). The time courses of the excretion profiles showed good correlation with the corresponding absorption profiles. The mean excretion rate was 0.27 % of the absorbed kallikrein. Renal excretion plays therefore only a secondary role in the elimination of PPK from serum.

Transsudation of kallikrein into seminal plasma could be definitly not be detected at a lower detection limit of 10 pg/assay. Corresponding to the absorption and excretion profiles specimen collection at 8h after oral application of kallikrein should be optimal. We conclude therefore that PPK cannot cross the serum-seminal barrier. In vitro kallikrein stimulates sperm metabolism and sperm motility (12, 13). Accordingly it was speculated that PPK is transsudated into the seminal plasma causing the mentioned effects. However, our results indicate not a direct action but an indirect action via increase of spermatogensis and/or sperm transport. The absorbed amounts of PPK are rather low but kallikrein acting as kininogenase liberates manifold quantities of kinin (14) - the terminal effector of the kallikrein-kinin system. Therefore the concentrations of PPK we found in serum after intestinal absorption appear to be sufficient for exerting a possible effect on the target cells within the male gonads. Porcine pancreatic kallikrein is eliminated from serum in a few hours (not shown). Excretion of absorbed kallikrein by the kidney plays hereby only a secondary role (Tab. 2). Hence PPK is possibly eliminated by diffusion into and/or adsorption in different body compartiments - i.e. the male gonads.

In gel filtration experiments with serum of volunteers kallikrein was eluted in one single peak corresponding to a molecular mass of approximately 82 kDa. This might indicate that most of the intestinally absorbed kallikrein is bound to a plasma protein, probably α_1-proteinase inhibitor (α_1-antitrypsin). Possibly PPK (mol. mass 35 kDa (9)) is inhi-

bited after intestinal absorption by α_1-proteinase inhibitor
(mol. mass 54 kDa). The so formed high molecular complex
elutes in the gel filtration with a retention time corresponding to 82 kDa. Gel filtration is a time consuming method
and moreover these experiments could only be done after
following intestinal absorption. Hence there is enough time
for the formation of the PPK-α_1-PI complex, which takes
several hours under in vitro conditions(15).

CONCLUSIONS

Porcine pancreatic kallikrein is absorbed intestinally in
unaltered form and is slowly inhibited in serum probably by
α_1-proteinase inhibitor. The absorbed amount of PPK is
sufficient to exert a possible effect in enzymatically
active form on the target cells in the male gonads for
several hours. For the elimination of kallikrein from serum
renal excretion plays only a minor role.

REFERENCES

1. Schill, W.-B., Kininogenases, Kallikrein, Physiological
    Properties and Pharmacological Rationale (Haberland,
    G.L., Rohen, J.W., Suzuki, T., Hrsg.), S. 251-280,
    Schattauer, Stuttgart (1977).

2. Schill, W.-B., Arch. Androl. 2, 163-170 (1979).

3. Fink, E., Geiger, R., Witte, J., Biedermann, S.,
    Seifert, J., Fritz H., Enzymatic release of vasoactive
    peptides (Gross, S., Vogel, E., Hrsg.), S. 101-115,
    Raven, New York (1980).

4. Miska, W., Geiger, R., J. Clin. Chem. Clin. Biochem.,
    25, 23-30 (1987).

5. Geiger, R., Miska, W., J. Clin. Chem. Clin. Biochem.,
    25, 31-38 (1987).

6. Miska, W., Geiger, R., Biol. Chem. Hoppe-Seyler, 369, 407-411 (1988).

7. Miska, W., Geiger, R., J. Biolum. Chemilum. 4, 119-128 (1989).

8. Geiger, R., Miska, W., Meth. Enzymol., 163, (1988).

9. Fritz, H., Fiedler, F., Dietl, T., Warwas M., Truscheit, E., Kolb, H.J., Mair, G., Tschesche, H., Kininogenases. Kallikrein (Haberland, G.L., Rohen, J.W., Suzuki, T., Hrsg.), 4. Aufl., S. 15-28, Schattauer, Stuttgart (1977).

10. Miska, W., Geiger, R., Bioluminescence and Chemiluminescence: Current Status (Stanley, E.P., Kricka, L.J., Hrsg.), S. 183-186 (1990).

11. Fink, E., Seifert, J., Güttel, L., Fresenius Z. Anat. Chem., 290, 183 (1978).

12. Schill, W.-B., Haberland, G.L., Hoppe-Seyler's Z. Physiol. Chem., 355, 229-231 (1974).

13. Schill, W.-B., Haberland, G.L., Klin. Wochenschr., 53,, 73-79 (1975).

14. Geiger, R., Proteinases and their Inhibitors (Turk, V., Vitale, Lj., Hrsg.), S. 353-376, Mladinska Knjiga-Pergamon Press, Ljubljana (1981).

15. Geiger, R., Stuckstedter, U., Clausnitzer, B., Fritz H., Hoppe Seyler's Z. Physiol. Chem., 362, 317-325.

16. Miska, W. and Schill, W.-B., Arzneim.Forsch./Drug Res., 41(II), 1061-64, (1991).

AAS 38/II
Recent Progress on Kinins
© 1992 Birkhäuser Verlag Basel

THE REGULATING INTERRELATIONSHIP OF SOME SERINE PROTEINASES
FROM LEUKOCYTE WITH THE HUMAN PLASMA KALLIKREIN-KININ SYSTEM

Vera L. Dotsenko, Elena A. Neshkova,
Galina A. Yarovaya.

Department of Biochemistry, Central Institute for
Advanced Training of Physicians, Moscow, USSR

INTRODUCTION

Activation of the plasma kallikrein-kinin system (KKS) is
generally coincident in time with inflammation (Colman and Wong,
1979; Burch et al 1989). This activation is essential for formation
of the inflammative focus and may be considered as a crucial moment
in the regulation of other plasma proteolytic systems, such as
clotting, fibrinolysis, the renin-angiotensin and the complement
systems (Colman and Wong 1979; Colman 1984; Ghebrehiwet et al 1981;
Goldsmith 1980; Kaplan et al 1976).

It is not yet clear which factors in activated leukocytes are
responsible for KKS activation. Melmon and Cline (1968), as well
as Wasi et al (1978), insisted that cell kininogenase releases
vasoactive peptides from plasma kininogene. Newball et al (1975,
1978) reported the presence in basophils of an enzyme, released by
the IgE-mechanism and capable of activating Hageman factor. As for
neutrophils it is unknown whether there are any enzymes in them
capable of activating the key enzymes of plasma KKS. However in
our earlier papers we have demonstrated not only the activating
(Dotsenko et al 1987) but also the inactivating effect (Dotsenko
et al 1989) of leukocytes on human Hageman factor. Discrepancy of
results obtained is partly due to the complex composition of the
cell enzyme extracts.

In this study we have made an attempt to characterize the new
leukocyte membrane proteinase and to elucidate the effect of
leukocyte serine granule proteinases (elastase and cathepsin G)
and of this leukocyte membrane trypsin-like proteinase on key KKS
enzymes (Hageman factor and kallikrein) and on their precusors.

MATERIALS AND METHODS

Obtaining of leukocyte extracts and purification of elastase and cathepsin G

Initial material for the extracts was prepared by the usual procedure (i.e. by leukocyte sedimentation in Dextran T-500) with some modifications (Dotsenko et al 1992). The specific activity of the leukocyte elastase, obtained with MeO-Suc-Ala-Ala-Pro-Val-pNA was 20-25 $\mu mol \cdot min^{-1} \cdot mg^{-1}$. There were three isoforms of elastase in the elastase preparation with 26,300, 27,800 and 28,900 D. The isolated and purificated Cathepsin G had a specific activity of 20-40 μmol $BTEE \cdot min^{-1} \cdot mg^{-1}$.

Preparation and isolation of a latent trypsin-like proteinase from the leukocyte membrane extract

Leukocyte membrane extract was prepared by the method of Wintroub et al (1974, 1977) with slight modification.

Supernatant was filtrated through a Sephadex G-100 column with a total volume of 50 ml and equilibrated with 0,01M Tris-HCl buffer, pH 8,0, with 1M NaCl. The fraction volume was 0,8-1,0 ml; elution rate, 3,0 ml per hour. The activities thus determined were: BAEE-esterase (trypsin-like), BTEE-esterase (chymotrypsin-like), MeOSucAAPVpNA-amidase (elastase-like), kininogenase (with HMW-kininogen as substrate); and finally the ability of the fractions to activate Hageman factor and prekallikrein was determined. The fractions with BAEE-esterase and kininogenase activities were pooled and kept at $-20^{\circ}C$.

Isolation of neutrophils and their subcellular fractionation

Leukocytes, obtained from 3 doses of leukocyte mass (each dose - from 500 ml of fresh donor's blood) were resuspended in Krebs-Ringer buffer (121 mM NaCl, 4,9 mM KCl, 1,2 mM KH_2PO_4, 1,2 mM $MgSO_4$, 16,5 mM Na_2HPO_4, pH 7,4), containing 2 mg/ml glucose. Subsequent isolation of neutrophils was carried out by the method of Record et al (1985) in Percoll gradient.

Isolation and purification of human plasma prekallikrein

Prekallikrein was isolated from fresh donor's blood by chromatography of the serum on QAE and CM-Sephadex (Kawiak et al, 1984). Prekallikrein preparation was found to have a potential specific activity of 0,8-2,0 $U \cdot mg^{-1}$ (U, the unit of activity is defined as the quantity of enzyme which splits 1 $\mu mole$ BAEE for 1 min).

Isolation and purification of human Hageman factor

Hageman factor (inactive form) was purified from fresh donor's blood in 3-4 steps by ion exchange and gel chromatography of the serum (Dotsenko et al 1987). Hageman factor preparations used had a potential specific activity of 1-2 $U \cdot min^{-1} \cdot mg^{-1}$

Gordox-activating test

This test was carried out in 3 ml cuvette, containing 5-20 μl of the assayed fraction, 1,9 ml of 0,05M Tris-HCl buffer, pH 8,0, and 1,0 ml of BAEE (or other substrates) (1,5 10^{-3}M) at 37°C. Prior to assay 50-100 μl of Gordox were added to the cuvette and quickly mixed up; sample density was registered automatically in a Hitachi Model U-3200 spectrophotometer (Japan) every 0,1 min during 3-5 min. The activity was estimated from the maximal density increase in the first 0,1-0,3 min.

RESULTS AND DISCUSSION

1. Leukocyte elastase inactivates human plasma Hageman factor, prekallikrein, and their active forms

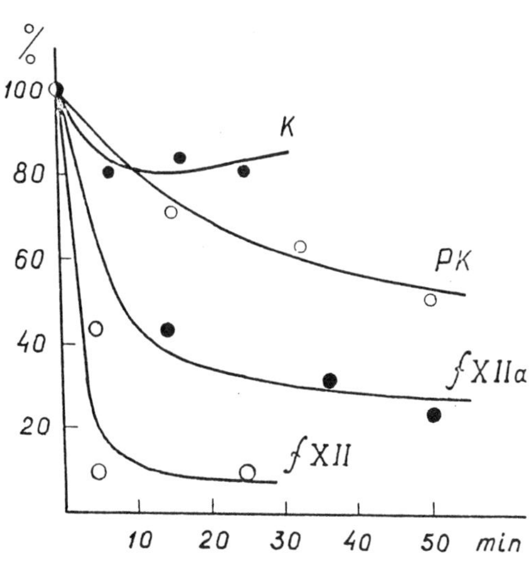

Fig. 1. Effect of elastase on native Hageman factor, prekallikrein and their active forms (residual activity in % of initial versus the time of incubation)

As already demonstrated, the leukocyte extract not only activated but also inactivated human Hageman factor (Dotsenko et al 1989), therefore it was of interest to elucidate the effect of well known leukocyte granule serine proteinases (elastase and cathepsin G) on key enzymes of the kallikrein-kinin system.

The results of the action of leukocyte elastase on native Hageman factor, prekallikrein and their active forms are presented in Fig. 1. In the absence of elastase both the native and trypsin-activated factors fully retained their total activities. However, 10-min incubation of elastase with this enzyme led to a 90% and 50% inactivation of the native and activated forms respectively.

Study of dose-dependent effect of elastase demonstrated that 1 mU of elastase inactivated within 1 min the 1,1 mU·min^{-1} of the potential and 0,8 mU·min^{-1} of the actual Hageman factor's activity. The same amount of elastase inactivated 2,6 mU of prekallikrein and 2,7 mU of kallikrein within 45 min incubation. These results indicate that destroying elastase activity towards prekallikrein and kallikrein was about 20 times lower than it was towards Hageman factor.

2. Leukocyte cathepsin G inactivates Hageman factor but not prekallikrein and kallikrein

Similar to elastase cathepsin G did not activate either prekallikrein or Hageman factor. Incubation of increasing quantities of cathepsin G (37, 93, 186 and 373 mU) in samples that contained 6,7 mU of prekallikrein and kallikrein influenced neither the activity of this plasma enzyme nor the activity of its precusor (Fig. 2B).

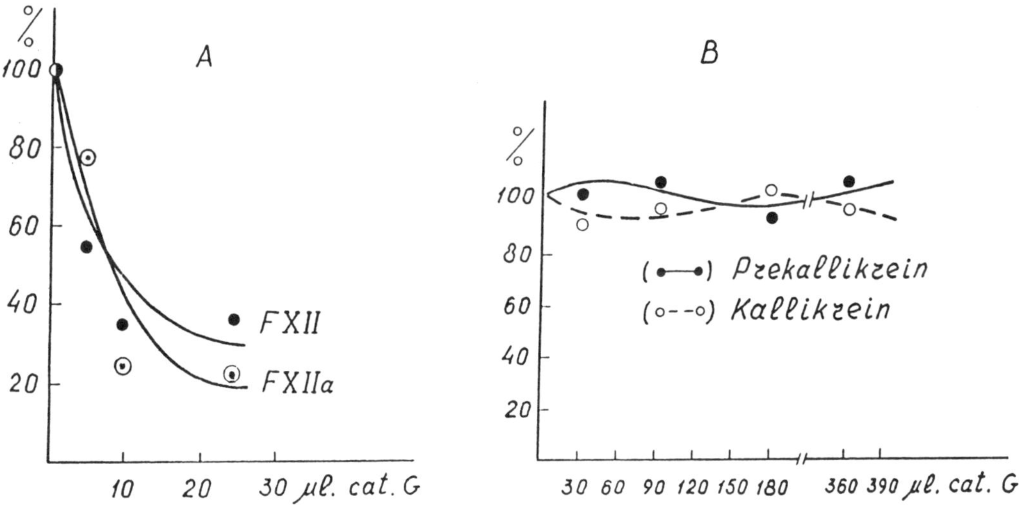

Fig. 2. Effect of cathepsin G on native and activated Hageman factor (A), on prekallikrein and kallikrein (B) (residual activity in % of initial versus the quantities of enzymes)

Hageman factor (both native and activated) was less stable under the action of cathepsin G than was prekallikrein and kallikrein: 4,1 mU of cathepsin G for 10 min of incubation at 37°C inactivated 68% (5 mU·min^{-1}) of the native and 72% (4,2 mU·min^{-1}) of the activated factor (Fig. 2A).

3. Proteinase(s) with the Hageman factor-activating, BAEE-esterase, and kininogenase activities was demonstrated in the leukocyte membrane

At the very first steps of research, we used the advantage of the simple and time-saving method of Wintroub et al (1974, 1977) for the isolation of leukocyte membrane fraction and receiving the extracts: 100 xg centrifugation of leukocyte homogenate with following slight sonication and extraction of the proteins for 1 hour by the use of 0,01M Tris-HCl buffer, pH 7,4, with 1M NaCl. The pellet consisted of membrane pieces and cell debrises with high content of membrane material that was confirmed by 5-nucleotidise test activity (Wintroub et al 1974).

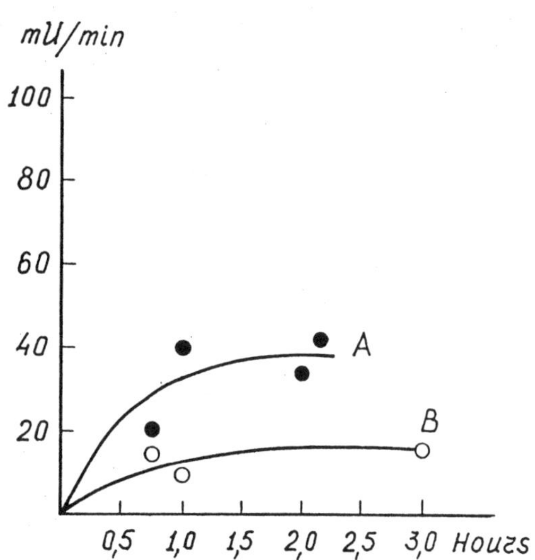

Fig. 3. Prekallikrein-activating activity of Hageman factor in control (o——o) and after its incubation with 100 xg fraction extract (●——●)

The extract with the protein concentration of 20-30 mg/ml revealed the appreciable BAEE- and BTEE-esterase activities: 0,911 and 0,648 μmol min^{-1}· ml^{-1}, respectively. The elastase-like activity was considerably lower: 0,032 μmol·min^{-1}· ml^{-1}.

It has been demonstrated that the BAEE-esterase activity was not stable in the extract but its value was slightly growing during storage at 4°C.

The kininogenase reaction with human plasma high molecular weight kininogen as substrate showed the ability of the extract to release bradykinin: for 30 min of incubation 1 ml of extract released 575 ng-equivalents of bradykinin.

The data obtained showed that the leukocyte extract possesses the Hageman factor activating ability. Fig. 3 demonstrates the activation of Hageman factor in incubation mixture, containing 1 ml of native factor (with potential activity of 1,13 U·min^{-1}· ml^{-1}), 0,3 ml of 0,5M Tris-HCl buffer, pH 8,0, and 40 μl of membrane extract. The control incubation mixture did not contain the membrane extract. Both mixtures were incubated for 2 h at 37°C and 0,1 ml aliquots were taken at regular time intervals to determine their prekallikrein-activating activity. The Hageman factor activating curve shows the excess of factor activity (curve A) above control factor activity (curve B) within the first hour of incubation. After the 2 h incubation the activity has been grown to 40,3 mU· min^{-1} which was about 45,5% of possible factor activity. There was also some activation of Hageman factor in control, but it did not exceed 10-15% of initial potential activity.

4. Phenomenal increasing of the BAEE-esterase activity of leukocyte membrane proteinase under the action of tissue proteinase inhibitor (Kunitz type)

The low level of BAEE-esterase activity of membrane protein extract sharply elevated to that as high as 40-60 μmol BAEE min^{-1}· ml^{-1} during 0,1-0,2 min after bringing in cuvette some quantities of Trasylol, Gordox or Kontrical.

The very high activity was changed during 1-2 min for moderate values and after that the activity fell down to 0,1-0,3 μmol min^{-1} ml^{-1} within 6-10 min.

The curves of the dependence between BAEE-esterase activity of proteinase (in μmol· min^{-1}· ml^{-1}) and the quantities of Kunitz type inhibitor bringing in specimen (in μl) were submitted in Fig. 4. After measuring of the initial activity the volume of inhibitor indicated on the axis was introduced to the cuvette. After fast mixing the change of density was registered in spectrophotometer Hitachi Model U-3200 during 3-5 min with time interval 0,1 min.

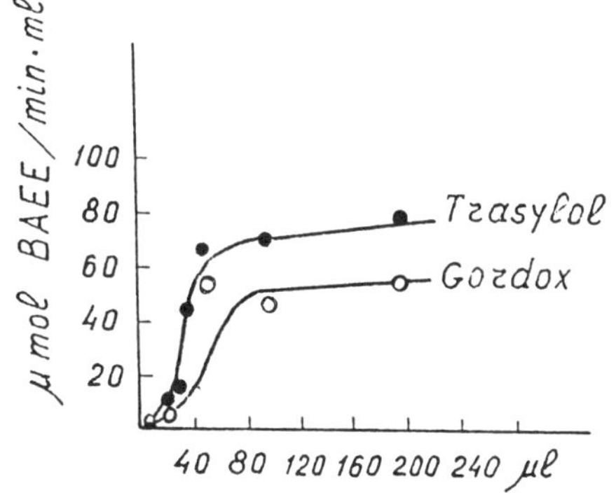

Fig.4. Activation of latent leukocyte membrane proteinase (in mol BAEE/min ml) under the action of the tissue Kunitz inhibitor (in μl of preparations of Trasylol and Gordox).

5. Substrate and inhibitor analysis characterized the leukocyte membrane BAEE-esterase as latent trypsin-like proteinases

All substrates that have been tested with activated proteinase were listed in the Table 1. As will be seen from the table, the highest susceptibility to the activated enzyme was in the case of arginine and lysine esters and nitroanilides but not of valine, alanine and tyrosine esters and nitroanilides. It is very difficult to estimate by the usual methods the kinetic constants of enzymes reactions because of short duration of this activity, but it is

Table 1. Substrate specificity of activated leukocyte membrane proteinase

Substrate	Activity (μmol/min·ml)	Substrate	Activity (μmol/min·ml)	Substrate	Activity (μmol/min·ml)
1. BAEE	245.7	5. Bz-Pro-Phe-Arg-pNA	0.98	8. MeOSuc-Ala-Ala-Pro-Val-pNA	0.0
2. TLME	263.3	6. Bz-Ile-Glu-Gly-Arg-pNA	4.9	9. T-Boc-Ala-ONp	0.0
3. BTEE	0.0	7. Z-Gly-Pro-Arg-pNA	4.9	10. Suc-Ala-Ala-Ala-pNA	0.0
4. H-Pro-Phe-Arg-pNA (with mannitol)	5.5				

Table 2. The substances tested as the leukocyte membrane proteinase activator

Substance	Activation (%)	Substance	Activation (%)	Substance	Activation (%)
1. Tissue Kunitz inhibitor	100	7. Pancreatic elastase	0.0	13. Cystein	0.0
2. Protamine sulphate	58.7	8. Leukocyte elastase	0.0	14. Human plasma albumin	0.0
3. Human plasma kallikrein	15.1	9. Cathepsin G	0.0	15. Heparin	0.0
4. Ampholines pH 7-9	7.8	10. Human plasma prekallkrein	0.0	16. 4-amino-benzamidine	0.0
5. Trypsin	0.0	11. HMW-kininogen	0.0	17. Benzamidine	0.0
6. Tissue kallikrein	0.0	12. Dextran sulphate	0.0		

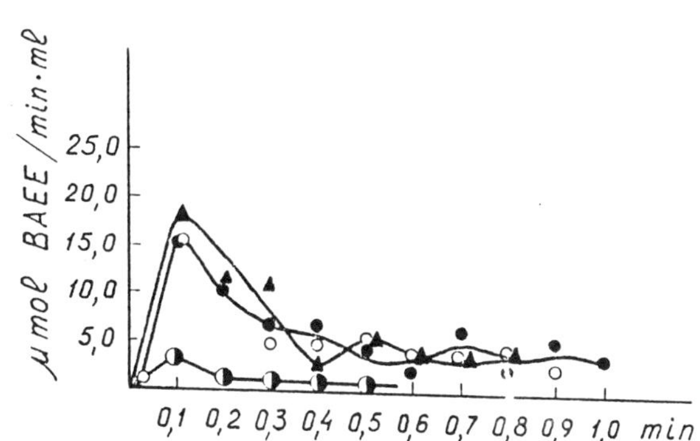

Fig. 5. Activation of latent leukocyte membrane trypsin-like proteinase (in μmol BAEE/min ml) under the action of Gordox in the presence of SBTI (o——o), ovomucoid (●——●), DFP (◑——◑) and without any inhibitor (▲---▲)

obvious that the small molecules of modified aminoacids (BAEE and TLME) are preferable to three- or tetrapeptides.

Both protein inhibitors of trypsin and trypsin-like proteinases as SBTI, ovomucoid and also ε-ACA (0,2 mg/ml) and EDTA (0,003M) did not prevent the activation of membrane proteinase under the action of Trasylol. But preliminary incubation of latent proteinase with 0,13M DFP for 10 min and the presence of $6,6 \times 10^{-3}$M DFP in the specimen during Trasylol action, prevented the elevation of the activity.

The curves of activating effect of Trasylol on leukocyte membrane proteinase in the presence of SBTI, ovomucoid and DFP are demonstrated in Fig.5. Depression of the arising activity (or preventing of the activating) by DFP incontrovertibly testified to the presence of serine in the active centre of the membrane proteinase. The probable reason of failure with another inhibitors may be accounted for the short time of proteinase living.

6. Strongly pronounced alkaline properties of the molecules are evidently the main characteristics of activators for latent membrane proteinase

The activation of the latent membrane proteinase occured not only under the action of pharmacological preparations of inhibitor, but also under that of inhibitor heated to 100°C.

The curve obtained was presented in Fig. 6. As it appears from these data, Gordox increased its activating ability for the first 3-5 hours of heating at 100°C. It should be mentioned that the inhibitory properties of preparation gradually decreased during heating, and after 5 hours of heating the quantity of aggregated proteins in preparation was increased and became visible.

Besides alkaline Kunitz inhibitor, other substances as well play the role of the leukocyte membrane proteinase activator:

protamine sulfate, human plasma kallikrein and alkaline ampholines.

Table 2 presents the list of substances tested as possible activators of this proteinase. Comparison of their properties emphasized the probable significance of polycationic nature of activators.

7. Neutrophil membrane contains the latent trypsin-like proteinase.

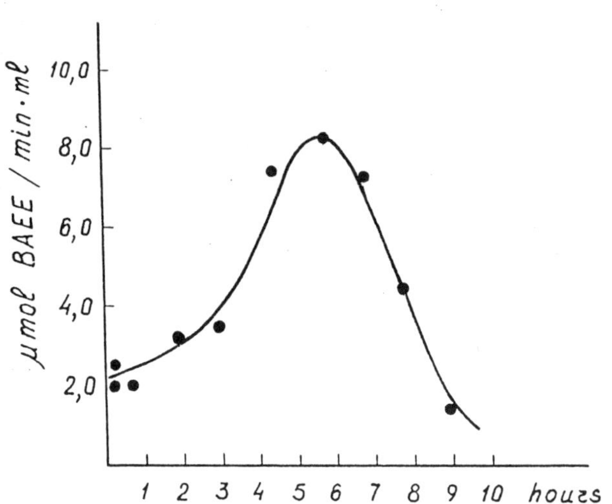

Fig. 6. Activation of leukocyte membrane trypsin-like proteinase (in µmol BAEE/min·ml) under the action of thermal worked up Gordox. The time of thermal working up (100°C) on the axis of absciss.

Subcellular fractionation of homogenized polymorphonuclear neutrophils in Percoll gradient gave an opportunity to receive the membrane fraction strictly separately from granule fraction.

Fig. 7 demonstrated the activities of these fraction from the top of gradient, where the external plasmatic membrane vesicles are localized, to the bottom, with granule fraction. Alkaline phosphatase, as the marker of membrane fraction, coincided with slight BAEE-esterase activity and Trasylol-activating phenomenon. The data obtained confirmed the results of Record et al (1985), who have demonstrated the localization of membrane fraction in the first 1-4 fractions with more specific marker 5'nucleotidise. The granule fractions in our experiments did not contain any BAEE-esterase activity, did not demonstrate trasylol-activating phenomenon and these fractions in the bottom of gradient are rich in elastase activity.

8. The localization on the chromatographic protein curve of the latent trypsin-like proteinase coincided with kininogenase and Hageman factor activating activities but it separated from chymotrypsin-like and elastase-like activities

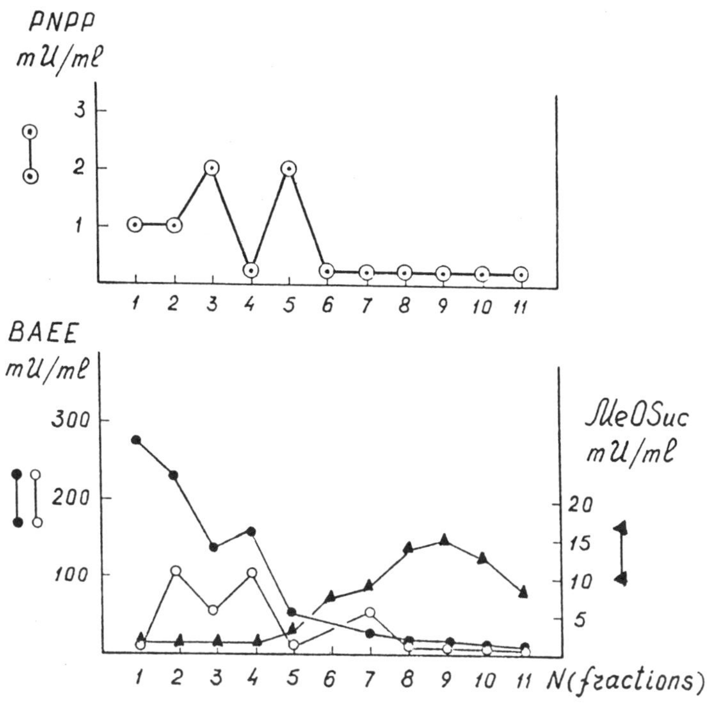

Fig. 7. Enzymatic activities of subcellular fractions of neutrophils (Percoll gradient).
o——o BAEE-esterase activity (nmol/min ml); ●——● BAEE-esterase activity excited by Trasylol; ▲——▲ MeOSucAAPVpNA-amidase elastase-like activity; ⊙——⊙ activity of alkaline phosphatase (nmol PNPP/min ml)

The elution curve, obtained in chromatografic experiment on the Sephadex G-100, is demonstrated in Fig. 8 (A, curve 1). The fractions in the first peak revealed only traces of BAEE-esterase activity (Fig. 8, A, curve 2; Fig 8, E, curve 1), which appreciably grew under the action of plasma kallkrein (Fig. 8, A, curve 3) and Gordox (Fig. 8, E, curve 2). This protein peak contained kininogenase (Fig. 8, C) and Hageman factor-activating activities (Fig. 8, D).

Elastase-like and chymotrypsin-like activities were separated from the first protein peak and were eluted with the volume corresponding to 30 kD.

CONCLUSION

1. The results presented evidence for the inactivating action of serine leukocyte granule proteinases, elastase and cathepsin G, on the key enzymes of kallikrein-kinin systems, i.e. Hageman factor and prekallikrein. It has been shown that prekallikrein and kallikrein are about 20 times more stable than Hageman factor under

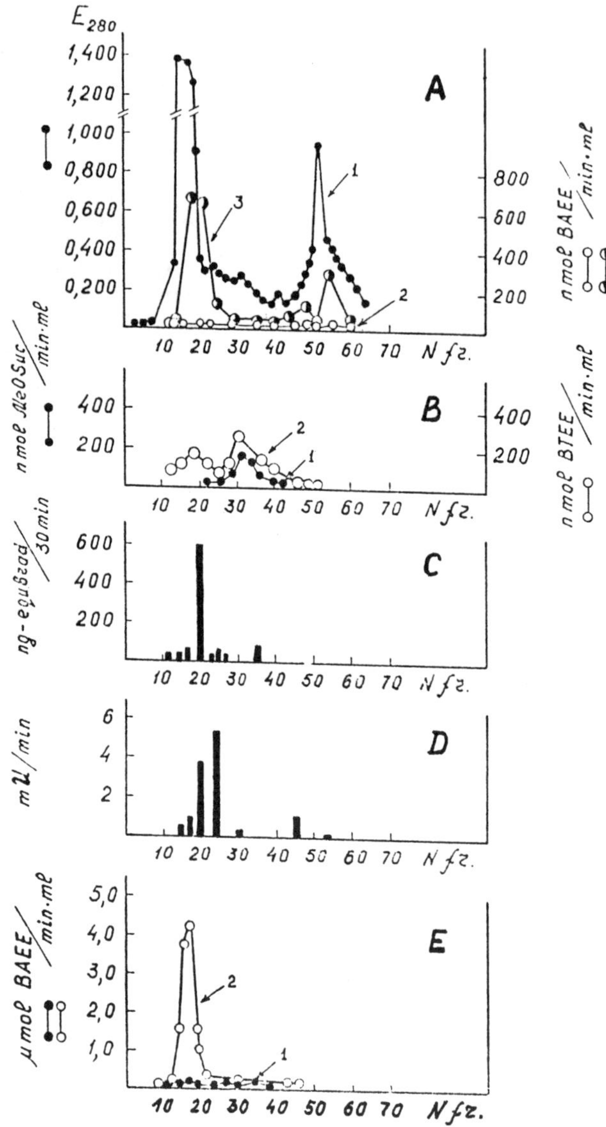

Fig. 8. Separation of leukocyte membrane proteinase on Sephadex G-100. A – ●——● A_{280} (curve 1); o——o the initial activity in nmol BAEE/min·ml (curve 2); ●——● the activity after incubation with plasma kallikrein in nmol BAEE/min·ml (curve 3); B – ●——● the activity in nmol MeOSuc/min·ml (curve 1); o——o the activity in nmol BTEE/min·ml (curve 2); C – kininogenase activity; D – Hageman factor-activating activity; E – ●——● the initial activity in μmol BAEE/min·ml (curve 1); o——o Trasylol excited activity in μmol BAEE/min·ml (curve 2)

the action of elastase and are not inactivated by cathepsin G.

2. We succeded in identification and initial separation of the latent trypsin-like leukocyte membrane proteinase with kininogenase and Hageman factor activating activities. Its esterase and amidase

activities with arginin and lysine substrates were enormously but temporarily increased under the action of substances with poly-cationic molecules, such as Trasylol, protamine-sulfate and alkaline Ampholines.

This proteinase was identified in external membrane of neutrophil polymorphonuclear leukocytes.

3. The presence of this trypsin-like membrane proteinase which activates Hageman factor raised the question about its role in cell-plasma interrelationship and in activation of the Hageman factor depending systems. Further studies are necessary to clarify whether this proteinase is a kind of secretary protein or whether it is structurally bound to leukocyte membrane. This proteinase may probably play an important role in physiology of leukocyte itself.

ACKNOWLEDGEMENTS

We are grateful to managers of the firm "Pharmacia LKB Instruments" for placing at our's disposal the high quality instruments.

REFERENCES

1. Baugh RJ, Travis J. Human leukocyte granule elastase: rapid isolation and characterization. Biochem 1976; 15: 836-841.

2. Burch RM, Connor JR, Tiffany CW. The kallikrein-kininogen-kinin system in chronic inflammation. Agents and Actions 1989; 27: 258-260.

3. Colman RW, Wong S. Kallikrein-kinin system in pathological conditions. In: Handbook of Experimental Pharmacology (Erdös EG, editor). Berlin: Springer-Verlag, 1979; XXV. Suppl: 569-607.

4. Colman RW. Perspectives: surface-mediated defence reactions. The plasma contact activation system. J Clin Invest 1984; 73: 1249-1253.

5. Dotsenko VL, Nenasheva NM, Neshkova EA, Morozova NA, Yarovaya GA. Mechanism of activation of the kallikrein-kinin system in plasma of patients with atopic allergic diseases. In: Advances in Experimental Medicine and Biology, Kinin V (Abe K, Moriya H, Fumii S, editors). New York: Plenum Press 1989; part B: 515-521.

6. Dotsenko VL, Neshkova EA, Yarovaya GA. Leukocyte proteinases as a regulating factor for the kallikrein-kinin systems of human plasma. 1. Elastase and cathepsin G. Biomed Sci 1992; 3.

7. Dotsenko VL, Serova NI, Logunov AJ, Lebkova NP, Yarovaya GA. On the
    activation of kallikrein-kinin system in human blood plasma under
    conditions of gastroduodenal ulcer. Voprosy Meditsinskoi Khimii
    1987; 33 (4): 104-109.

8. Edbring K, Schmidt W, Fuchs G, Havemann K. Demonstration of
    granulocytic proteases in plasma of patients with acute leukemia
    and septicemia with coagulation defects. Blood 1977; 49: 219-231.

9. Ghebrehiwet B, Silverberg M, Kaplan AP. Activation of the classical
    pathway of complement by Hageman factor fragment. J Exp Med 1981;
    153: 665-676.

10. Goldsmith GH. Contact-activated fibrinolysis: role of surface
    concentration and high-molecular-weight kininogen. J Lab & Clin Med
    1980; 96: 564-566.

11. Kaplan AP, Meier HL, Mandle R. The Hageman factor dependent
    pathways of coagulation fibrinolysis and kinin generation. Seminar
    Thrombosis Haemostasis 1976; 3: 1-26.

12. Kawiak J, Kawalec M, Dotsenko VL, Yarovaya, GA. Purification of
    human serum prekallikrein; some properties of the purified
    proenzyme and its stability. Clin Chim Acta 1984; 141: 287-292.

13. Melmon KL, Cline MJ. The interaction of leukocytes and kinin
    system. Biochem Pharmacol (Suppl) 1968; 28: 271-275.

14. Newball HH, Talamo RC, Lichtenstein LM. Release of leukocyte
    kallikrein mediated by IgE. Nature 1975: 254-635.

15. Newball HH, Revak SD, Cochrane CG, Griffin JH, Lichtenstein LM.
    Activation of human Hageman factor by a leukocytic protease. In:
    Advances in Experimental Medicine and Biology, Kinin II. New York:
    Plenum Press, 1978; 120, part B: 139-152.

16. Record M, Laharraque P, Fillola G, Thomas J, Ribes G, Fontan P,
    Chap H, Corberand J. A rapid isolation procedure of plasma
    membranes from human neutrophils using self-generating Percoll
    gradient. Biochim Biophys Acta 1985; 819: 1-9.

17. Wasi S, Movat HZ, Pass E, Chan YYC. Production, conversion and
    destruction of kinins by human neutrophils leukocyte proteases. In:
    Neutral Proteases of Human Polymorphonuclear Leucocytes (Havermann
    K, Janoff A, editors). 1978: 245-260.

18. Wintroub BU, Coetzl EJ, Austen KF. A neutrophil-dependent pathway
    for the generation of a neutral peptide mediator. J Exp Med 1974;
    140: 812-824.

19. Wintroub BU, Coetzl EJ, Austen KF. A neutrophil-dependent pathway
    for the generation of a neutral peptide mediator; II. Subcellular
    localization of the neutrophil protease. Immunology 1977; 33: 41-
    50.

TISSUE KALLIKREIN CLEARANCE BY THE LIVER –

EFFECT OF PLASMA COMPONENTS ON KALLIKREIN UPTAKE BY CULTURED RAT HEPATOCYTES

K. Aoki, M. Kamada, M. Ikekita, K. Kizuki and H. Moriya

Department of Biochemistry, Science University of Tokyo,
12 Ichigaya-Funakawara-machi, Shinjuku-ku, Tokyo 162, Japan

SUMMARY: Rat urinary kallikrein (RUK) injected intravenously to the rat rapidly disappeared from the blood circulation and mainly distributed to the liver. RUK was also incorporated to the primary cultured rat hepatocytes. The amounts of RUK incorporated into the hepatocytes increased by preincubation of RUK with rat plasma. These results and SDS-PAGE analysis suggested some plasma components may be involved in tissue kallikrein clearance in the blood.

INTRODUCTION

Tissue kallikrein exists in plasma of mammals as well as tissues such as pancreas and kidney (1). Some groups have reported that the origin of tissue kallikrein in plasma might be the submandibular gland (2) and/or kidney (3), but its origin and function are still vague. The level of active kallikrein in the plasma are very low (4) and a great part of the kallikrein forms complexes with binding proteins in the plasma (5). The formation of protease/protease-inhibitor complex in the plasma is considered to be important to the turnover of proteases in the blood circulation (6).

In the present study, we report studies on the metabolism of tissue kallikrein in rat blood and the effect of plasma components on the kallikrein uptake into primary cultured hepatocytes.

MATERIALS AND METHODS

<u>Materials and animals:</u> L-15 medium (Sigma Chemical Co., St. Louis, USA) was used at pH 7.4. Membrane filter (Sterivex-GV, 0.22 μm, Millipore Co.,

Bedford, USA) was used to sterilize the media. Rat urine was collected from housed male Wistar rats (Sankyo Laboratories Inc., Tokyo, Japan) in metabolic cages.

Purification of rat urinary kallikrein. RUK used as tissue kallikrein was purified according to the modified method of Takaoka et al. (7). The final preparation was homogeneous on SDS-polyacrylamide gel electrophoresis and its specific activity was 4.2 AU/A_{280}. One amidase unit (AU) was defined as the amount of enzyme that could hydrolyze 1 μmol of L-prolyl-L-phenylalanyl-L-arginine 4-methyl-coumaryl-7-amide per 1 min at 30°C, pH 8.0.

Labeling of RUK with ^{125}I. RUK (10 μg) was labeled with Na[^{125}I] (34 MBq, 37 GBq/ml, Amersham, Buckinghamshire, UK) by lactoperoxidase method (8) and the labeled RUK was separated from Na[^{125}I] by Bio-Gel P-30 gel filtration.

Primary culture of hepatocytes. Primary cultured hepatocytes were prepared by the modified method of Tanaka et al. (9). The liver of male Wistar rat (6-7 weeks old) was perfused with saline solution containing 0.05 %(w/v) collagenase (type I, Sigma) and 0.05 %(w/v) soybean trypsin inhibitor (SBTI, type I-S, Sigma). Dispersed hepatocytes were separated from other cells by centrifugation. The prepared hepatocytes (1×10^6 cells) were cultured with L-15 medium containing 10 %(v/v) fetal bovine serum in a collagen-coated dish (9 cm^2, Iwaki Glass, Tokyo, Japan) for 4 h at 37°C. The cells were washed four times with phosphate-buffered saline (PBS) to remove unattached cells and serum. The hepatocytes were then cultured with L-15 medium containing 1×10^{-7} M insulin, 1×10^{-6} M dexamethasone and 1×10^{-9} M glucagon (Sigma) for 24 h at 37°C.

Assay for the amounts of uptake of RUK into primary cultured hepatocytes.
These hepatocytes were divided into two groups. One of them was assayed at 37°C and the other group was done at 4°C. The hepatocytes were washed three times with PBS and were added to L-15 medium containing insulin, dexamethasone, glucagon, 0.1 %(w/v) bovine serum albumin and various concentrations of ^{125}I-RUK. Each group was incubated for 30 min at 37°C or 4°C, respectively. The hepatocytes were washed four times with cold PBS and 0.5 N sodium hydroxide was added to the dishes to harvest the cells. Incorporated radioactivies in the cells were measured with γ-scintillation counter. The amounts of protein in the cells on the dishes also were measured by Hartree's method (10).

RESULTS AND DISCUSSION

Labeled RUK administered to the rat rapidly disappeared from the blood with a half-life of 9.7 min (Fig.1). Thirty-four percent of the administered radioactivity, however, was detected in the blood circulation at 60 min, suggesting that administered RUK may be degraded some organ(s) in the body and the metabolites may be released into the blood.

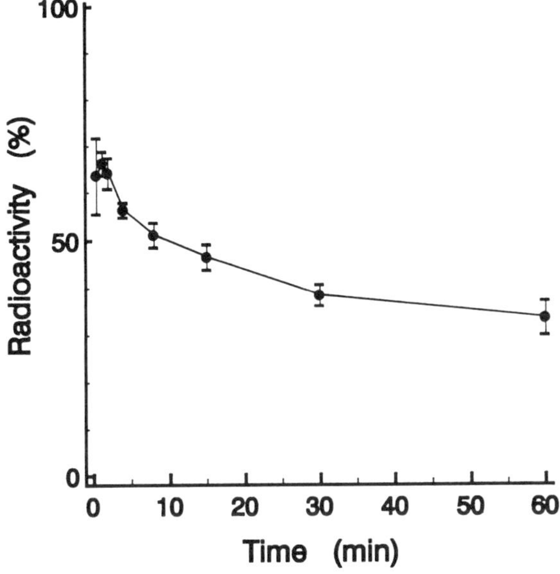

Fig.1 Disappearance of Intravenously Administered ^{125}I-RUK from Rat Blood Circulation. RUK (247 ng eq., 750,000 cpm) labeled with ^{125}I was intravenously administered to male Wistar rat. Blood samples were collected by heparinaized syringes from the carotid artery at the indicated period after the administrations. Data are the means ± S.E. of four experiments.

Figure 2 shows the distribution of ^{125}I-RUK that disappeared from the blood circulation. Twenty-two percent of the radioactivity was detected in the liver at 15 min after the administration of ^{125}I-RUK and then decreased gradually. The radioactivity in the kidney, spleen and urine was only 2.8, 0.7 and 0.2 %, respectively, at 15 min. These results showed that tissue kallikrein disappearance from the blood circulation was mainly due to uptake into the liver. It is possible that the primary origin of tissue kallikrein excreted into the urine was not tissue kallikrein in the blood. We could detect 72 % of the radioactivities of the administered RUK in the blood, liver, kidney, spleen, and urine at 15 min after the administration. The remaining radioactivity might diffuse via capillary circulation into the whole body, but it is not elucidate at this time.

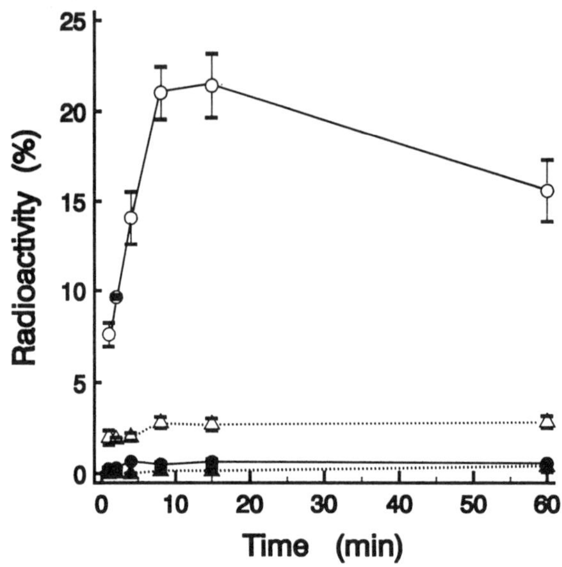

Fig.2 Distribution of ^{125}I-RUK Administered to the Rat. ^{125}I-RUK (247 ng eq., 750,000 cpm) was intravenously administered to male Wistar rats.   Then, the liver (O), kidneys (△) and spleen (●) were excised from the rats at the indicated period after the administration of ^{125}I-RUK.   Each tissue was homogenized with 0.1 N sodium hydroxide solution for measurement of radioactivity.   The radioactivity of the urine (▲) collected at the indicated periods was also measured.   Data are the means ± S.E. of three experiments.

We also investigated the uptake of tissue kallikrein into primary cultured rat hepatocytes and the effects of rat plasma on kallikrein uptake. The hepatocytes incorporated ^{125}I-RUK at more than 30 ng/ml RUK concentration in the medium.   The amounts of ^{125}I-RUK incorporated by the hepatocytes depended on the concentration of RUK in the medium (Fig.3, triangles).   When ^{125}I-RUK preincubated with rat plasma was added to the cultured medium of the hepatocytes, the uptake by hepatocytes was observed at about 10 ng/ml RUK concentration (Fig.3, circles).   The amount of plasma-treated ^{125}I-RUK in the hepatocytes was higher than that of non-treated ^{125}I-RUK in the hepatocytes at each concentration of RUK. The treatment of tissue kallikrein with rat plasma resulted in increased amounts of tissue kallikrein in the hepatocytes at the same concentrations of kallikrein in the medium, suggesting that some components in rat plasma accelerated tissue kallikrein incorporation by the hepatocytes.

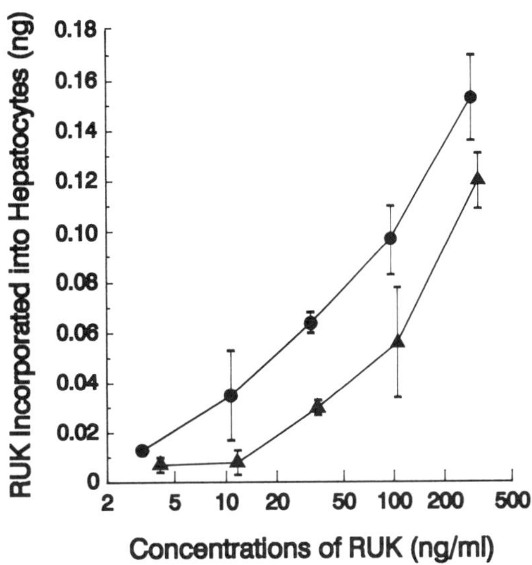

Fig.3 Uptake of ^{125}I-RUK by Primary Cultured Rat Hepatocytes. The Hepatocytes were cultured with the medium containing various concentrations of non-treated (▲) or plasma-treated (●) ^{125}I-RUK. Plasma-treated ^{125}I-RUK was prepared by incubation of ^{125}I-RUK (1122 ng eq., 5,935,000 cpm) with rat plasma (2 ml) for 24 h at 37°C. Hepatocytes were divided into two groups and were incubated for 30 min at 37°C or 4°C each other. Points indicate the difference between the amounts of kallikrein detected in the hepatocytes at 37°C and those at 4°C. Data are calculated as the amount of kallikrein incorporated by the hepatocytes per ng of cellular protein and are the means ± S.E. of four experiments.

We incubated ^{125}I-RUK with rat plasma or serum and these incubation mixtures were analyzed by SDS-PAGE. As shown in figure 4, a 38 kDa band corresponding to ^{125}I-RUK rapidly shifted to three higher mass labeled bands (a 94 kDa main band and two sub-bands), indicating that RUK formed the complexes with some components in rat plasma as well as serum. The formation of a 94 kDa complex was very fast: the complex was main complex. The molecular mass of the plasma component forming the 94 kDa complex with

K. Aoki et al.

RUK (38 kDa) was calculated to be about 56 kDa. Judging from its molecular mass, this plasma component may be α_1-antitrypsin (54 kDa) (11) or kallikrein-binding protein (60 kDa) (12). It is known that trypsin forms a complex with α_2-macroglobulin and that this complex is rapidly incorporated into hepatocytes from circulation (6). We conclude that tissue kallikrein in the plasma may bind to plasma components such as α_1-antitrypsin or kallikrein-binding protein and are incorporated into hepatocytes by a similar mechanism. Borges et al. reported that horse urinary and pig pancreatic kallikrein were incorporated into perfused rat liver by carbohydrate-binding receptors while rat urinary kallikrein was not incorporated (13, 14). These results indicate that tissue kallikreins purified from other species are recognized by the carbohydrate-binding receptors on the rat hepatic cells. On the other hand, from our results, we speculate that complex formation with plasma components may play a more important role than a carbohydrate-specific recognition system for the clearance of rat tissue kallikrein in rat liver.

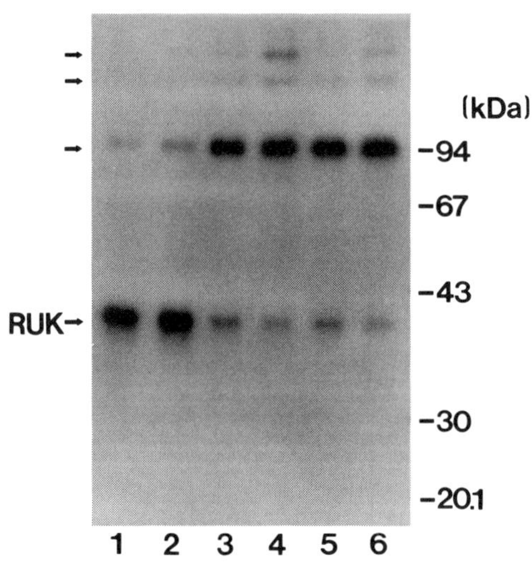

Fig.4 Electrophoretogram of ^{125}I-RUK Incubated with Rat Plasma or Serum. Each 83 ng of ^{125}I-RUK was incubated with 20 µl of rat plasma (lane 1,3,5) or 20 µl of rat serum (lane 2,4,6) for 0 (lane 1,2), 8 (lane 3,4) and 60 min (lane 5,6). SDS-polyacrylamide gel (10%) electrophoresis was performed by the method of Laemmli (15). Detection was carried out by autoradiography.

Plasma-treated RUK was incorporated into hepatocytes at one fourth or one fifth the rate of kallikrein at concentrations which were required (Fig. 3). This suggested that the liver preferentially took up tissue kallikrein to have formed the complexes in normal state. In case of diseases such as acute pancreatitis, the amount of human tissue kallikrein in blood is 2.5 times more than in controls (16). When the amount of tissue kallikrein in blood is elevated, the hepatocytes also may take up tissue kallikrein that is not bound to the plasma components.

CONCLUSION

We showed that the main organ is the liver on the clearance of tissue kallikrein in blood circulation and tissue kallikrein was incorporated into hepatocytes using the primary cultured cell system. Furthermore, we found that plasma-treatment of tissue kallikrein accelerated uptake of tissue kallikrein by the hepatocytes.

ACKNOWLEDGMENT

This work was supported in part by grants from the Ministry of Education, Science and Culture of Japan. We thank Dr. Hiroaki Kato, Medical Research Institute, Tokyo Medical and Dental University, for helpful technical advice.

REFERENCES

1. Rabito SF, Amin V, Scicli AG, Carretero OA. Glandular kallikrein in plasma and urine: evaluation of a direct RIA for its determination. In: Advances in Experimental Medicine and Biology, vol. 120A. Fujii S, Moriya H, Suzuki T, editors. New York: Plenum Press, 1979: 127–142
2. Lawton WJ, Proud D, Frech ME, Pierce JV, Keiser HR, Pisano JJ. Characterization and origin of immunoreactive glandular kallikrein in rat plasma. Biochem Pharmacol 1981; 30:1731.
3. Roblero J, Croxatto H, Garcia R, Corthorn J, De Vito E. Kallikrein activity in perfusates and urine of isolated rat kidneys. Am J Physiol 1976; 231:1383.
4. Geiger R, Stuckstedte U, Clausnitzer B, Fritz H. Progressive inhibition of human glandular (urinary) kallikrein by human serum and identification of the progressive antikallikrein as α_1-antitrypsin (α_1-protease inhibitor). Hoppe-Seyler's Z Physiol Chem 1981; 362:317.
5. Johansen L, Nustad K, Berg T, Pierce JV. Excess antibody immunoassay for rat glandular kallikrein. measurement of kallikrein complexed with inhibitors and in plasma. J Immunol Methods 1984; 69:253.
6. Davidsen O, Christensen EI, Gliemann J. The plasma clearance of human α_2-macroglobulin-trypsin complex in the rat is mainly accounted for by uptake into hepatocytes. Biochim Biophys Acta 1985; 846:85.

7. Takaoka M, Okamura H, Iwamoto T, Ikemoto C, Mimura Y, Morimoto S. Purification to apparent homogeneity of inactive kallikrein from rat urine. Biochem Biophys Res Commun 1984; 122:1282.
8. Shimamoto K, Chao J, Margolius HS. The radioimmunoassay of human urinary kallikrein and comparisons with kallikrein activity measurements. J Clin Endocrinol Metab 1980; 51:840.
9. Tanaka K, Sato M, Tomita Y, Ichihara A. Biochemical studies on liver functions in primary cultured hepatocytes of adult rats. J Biochem 1978; 84:937.
10. Hartree EF. Determination of protein: a modification of the Lowry Method that gives a linear photometric response. Anal Biochem 1972; 48:422.
11. Chao S, Chai KX, Chao L, Chao J. Molecular cloning and primary structure of Rat α_1-antitrypsin. Biochemistry 1990; 29:323.
12. Chao J, Chai KX, Chen L, Xiong W, Chao S, Woodley-Miller C, Wang L, Lu HS, Chao L. Tissue kallikrein-binding protein is a serpin. J Biol Chem 1990; 265:16394.
13. Borges DR, Kouyoumdjian M, Prado ES, Prado JL. Receptor-mediated clearance of tissue kallikreins by rat liver. In: Advances in Experimental Medicine and Biology, vol. 198A. Greenbaum LN, Margolius HS, editors. New York: Plenum Press, 1986: 235-239.
14. Kouyoumdjian M, Borges DR, Prado ES, Prado JL. Identification of receptors in the liver that mediate endocytosis of circulating tissue kallikreins. Biochim Biophys Acta 1989; 980:299.
15. Laemmli UK. Cleavage of structual proteins during the assembly of the head bacteriophage T4. Nature 1970; 227:680.
16. Shimamoto K, Mayfield RK, Margolius HS, Chao J, Stroud W, Kaplan AP. Immunoreactive tissue kallikrein in human serum. J Lab Clin Med 1984; 103:731.

KALLIKREIN-KININ SYSTEM IN THE ANGIOGENESIS

M.A.N.D. Ferreira, S.P. Andrade, J.L. Pesquero, M.H. Feitosa, G.M.R. Oliveira,
[1]E. Rogana, [2]J.C. Nogueira and W.T. Beraldo[*]

Department of Physiology and Biophysics, [1]Department of Biochemistry and
Immunology, [2]Department of Morphology, Federal University of Minas Gerais,
Belo Horizonte, 31270, Brazil.

SUMMARY: Using the bioassay to investigate the presence of mediators in the
angiogenesis exudate to explain its property to cause vascular permeability and fall
in the blood pressure we found the presence of histamine, bradykinin,
prostaglandin E_2 and angiotensin in the exudate. Howewer, the role of these
mediators in the angiogenesis process needs to be investigated.

INTRODUCTION

As it was found that the exudate of angiogenesis causes increase of vascular
permeability and fall in the blood pressure (1), we decided to investigate the
presence of pharmacological mediators in the exudate.

MATERIALS AND METHODS

Sponge implants - Male Wistar rats weighing 200-300 g were used. Polyester
sponge was used as matrix for vessel growth. In order to get exudate fluid of
angiogenesis a circular polyester sponge disc with a central cannula was implanted
subcutaneously (2).

---

[*] Corresponding Author

Vascular Permeability - To test the activity of the exudate upon vascular permeability, the conventional blue test was performed in the abdominal wall of rats (200-300 g), injecting intravenously 0.7 ml of a 0.8 % solution of Evans blue in Tyrode and 0.1 ml of the exudate intradermally.

Blood pressure - Wistar rats of both sexes (200-300 g) were anesthetized with thiopental. One end of polyethylene tubing filled with heparin was inserted into the left carotid artery and a similar cannula inserted into the femoral vein. Blood pressure and respiratory movements were recorded on a Hewllet-Packard polygraph (model 7754-A).

Bioassay - Different smooth muscle preparations were used to identify pharmacological mediators since they can solve problems that could not be solved by purely biochemical means (3). The following preparations were used: rat blood pressure, vascular permeability in the skin of rat, isolated guinea-pig ileum, isolated rat duodenum and chick rectum. The rat duodenum and guinea-pig ileum were suspended in 5 ml bath Tyrode solution at 37° C and chick rectum in Krebs solution at 40° C. Isotonic contractions or relaxations of all preparations were recorded with a frontal writing lever (ten times magnification). The sensitivity was similar to that of isometric responses recorded with a Grass force displacement transducer (FTD 3C) and polygraph used for comparison.

Chromatography - The exudate was applied on gel filtration chromatography utilizing a Sephadex G-15 column. The material was eluted with 50 mM sodium phosphate buffer (pH 7.4) being the optical density of fractions determined at 214 and 280 nm. The activity of collected fractions was verified using bioassays.

Chemicals - Evans blue (Baker), chymotrypsin, from bovine pancreas 3x crystallized, 17- β estradiol were purchased from Sigma Co., bradykinin (Sandoz S.A.), prostaglandin E_2, prostaglandin $F_{2\alpha}$ (Sigma Co.). Angiotensin and saralasin were synthetized by Paiva and Juliano, Escola Paulista de Medicina, São Paulo, Brazil.

RESULTS

Vascular permeability - The capacity of exudate to produce vascular permeability with extravasation of dye was tested in the skin of the rat. Figure 1 shows that all the exudates tested caused extravasation of the Evans blue dye. Simple measurement of the diameter of the area shows that the exudate of the first, third, and fourth days after the sponge implant, induced capillary permeability with extravasation of the dye.

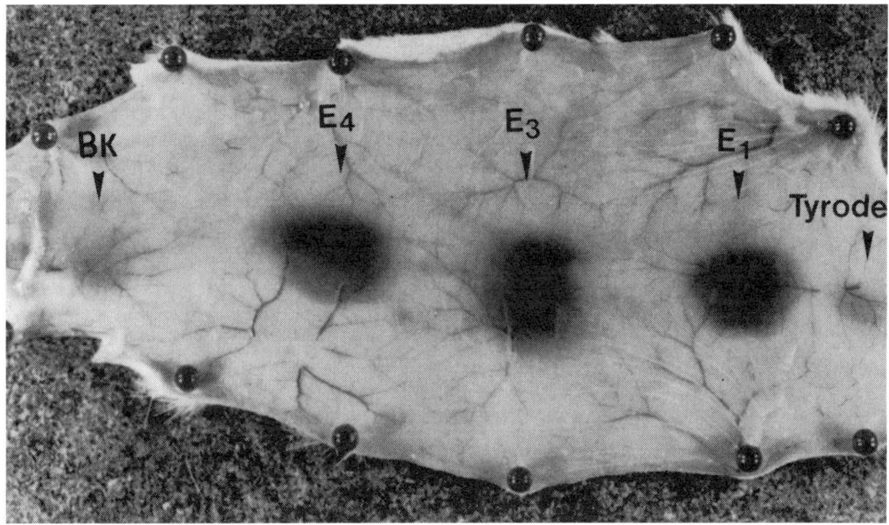

Fig. 1. Effect of the exudate of the angiogenesis in capillary permeability. E_1, E_3 and E_4 = 0.1 ml intradermally injected exudate after first, third and fourth day of sponge implant. Tyr=0.1 ml Tyrode; BK=0.1 ml (6 mg) bradykinin.

Effect of exudate on blood pressure - The vasodilating effect caused by the exudate induced us to test the exudate on the blood pressure. Figure 2 shows the effect of exudate on the blood pressure and respiratory movement of the rat. The injection of 50 mg of lyophilised exudate caused fall in the blood pressure and a progressive decrease of the respiratory movements and apnea killing the animal in 30 min.

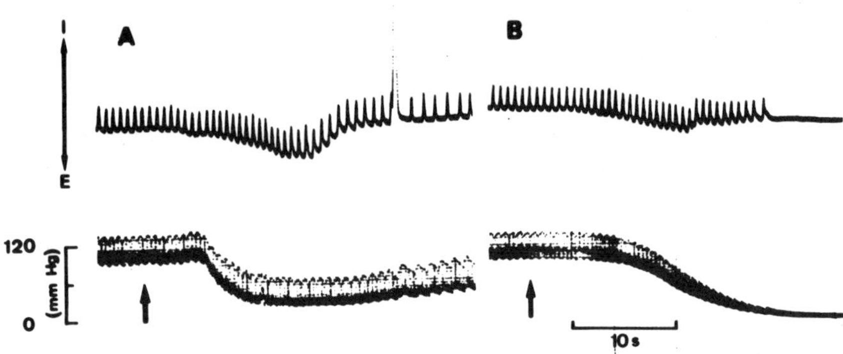

Fig. 2. Cardiovascular and respiratory effects elicited by intravenous injection of the angiogenesis exudate. A rat (250g) was anesthetized with thiopental. Upper tracings: respiratory movements (I=inspiration; E=expiration). Lower tracings: arterial blood pressure. B: 3 min after A. The arrow in A indicate intravenous (iv) injection of 10 mg of bradykinin. The arrow in B indicates iv injection of 50 mg of liophylized exudate, obtained after 2 days of sponge implant in another rat.

In view of the effect of exudate on vascular permeability and blood pressure, we decided to investigate the presence of pharmacological mediators in the exudate responsible for increasing vascular permeability and fall in the blood pressure. For that purpose we used isolated smooth muscle preparation.

As histamine produces vasodilatation, increases vascular permeability and hypotension, the presence of histamine in the exudate was tested using the isolated guinea-pig ileum. The guinea-pig ileum contracts to extremely low concentration of histamine. In five experiments it was found histamine in the exudate. To identify histamine an anti-histamine was used.

Since the antagonist of histamine did not completely block the contraction caused by exudate, others mediators should be involved in the guinea-pig ileum contraction. So, we decided to test the exudate on the rat duodenum, for this preparation is insensitive to histamine and very sensitive to bradykinin, prostaglandin E_2 and 5-hydroxytriptamine.

Rat Duodenum - In order to test the presence of bradykinin in the exudate we used the rat duodenum and rat stomach strip, for bradykinin is only mediator that causes relaxation of the duodenum and contraction of the rat stomach (3,4) and histamine has no effect, as we observed in our experiments. Figure 3 shows that the exudate induced relaxation of the duodenum as bradykinin; prostaglandin E_2 caused relaxation followed by contraction; 5-hydroxytriptamine caused contraction and histamine showed no effect. The rat duodenum relaxes in the presence of bradykinin, whereas most of other isolated organs contract. These experiments suggest the presence of bradykinin in the exudate. So far using isolated organs, we could detect the presence of histamine and bradykinin in the angiogenesis exudate. On the other hand, 5-HT can be discarded when these preparations were used.

Chick rectum - The chick rectum preparation is very sensitive to prostaglandins and does not respond to bradykinin, angiotensin, histamine serotonin and S-R-S (5,6,7,8). The exudate when added to the bath containing the chick rectum preparation produced contraction, as well as prostaglandin (PGE_2), but bradykinin had no effect (Figure 3). In order to ascertain if the prostaglandin was being syntethized during the contact of the exudate with the preparation, the exudate was added to the bath containing the chick rectum preparation after previous addition of indometacin into the Krebs liquid in which the preparation was suspended. Preliminary results showed that indometacin did not alter the response of the preparation to the exudate, reinforcing the presence of prostaglandin already in the exudate, independent of its synthesis during the action of the exudate on the chick rectum.

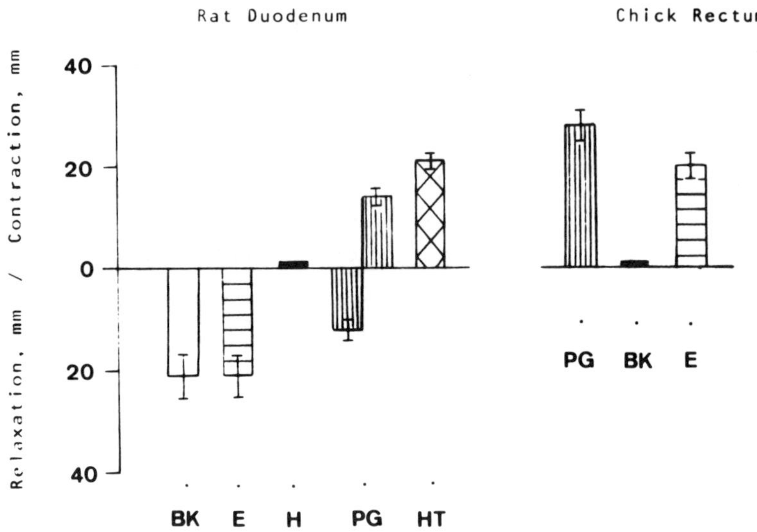

Fig. 3. Effect of the angiogenesis exudate on the isolated rat duodenum and chick rectum. On the rat duodenum: BK=10 ng bradykinin; E=100 ml exudate; H=0.2 mg histamine; PG= 8 mg prostaglandin E2; HT= 4 mg serotonin. On the chick rectum: PG= 0.5 mg prostaglandin E2; BK=10 mg bradykinin; E= 300 ml exudate. Data are mean ± SD of 5 experiments.

Notwithstanding the relaxation caused in the rat duodenum by the exudate, suggesting the presence of bradykinin, we decided to incubate chymotrypsin with the exudate since it was demonstrated bradykinin inactivation when incubated with chymotrypsin (9,10). Howewer, when the exudate was incubated with chymotrypsin, the relaxation was reduced but a strong contraction of the duodenum appeared. We also observed that when the same amount of exudate incubated with chymotrypsin was repetitively added to the organ bath at 2 min intervals, the high of the contraction gradually decrease, whereas the relaxation increased. It has been demonstrated the liberation of angiotensin II when rat plasma was incubated with chymotrypsin (11). On the other hand, angiotensin II caused tachyphylaxis when added to differents smooth muscle preparations (12,13). So, the result of the exudate incubation with chymotrypsin suggests the presence of angiotensinogen in the exudate, as observed by Fernandez et al (14).

In order to test this possibility, we added saralasin into the perfusing bath before the addition of the incubate (exudate and chymotrypsin). Figure 4 shows the results of these experiments demonstrating the inhibition of contraction, reinforcing the relaxation of the duodenum caused by the exudate incubated with chymotrypsin. As far as the relaxation is concerned, in part it is due to bradykinin present in the exudate.

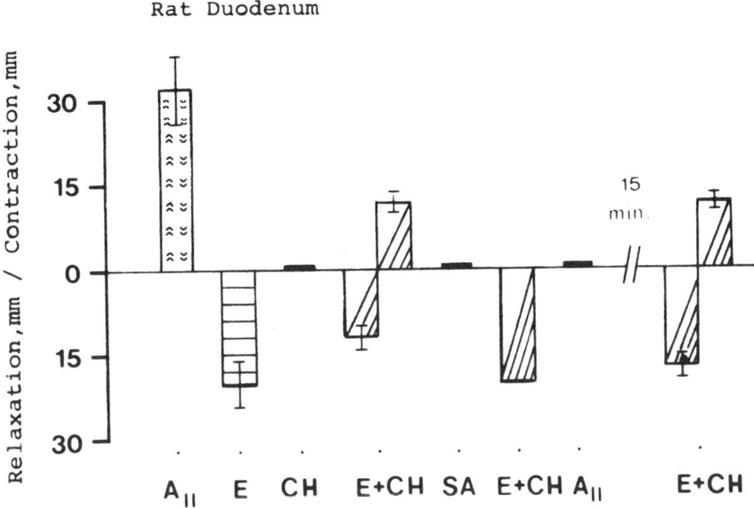

Fig. 4. Liberation of angiotensin II by chymotrypsin incubated with exudate. A$_{II}$= 40 ng angiotensin II; E= 100 ml exudate; CH= 30 chymotrypsin units; E+CH= 100 ml exudate incubated with 30 chymotrypsin units for 10 min. SA= 10 ng saralasin. The contractile response of the incubated (E+CH) appeared again after 15 min interval of the last addition of angiotensin II. Data are mean ± SD of 5 experiments (except when saralasin was used).

Chromatography - The exudate of the third day after sponge implant was applied on a gel filtration chromatography utilizing a Sephadex G-15 column, eluted with 40 mM sodium phosphate buffer (pH 7.4) containing 1 mM EDTA. The activity of the collected fractions was tested using rat uterus bioassay. Only fraction 42 (Figure 5) presented oxytocic activity. This fraction corresponds to a peptide presenting a molecular weight around 1000 daltons which may be bradykinin, that was confirmed by the results obtained when rat duodenum was used (Figure 3).

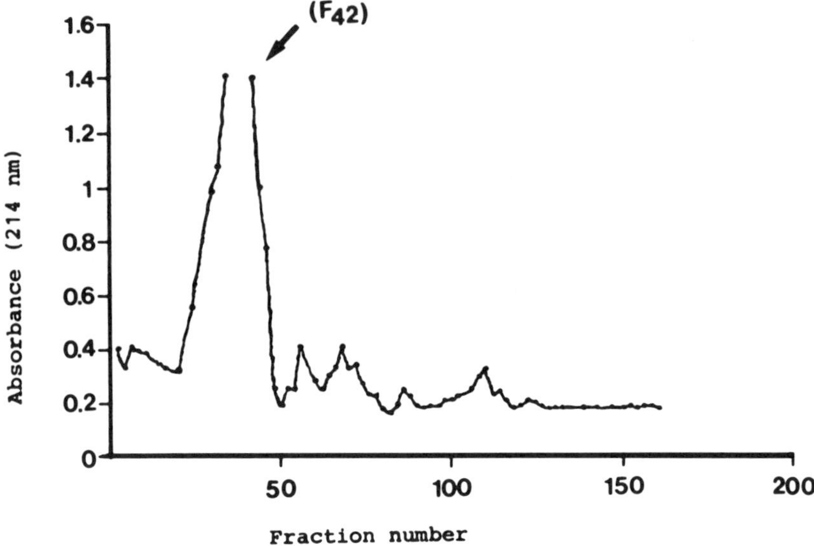

Fig. 5. Gel filtration chromatography (Sephadex G-15) of the angiogenesis exudate

DISCUSSION

It was observed the presence of T-kininogen and kinin in sponge induced exudate in rats (15). In experiments using different smooth muscle preparations for bioassay (3), we found on the angiogenesis exudate, kinin, histamine and prostaglandin E_2. The incubation of the exudate with chymotrypsin released angiotensin II, demonstrating the presence of angiotensinogen in the exudate (11,1).

The increase of vascular permeability and fall in the blood pressure of the rat probably are due to the presence of histamine and bradykinin in the exudate. The role of these mediators in the angiogenesis process still needs more investigation.

CONCLUSIONS

Using bioassay in different smooth muscle preparation, rat blood pressure and vascular permeability in the rat skin, we found in the rat angiogenesis exudate the presence of histamine, bradykinin, prostaglandin E_2 and angiotensinogen. However, the role of these mediators in the angiogenesis process still has to be investigated.

ACKNOWLEDGMENTS

Supported by FAPEMIG, CNPq, PRPq-UFMG and FINEP. We are much indebted to Prof. I. F. Heneine, for critically reading this manuscript.

REFERENCES

1. Ferreira, MAND. Mediadores farmacológicos no processo da angiogênese. M Sc Thesis, 1990.
2. Andrade, SP, Fan, TPD, Lewis GP. Quantitative *in vivo* studies on angiogenesis in a rat sponge model. Br J Pharmacol 1987; 60: 755-766.
3. Vane, JR. The use of isolated organs for detecting active substances in the circulating blood. Br J Pharmacol 1964; 23: 360-373.
4. Horton EW. Human urinary kinin excretion. Br J Pharmacol 1959; 14: 125-132.
5. Regoli D, Vane JR, A sensitive method for the assay of angiotensin. Br J Pharmacol 1964; 23: 351-359.
6. Ferreira, SH, Vane JR. Prostaglandins: their disappearence from release in the circulation. Nature 1967; 216: 868-873.
7. Campanha VP. Presença de material cinina-símile em perfusato dos ventrículos cerebrais de coelhos submetidos à hipertermia. M Sc. Thesis, 1976.
8. Sanchez JF. Características farmacológicas do fator hiperalgésico de macrofagos (FHM) e sua presença na resposta inflamatória aguda. Ph.D. Thesis, 1986.

9. Boisonnas RA, Guttman S, Jacquenoud RA. Synthèse de la L-arginyl L-prolyl-L-prolylglycil L-phenylalanyl L-seryl L-prolyl L-phenylalanyl L-arginine, un nonapetide portant les proprietés de la bradykinine. Helv Chim Acta 1960; 43: 1349-1358.

10. Elliott DF, Lewis GP Horton EW. The structure of bradykinin, a plasma kinin of blood. Biochem Biophys Res Comm 1960; 3: 87-91.

11. Hiraichi E, Schiripa LN, Yamanoye N, Abdalla FMF, Picarelli ZP Ação da quimotripsina (Qt) na pressão arterial (PA) de rato. In: Reunião Anual da Federação das Sociedades de Biologia Experimental, 4 1989, Caxambú, Ribeirão Preto: Regis Summa, 1989, p. 69.

12. Khairallah PA, Page IH, Bumpus FM, Turker RK. Angiotensin tachyphylaxis and its reversal. Cir Res 1966; XIX: 247-254.

13. Oshiro MEM, Miasiro N, Paiva TB, Paiva ACM. Angiotensin tachyphylaxis in the isolated rabbit aorta. Bl Ves 1984; 21: 72-79.

14. Fernandez LA, Twickler J, Mead A. Neovascularization produced by angiotensin II. J Lab Clin Med 1985, 105 (2): 141-145.

15. Damas J, Adam A, Bourdon V, Remacle-Volon G. Presence of T-kininogen and kinin in sponge induced exudates in rats. Br J Pharmacol 1989; 97: 1343-1349.

TISSUE KALLIKREIN AND THE EFFECT OF BROMOCRIPTINE IN HUMAN PROLACTIN AND GROWTH HORMONE-SECRETING PITUITARY ADENOMAS

T.H. Jones[*], C.D. Figueroa[**], C.M.L. Smith[+], K.D. Bhoola[**]

[*]University Department of Medicine, Northern General Hospital, Herries Road, Sheffield, S5 7AU, [+]Department of Neuropathology, Royal Hallamshire Hospital, Sheffield and [**]Department of Pharmacology, University of Bristol, BS8 1TD, UK

SUMMARY: Tissue kallikrein (TK) is present and co-localises with prolactin producing cells in human prolactinoma and mixed growth hormone (GH) and prolactin-secreting pituitary adenomas.   TK immunoreactivity was reduced or absent in these types of adenomas from patients who had received the dopamine agonist, bromocriptine before surgery. Pure GH secreting adenomas had no TK immunoreactivity.

INTRODUCTION

Adenomas of the pituitary gland comprise approximately seven percent of patients presenting with intracanial tumours. The commonest type of pituitary adenoma is the prolactinoma which may present clinically with disturbance of menstrual function, infertility, galactorrhoea or loss of libido and/or headache and visual impairment secondary to an expanding tumour. Adenomas, which cause the clinical conditions of gigantism and acromegaly, are less common and may occur as pure GH or mixed GH and prolactin-secreting tumours.   Prolactin secretion is mainly under a tonic inhibitory control by hypothalamic dopamine but release can be stimulated by oestrogen. The dopamine agonist, bromocriptine is effective in the majority of cases in normalising serum prolactin levels and reducing tumour size in prolactinoma patients. In 20-30% of patients with GH-secreting adenomas bromocriptine can inhibit GH release but has little effect on tumour mass.

TK is present in the rat anterior pituitary gland (1,2) and has been located to the lactotrophs, the prolactin-secreting cells (3). There is a distinct sex-linked difference with levels of TK being twenty-fold greater in female anterior pituitaries (4). TK mRNA is present in the rat anterior pituitary (5). The expression of the TK mRNA and TK is stimulated by oestrogen (6,7,8,9) and inhibited by dopamine (9,10,11). Bromocriptine markedly attenuates oestrogen-induction of TK (11).

Oestrogen-induced rat prolactinomas have enhanced TK mRNA expression (12) and a 250-fold increase in TK content compared to normal female pituitary glands (11). When oestrogen is initially administered to these rats, the rise in TK content parallels the increase in prolactin over the first five weeks of treatment. After this period levels of TK stablise although prolactin synthesis continues to rise (13). Bromocriptine treatment or oestrogen withdrawal inhibits TK mRNA and protein synthesis (12). We have previously reported that there is considerable TK immunoreactivity and co-localisation of the enzyme with prolactin in human prolactinoma cells (14). This present study examines TK immunoreactivity in GH-secreting and mixed GH and prolactin-secreting adenomas, and also investigates the effect of pre-operative bromocriptine therapy on TK in prolactin and GH-secreting adenomas.

MATERIALS AND METHODS

Pituitary adenoma tissue from 27 patients with GH-secreting adenomas was examined immunocytochemically for TK and the anterior pituitary hormones (GH, prolactin, ACTH, TSH, LH, FSH) The clinical data is presented in Table 1. In addition, 6 prolactinomas, 2 mixed GH/prolactin-secreting and 5 GH-secreting adenomas from patients who had had bromocriptine therapy of varying dose and duration were studied (Tables 1 and 2). Tissue removed after routine surgery was fixed in formol saline (10% v/v) at room temperature for 24-48 hours. The tissue blocks were dehydrated in a graded series of ethanol and embedded in paraffin wax. Sections, 5μm thick, were mounted on glass slides coated with poly-lysine. Immunostaining for tissue kallikrein and anterior pituitary hormones was performed as previously described (14).

RESULTS

GH-secreting adenomas: TK immunoreactivity was present in 14 of the 27 adenomas investigated. The adenomas could be classified into three groups (i) prolactin and TK immunopositivity associated with clinical hyperprolactinaemia (Table 1; [adenomas 1 to 6]) (ii) prolactin and TK immunopositivity with normal serum prolactin levels (4 had <1% of cells staining [7-9 and 11-14]) (iii) no prolactin or TK immunoreactivity [15-27]. There was a close correlation in individual adenomas between numbers of cells staining for prolactin and TK but no relationship between TK and GH. TK immunoreactivity was located to the Golgi region (Figure 1). Patient 10 had received pre-operative bromocriptine

Table 1. Tissue kallikrein, prolactin and GH immunoreactivity and clinical data of GH-secreting adenomas

Patient	Age	Sex	Serum Prolactin mIU/l	Mean Serum GH mIU/l	% cells within adenomas immunostaining for		
					TK	Prolactin	GH
1	35	F	965	120	65	77	0
2	16	M	37900	29.2	60	77	2
3	50	M	4686	78	50/10[+]	70/15[+]	37
4	29	F	2409	14[*]	30	45	19
5#	30	M	6357	1.5[*]	30/6[+]	35/11[+]	80
6	50	M	>2000	130.6	15	28	58
7	57	F	261	28	10	15	72
8	66	M	178	122	7	16	63
9	36	M	257	39[*]	2	8	64
10#	25	F	3379	9.6	<1	<1	52
11#	36	F	463	27.8	<1	2	9
12	34	M	n/a	380[*]	<1	5	85
13	67	F	187	18	<1	<1	70
14#	40	M	95	19.4	<1	2	90
15	26	F	n/a	338	<1	0	94
16	36	M	952	75.4	0	0	90
17	23	M	374	29.5	0	0	50
18	48	F	n/a	80.8	0	0	87
19	44	F	941	26.8	0	0	48
20#	53	M	127	39.3	0	0	45
21	49	F	158	24.5	0	0	86
22	64	F	367	7.3[*]	0	0	73
23#	28	F	n/a	210.8	0	0	64
24	49	M	n/a	178.8	0	0	90
25	54	F	106	57.3	0	0	99
26#	35	M	669	17.6	0	0	82
27	36	M	106	81.5	0	0	96

Those patients who had received pre-operative bromocriptine therapy. The mean serum GH is taken as the mean level during a 75g oral glucose tolerance test (OGTT). [*]GH levels are random single measurements where no OGTT was performed. Normal GH <5mIU/l, prolactin 60-550mIU/l. n/a = not assayed. [+] Regions tumour tissue varied in prolactin and TK immunopositivity. The mild hyperprolactinaemia in patients whose adenomas had negative immunocytochemistry (patients 16,19,26) is most likely to be secondary to compression of the pituitary stalk by the adenoma. No significant immunoreactivity of any other anterior pituitary hormones (ACTH, LH, FSH, TSH) was present in any of the adenomas.

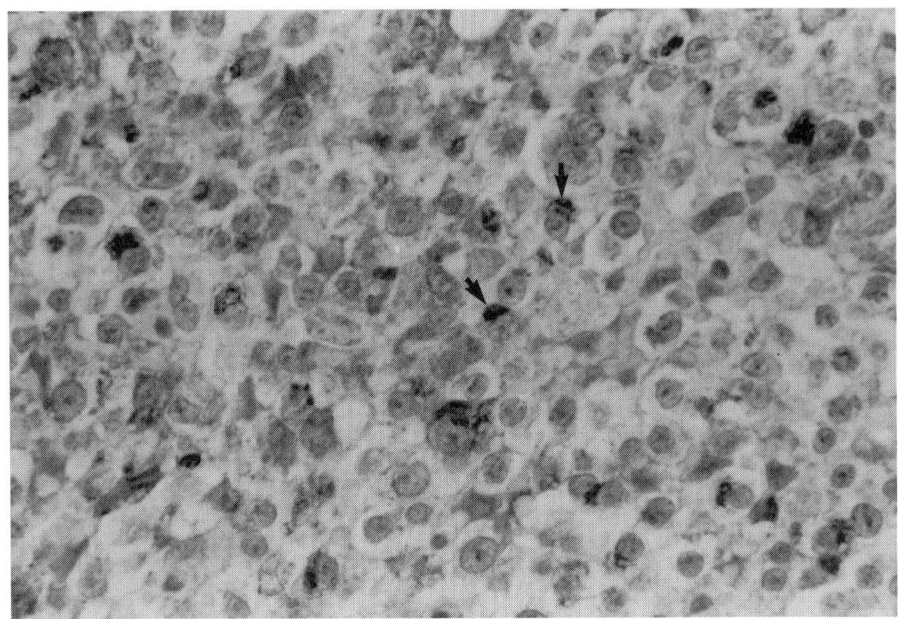

Figure 1.   Tissue kallikrein immunopositivity in a mixed prolactin/GH-secreting adenoma. TK present in Golgi region of cells (arrowed). (x 800).

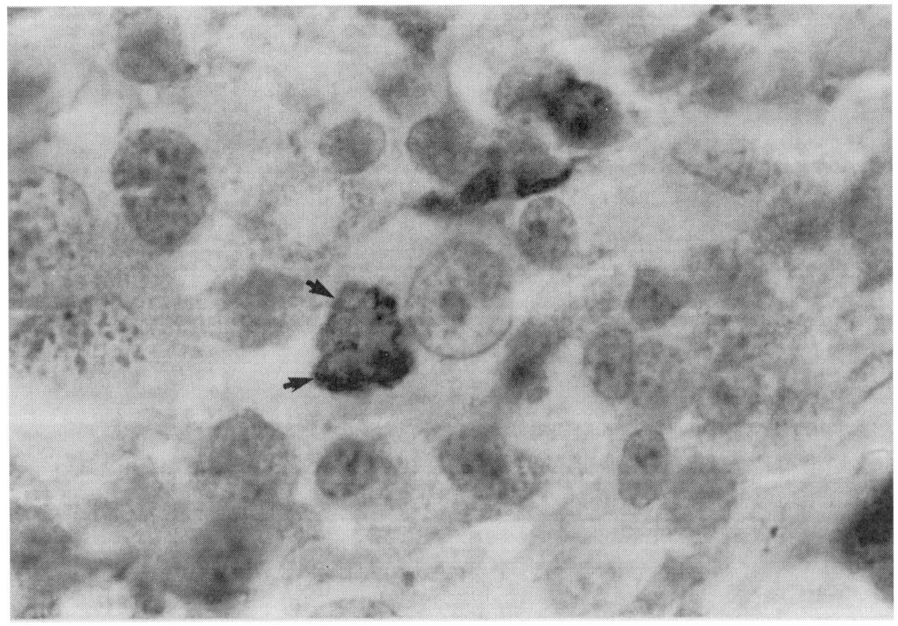

Figure 2.   Effect of bromocriptine on TK in a prolactin-secreting adenoma showing 'blob' formation (arrowed) which may represent an involuting Golgi apparatus. (x 2000).

(serum prolactin measured before bromocriptine) which explains very sparse TK and prolactin immunoreactivity (see below).

Effect of bromocriptine therapy: Cumulated data from previous work on prolactinomas from patients who had not received bromocriptine show that $81.9 \pm 21.7\%$ SD (n=14) cells were immunopositive for prolactin and $76.1 \pm 21.5\%$ for TK. In the prolactinomas (Table 2;[28-33]), three patients had received bromocriptine for less than one week, of which only one adenoma [30] from this group showed relatively lower immunostaining than the untreated group although there was no change in intracellular distribution of TK. Adenomas from patients treated for a longer period showed either a marked reduction in prolactin and TK and a change in the intracellular distribution of TK to a 'blob' adjacent to the nucleus [32] (Figure 2), or had no significant TK or prolactin present [31,33]. Seven patients with GH-secreting adenomas had received pre-operative bromocriptine. Of the two mixed GH/prolactin-secreting adenomas [7] one showed evidence of 'blob' formation and another [10] diagnosed on the basis of a very elevated serum prolactin prior to bromocriptine had only sparse TK and prolactin present (Table 2). Four of the remaining five GH-secreting adenomas with no pre-bromocriptine evidence of hyperprolactinaemia, had no prolactin or TK. The other adenoma [11] had reduced levels of GH (9%) compared to others with a small number of cells with TK and prolactin.

Table 2. Tissue kallikrein immunoreactivity in prolactin-secreting adenomas from patients treated with bromocriptine before surgery

Patient	Age	Sex	Serum Prolactin mIU/l	% cells immunostaining for TK	Prolactin	Duration of bromocriptine treatments (days)
28	22	F	9073	80	98	3*
29	22	F	21800	70	91	5*
30	45	M	4600	35	46	7*
31	35	F	4456	0	0	182
32	53	M	16794	35	50	42
33	33	M	17300	0	<1	14*
5	30	M	6357	30/6+	35/11+	42
10	25	F	3379	<1	<1	140

* Bromocriptine (15mg/day) given before surgery to reduce tumour vascularity.
+ see Table 1. In other patients dose of bromocriptine between 7.5mg and 15mg per day.

DISCUSSION

In both prolactinomas and mixed GH/prolactin-secreting adenomas there is a unique relationship between prolactin and TK. This strongly implies a role for TK in prolactin synthesis and release in humans as well as in the rat. The exact function of TK is unclear but there is preliminary in vitro evidence, in the rat, that it may be involved in the intracellular processing of the prolactin molecule before secretion (15,16). This is supported by its intracellular location in the Golgi apparatus. Alternatively, TK may regulate excessive production of prolactin. The serine protease inhibitior, tripeptide aldehyde t-butyloxycarbonyl-DPhe-Pro-Arg-H (BOC-dPPA) is a potent inhibitor of prolactin, GH (20), corticotrophin and beta-endorphin release in vitro (21). Kinins may have an autocrine or paracrine action in the pituitary, as both kallidin and bradykinin can stimulate prolactin secretion in vitro (17,18,19). Bradykinin can stimulate GH release from the anterior pituitaries of adult female rats (17) although has no effect in younger rats (18).

Bromocriptine reduces TK immunoreactivity in prolactinomas and this is paralleled by a decrease in prolactin immunopositivity. It is likely that the mechanism by which bromocriptine reduces TK content is by inhibiting TK mRNA expression as it is known to do so in the rat pituitary. The intracellular 'blob' induced by bromocriptine may represent an involuting Golgi apparatus.

It is unclear whether or not TK plays a role in the pathogenesis of these tumours. TK may be present just to process the prolactin molecule, however, the enzyme may be potentially be involved in the activation of growth factors and synthesis of kinins (22). TK and kinins can also stimulate angiogenesis and control vascular blood flow which may be important in pituitary tumour pathogenesis. Kinins have mitogenic properties and we have recently demonstrated that kallidin can stimulate the phosphoinositide second messenger system and hormone release from some pituitary adenomas (T.H. Jones unpublished observations).

REFERENCES

1.   Powers CA, Nasjletti A. A novel kinin-generating protease (kininogenase) in the porcine anterior pituitary. J Biol Chem 1982; 257-5594-98.

2.   Powers CA, Nasjletti A. A kininogenase resembling glandular kallikrein in the intermediate lobe of the rat pituitary. Endocrinol 1983; 112:1194-1200.

3.   Vio CP, Roa JP, Silva R, Powers CA. Localization of immunoreactive glandular kallikrein in lactotrophs of the rat anterior pituitary. Neuroendocrinol 1990; 51:10-14.

4.   Powers CA, Nasjletti A. A major sex difference in kallikrein-like activity in the rat anterior pituitary. Endocrinol 1984; 114:1841-44.

5.   Fuller PJ, Clements JA, Whitfield PJ, Funder JW. Kallikrein gene expression in the rat anterior pituitary. Mol Cell Endocrinol 1985; 39:99-105.

6.   Hatala MA, Powers CA. Dynamics of estrogen induction of glandular kallikrein in the rat anterior pituitary. Biochem Biophys Acta 1987; 926:258-63.

7.   Chao J, Chao L, Swain CC, Tsai J, Margolius HS. Tissue kallikrein in rat brain and pituitary: Regional distribution and estrogen induction in the anterior pituitary. Endocrinol 1987; 120:475-482.

8.   Powers CA. Anterior pituitary glandular kallikrein: trypsin activation and estrogen regulation. Mol Cell Endocrinol 1986; 46:163-73.

9.   Clements JA, Fuller PJ, McNally M, Nikolaidis I, Funder JW. Estrogen regulation of kallikrein gene expression in the rat anterior pituitary. Endocrinol 1986; 119:268-73.

10.   Pritchett DB, Roberts JL. Dopamine regulates expression of the glandular-type kallikrein gene at the transcriptional level in the pituitary. Proc Natl Acad USA 1987; 84:5545-9.

11.   Powers CA, Hatala MA. Dopaminergic regulation of the estrogen-induced glandular kallikrein in the rat anterior pituitary. Neuroendocrinol 1986; 44:462-9.

12.   Fuller PJ, Matheson BA, MacDonald RJ, Verity K, Clements JA. Kallikrein gene expression in estrogen-induced pituitary tumours. Mol Cell Endocrinol 1988; 60:225-232.

13.   Hatala MA, Powers CA. Glandular kallikrein in estrogen-induced pituitary tumours: Time course of induction and correlation with prolactin. Cancer Res 1988; 48:4158-62.

14.   Jones TH, Figueroa CD, Smith C, Cullen DR, Bhoola KD. Characterization of a tissue kallikrein in human prolactin-secreting adenomas. J Endocrinol 1990; 124:327-31.

15.   Powers CA, Hatala MA. Prolactin proteolysis by glandular kallikrein: In vitro reaction requirements and cleavage sites, and detection of processed prolactin in vivo. Endocrinol 1990; 127:1916-27.

16.   Ho TWC, Balden E, Chao J, Walker AM. Prolactin (PRL) processing by kallikrein: Production of the 21-23.5K Prl-like molecules and inferences about PRL storage in mature secreting granules. Endocrinol 1991; 129:184-92.

17.   Drouhault R, Abrous N, David JP, Dufy B. Bradykinin parallels thyrotrophin-releasing hormone actions on prolactin release from rat anterior pituitary cells. Neuroendocrinol 1987; 46:360-4.

18.   Jones TH, Brown BL, Dobson PRM. Bradykinin stimulates phosphoinositide metabolism and prolactin secretion in rat anterior pituitary cells. J Mol Endocrinol 1989; 2:47-53.

19.   Jones TH, Brown BL, Dobson PRM. Kallidin-induced stimulation of inositol phosphate production and prolactin release in rat anterior pituitary cells. Acta Endocrinol (Copenh) 1990; 123:37-42.

20.   Rappay GY, Nagy I, Makara GB, Horvath GY, Karteszi M, Bacsy E, Stark E. Inhibition of growth hormone and prolactin secretion by a serine protease inhibitor. Life Sci 1984; 33:337-44.

21.   Barna I, Graf L, Makara GB, Rappay GY. A serine-protease inhibitor (Boc-D-Phe-Pro-Arg-H) inhibits the secretion of adrenocorticotropin- and beta-endorphin-immunoreactive peptides in vitro. Neuropeptides 1982; 3:65-70.

22.   Drinkwater CC, Evans BA, Richards RI. Kallikreins, kinins and growth factor biosynthesis. TIBS 1988; 13:169-72

THE EPIDERMAL GROWTH FACTOR PRECURSOR IN THE RAT KIDNEY SEEMS TO BE PROCESSED BY AN APROTININ SENSITIVE PROTEINASE

P.E. Jørgensen, E. Nexø, S.S. Poulsen and L. Raaberg

Institute of Medical Anatomy, Department B, University of Copenhagen, Department of Clinical Chemistry, Hillerød Central Hospital and Department of Clinical Chemistry, KH-University Hospital of Aarhus, DK-8000 Aarhus C, Denmark

SUMMARY: Epidermal growth factor (EGF) is synthesized as a membrane bound precursor in the rat kidney. The precursor seems to be processed by an aprotinin sensitive proteinase. Intravenous infusion of aprotinin reduces the urinary excretion of EGF by 85% and increases the amount of renal EGF. Kidney membranes incubated at 37°C release EGF and this release is inhibited by aprotinin.

INTRODUCTION

EGF is a 6 kDa peptide with a wide spectrum of activities both in vivo and in vitro (1,2). EGF is synthesized as a glycosylated membrane bound precursor with a molecular weight around 130 kDa (3-5). In the kidneys, mRNA for the EGF precursor has been demonstrated in the cells of the thick ascending limb of Henle and the early part of the distal convoluted tubule, and immuno-histochemical studies have shown EGF to be localized to the luminal cell membrane of these cells (6-9). Nanomolar amounts of EGF are excreted in the urine and the majority of this EGF is produced in the kidneys (10-13).

Together the above mentioned studies suggest an enzymatic processing of the EGF precursor in the kidneys. We have therefore studied the molecular weight forms of EGF in rat urine and the influence of aprotinin in vivo and in vitro on the excretion of EGF from the kidneys (10,14,16). The aim of the present paper is to review our current knowledge of the effect of aprotinin on the processing of the EGF precursor in the rat kidney.

MATERIALS & METHODS

<u>In vivo study:</u> Aprotinin was infused intravenously in femal wistar rats (20,000 KIU as a bolus injection followed by 10,000 KIU/h for 2.5 h). The effect of aprotinin on the amount and the molecular forms of urinary EGF, on the amount of protein and creatinine in urine and on EGF in the kidneys was examined (14). The renal uptake and excretion of aprotinin were examined in rats that received aprotinin mixed with trace amounts of ^{125}I labelled aprotinin. The TCA precipitability of the radioactivity in the urine was measured in order to examine the fraction of the radio-activity that represented intact ^{125}I-aprotinin. The localization of the labelled peptide in the kidneys was examined by auto-radiography as previously described (15).

    <u>In vitro study:</u> Kidneys from male wistar rats were homo-genized and a membrane preparation was produced. The release of EGF from the membranes was examined by incubation of the membranes at 37°C and at 4°C with and without aprotinin. The pH optimum of the EGF release from the kidney membranes at 37°C was determined and the molecular weight forms of EGF released from the membranes, were compared to the molecular weight forms of EGF in rat urine using gel filtration (16).

RESULTS

<u>In vivo study:</u> Intravenous infusion of aprotinin reduced the urinary excretion of EGF by 85% and increased the amount of EGF in the kidneys. The infused aprotinin did neither affect the volume of urine produced nor the urinary output of creatinine and protein. Both the 6 kDa molecular weight form of EGF which normally constitutes approximately 90% of urinary EGF and the 45 kDa EGF which normally constitutes approximately 10% of urinary EGF were excreted during the aprotinin infusion. However, the excretion of 6 kDa EGF was reduced by approximately 90% while the excretion of 45 kDa EGF only tended to be bisected. The

infusion of ^{125}I-aprotinin showed that during the 2.5 h of aprotinin infusion approximately 3000 KIU of aprotinin (7% of the administered amount of aprotinin) passed through the nephron and were excreted in the urine. Approximately 40% of the injected aprotinin was taken up by the kidneys at the end of the 2.5 h infusion period.

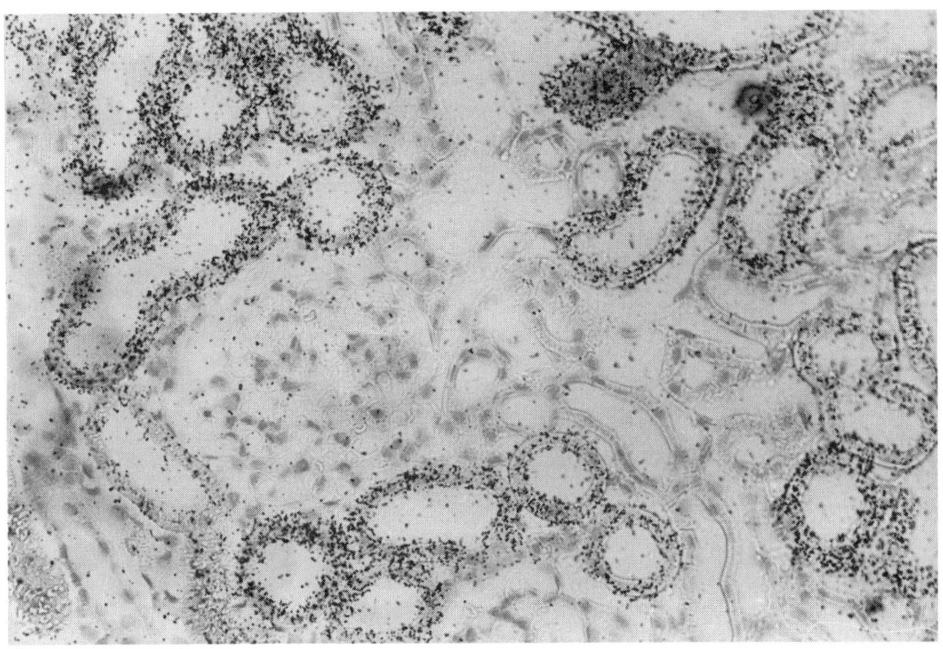

Figure 1. Autoradiography showed the ^{125}I-aprotinin to be located in the brush border as well as intracellularly in the proximal tubules. There was no distinct binding of ^{125}I-aprotinin in the distal tubules where the EGF-precursor is synthesized.

In vitro study: Increasing amounts of EGF were released from rat kidney membranes by enzymatic cleavage of the precursor when the membranes were incubated at 37°C. The EGF release was inhibited by aprotinin and by incubation at low temperature (4°C). The pH optimum of the reaction was 7.5-8.0. Gelfiltration showed that the EGF released from the kidney membranes consisted of the usual two molecular weight forms of urinary EGF: a 6 kDa

EGF and a 45 kDa EGF. The ratio between the amounts of the two
molecular weight forms of EGF released from the membranes was the
same as in urine.

DISCUSSION

Our studies (14,16) are the first to suggest that the EGF
precursor in the rat kidney is processed by an aprotinin
sensitive proteinase. We propose the following model for this
processing (Fig.2): the EGF precursor is a membrane bound protein
in the luminal cell membrane of the thick ascending limb of Henle
and the early part of the distal convoluted tubule. The EGF
moiety is located outside the cell in the tubular lumen and EGF
is excreted to the urine after extracellular cleavage of the
precursor.

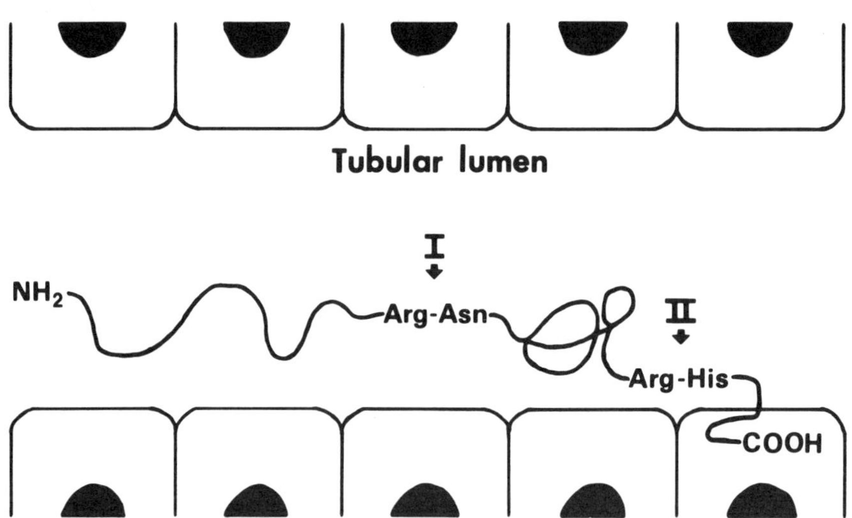

Figure 2. Figure illustrating the hypothesis of the EGF precursor
as a membrane bound protein in the luminal membrane of the distal
tubular cells with the EGF moiety located in the tubular lumen.
We propose an exctracellular processing of the precursor at I and
II followed by excretion of 6 kDa EGF in the urine. High
molecular weight forms of EGF are excreted in the urine if the
precursor is cleaved only at II.

The human EGF precursor consists of 1207 amino acids (3). The 53 amino acid EGF is flanked by 970 and 184 amino acids at its NH_2- and COOH-termini (3). A similar precursor has been demonstrated in the mouse and the 45 kDa weight form of EGF in rat urine contains an amino acid sequence that corresponds to a part of the precursor (4,10). The COOH-terminal part of the precursor contains a hydrophobic region and the precursor is a membrane bound protein (5). mRNA for the precursor is abundant in the cells of the thick ascending limb of Henle and in the early part of the distal convoluted tubule and by electron immunohisto-chemistry EGF immunoreactivity is localized to the luminal membrane of these cells (6,7,9). It has not been possible to demonstrate an intracellular processing of the precursor in kidney cells (6). However, proteolytic cleavage of the precursor followed by excretion of EGF in the urine is likely because high amounts of EGF are found in urine and the vast majority of this urinary EGF originates from the kidneys and not from plasma (11,12,13).

EGF is likely to be cleaved from the precursor by an arginine esterase. Both in man, mouse and rat the 53 amino acid EGF is cleaved from the precursor at Arg-Asn at the NH_2-terminal end and at Arg-His at the COOH-terminal end (3,4,17). Our studies (14,16) suggest that the EGF precursor in the rat kidney is processed enzymatically by an aprotinin sensitive proteinase. The in vitro study indicates that the processing enzyme is membrane associated because it is present in the membrane preparation. The intravenous infusion of ^{125}I-aprotinin in rats showed that small amounts of aprotinin was excreted in the urine. This means that aprotinin reached all parts of the nephron including the distal tubule where the EGF precursor is synthesized. By autoradiography the labelled aprotinin in the kidney was found in the proximal tubules but not in the distal tubules. If the EGF precursor processing enzyme is membrane bound it might be located in the distal tubules in a concentration too low for detection by autoradiography. Another possibility is that the enzyme is synthesized in the proximal tubules, perhaps as a brush border enzyme, and is then excreted into the urine to reach the EGF precursor in the more distal part of the nephron.

The processing enzyme has not yet been isolated. It is unlikely to be identical to the previously isolated mouse submaxillary EGF-binding protein with arginine esterase activity (18,19). The EGF-binding protein is able to cleave high molecular weight forms of human EGF to 6 kDa EGF (20), but it is not synthesized in the mouse kidney and it is unable to cleave preproEGF from mouse kidney membranes to 6 kDa EGF (21,22).

CONCLUSION

Aprotinin reduces the renal excretion of EGF in vivo and inhibits the enzymatic cleavage of the EGF precursor in kidney membranes in vitro suggesting that the EGF precursor in the rat kidney is processed by an aprotinin sensitive proteinase.

ACKNOWLEDGEMENT
The studies were supported by the Danish Cancer Society (89-060 & 90-022), by the Danish Medical Research Council (12-9312) and by the Danish Biotechnology Center for Neuropeptide Research. The photographical assistance of Mrs. Grazyna Hahn is warmly acknowledged.

REFERENCES

1.   Carpenter G, Wahl MI. The epidermal growth factor family. In: Peptide Growth Factors and Their Receptors I, Handb Exp Pharm 95/1. Sporn MB, Roberts AB, editors. Berlin: Springer Verlag, 1990: 69-171.

2.   Fisher DA, Salido EC, Barajas L. Epidermal growth factor and the kidney. Ann Rev Physiol 1989; 51:67-80.

3.	Bell GI, Fong NM, Stempien MM, Wormsted MA, Caput D, Ku L, Urdea MS, Rall LB, Sanchez-Pescador R. Human epidermal growth factor precursor: cDNA sequence, expression in vitro and gene organisation. Nucleic Acids Res 1986; 14:8427-8446.

4.	Scott J, Urdea M, Quiroga M, Sanchez-Pescador R, Fong N, Selby M, Rutter WJ, Bell GI. Structure of a mouse submaxillary messenger RNA encoding epidermal growth factor and seven related proteins. Science 1983; 221:236-240.

5.	Mroczkowski B, Reich M, Chen K, Bell GI, Cohen S. Recombinant human epidermal growth factor precursor is a glycosylated membrane protein with biological activity. Mol Cell Biol 1989; 9:2771-2778.

6.	Rall LB, Scott J, Bell GI, Crawford RJ, Penschow JD, Niall HD, Coghlan, JP. Mouse prepro-epidermal growth factor synthesis by the kidney and other tissues. Nature 1985; 313:228-231.

7.	Salido EC, Yen PH, Shapiro LJ, Fisher DA, Barajas L. In situ hybridization of prepro-epidermal growth factor mRNA in the mouse kidney. Am J Physiol 1989; 256:F632-F638.

8.	Poulsen SS, Nexø E, Olsen PS, Hess J, Kirkegaard P. Immunohistochemical localization of epidermal growth factor in rat and man, Histochemistry 1986; 85:389-394.

9.	Salido EC, Fisher DA, Barajas L. Immunoelectron microscopy of epidermal growth factor in mouse kidney. J Ultrastruc Mol Struc Res 1986; 96:105-113.

10.	Nexø E, Jørgensen PE, Thim L, Roepstorff P. Purification and characterization of a low and a high molecular weight form of epidermal growth factor from rat urine. Biochim Biophys Acta 1990; 1037:388-393.

11.	Mattila A-L, Viinikka L, Saario I, Perheentupa J. Human epidermal growth factor: renal production and abscence from plasma. Regul Pept 1988; 23:89-93.

12.	Jørgensen PE, Rasmussen TN, Olsen PS, Raaberg L, Poulsen SS, Nexø E. Renal uptake and excretion of epidermal growth factor from plasma in the rat. Regul Pept 1990; 28:273-281.

13.	Olsen PS, Nexø E, Poulsen SS, Hansen HF, Kirkegaard P. Renal origin of rat urinary epidermal growth factor, Regul Pept 1984; 10 37-45.

14.	Jørgensen PE, Raaberg L, Poulsen SS, Nexø E. The urinary excretion of epidermal growth factor in the rat is reduced by aprotinin, a proteinase inhibitor. Regul Pept 1990; 31:115-124.

15.   Jørgensen PE, Poulsen SS, Nexø E. Distribution of i.v. administered epidermal growth factor in the rat. Regul Pept 1988; 23:161-169.

16.   Jørgensen PE, Nexø E, Poulsen SS. The membrane fraction of homogenized rat kidney contains an enzyme that releases epidermal growth factor from the kidney membranes. Biochim Biophys Acta 1991; 1074:284-288.

17.   Dorow DS, Simpson RJ. Cloning and sequence analysis of a cDNA for rat epidermal growth factor. Nucleic Acids Res 1988; 16:9338.

18.   Taylor JM, Cohen S, Mitchell WM. Epidermal growth factor: high and low molecular weight forms. Proc Natl Acad Sci USA 1970; 67:164-171.

19.   Taylor JM, Mitchell WM, Cohen S. Characterization of the binding protein for epidermal growth factor. J Biol Chem 1974; 249:2188-2194.

20.   Hirata Y, Orth DN. Conversion of heigh molecular weight human epidermal growth factor (hEGF)/urogastrone (UG) to small molecular weight hEGF/UG by mouse EGF-associated arginine esterase. J Clin Endocrinol Metab 1979; 49:481-483.

21.   Drinkwater CC, Evans BA, Richards RI. Mouse glandular kallikrein genes: identification and characterization of the genes encoding the epidermal growth factor binding proteins. Biochemistry 1987; 26:6750-6756.

22.   Breyer JA, Cohen S. The epidermal growth factor precursor isolated from murine kidney membranes. J Biol Chem 1990; 265:16564-16570.

IMMUNOMODULATORS, INFLAMMATION AND LYSOSOMAL PROTEINASES OF MACROPHAGES

A. Safina, T. Korolenko, G.Mynkina, M.Dushkin[1] and
G. Krasnoselskaya

Institute of Physiology and Institute of Therapy[1], Siberian
Branch of the Russian Academy of Medical Sciences,Novosibirsk,
Russia

SUMMARY:Zymosan-induced stimulation of mononuclear phagocyte
system was used as a model for study of inflammation in vivo.
Zymosan administration to mice was followed by increase of macrophage enzyme markers β-N-acetylglucosaminidase and β-N-ace-
tylgalactosaminidase activity in liver and serum.Serum acid glucosidases secretion occured both after macrophage stimulation by
zymosan and macrophage depression induced by $GdCl_3$.Liver granulomatous inflammation resulted increased activity of liver cathepsin B and cathepsin L.There was no changes of cysteine proteinases studied in the case of macrophage depression by $GdCl_3$.The
role of lysosomal enzymes secretion in macrophage stimulation
and inflammation was discussed.

INTRODUCTION

Zymosan has been used for study of granulomatous inflammation in
vivo as well as macrophage stimulator in vitro (1).Zymosan-indu-
ced stimulation of mononuclear phagocyte system (MPS) is followed by the increased activity and secretion of macrophage lysosomal enzymes (2,3),which are able to activate different systems
(blood clotting, fibrinolysis and complement cascades) and promote tissue injury (4,5). The important role in this process be-
longs to lysosomal proteinases closely related to inflammation.
Liver cysteine proteinases activity during zymosan-induced MPS
stimulation was studied. The results were compared with the data obtained during macrophage depression by gadolinium chloride

(GdCl$_3$) (6).As a markers of macrophage activation β-N-acetylglu-
cosaminidase (NAGlu) and β-N-acetylgalactosaminidase (NAGal)
have been used,their activity increased up to several times in
such cases (3),especially serum secretion.

MATERIALS AND METHODS

Male mice CBA weighing 16-20 g were used.Zymosan (Olaine,Latvia)
was given i.v. as a single dose of 100 mg/kg b.w. GdCl$_3$ (a kind
gift of Prof. Hardonk M.J. and Prof.Bouma J.M.W.,The Netherlands)
was used in a dose of 20 μmoles per kg b.w. (6).Mice were sac-
rificed at 2 h, first and 5th days after a single zymosan or
GdCl$_3$ i.v. injections.The activity of lysosomal glucosidases was
determined using MUF-derivated substrates (Fluka,Switzerland,
Koch-Light, G.B. and IMBIMED, Russia) (7).Cysteine proteinases
were measured using the fluorogenic peptidyl substrates, Z-Arg-
Arg-NMec for cathepsin B, Z-Phe-Arg-NMec for cathepsin L (products of All-Union Institute of Molecular Biology, Koltsovo, Novosibirsk region) according to (8).The fluorescence was determined using Hitachi LTD model F-3000 spectrofluorimeter.

RESULTS AND DISCUSSION

Serum NAGlu and NAGal (in less degree acid phosphatase and
β-glucuronidase) secretion increased both after MPS stimulation
by zymosan (fig.1) and MPS depression induced by GdCl$_3$ (fig.1).
In both experiments the prominent elevation of marker macrophage
enzymes NAGlu and NAGal was noted. Surprisingly that significant
increase of glucosidases secretion occured in case of GdCl$_3$ administration (2 h, 1 day after) (fig.1).It is known that in zy-
mosan-treated group lysosomal enzymes secretion related to macrophage activation (1-3).In case of MPS depression uptake of ly-
sosomotropic agent GdCl$_3$ and macrophage overloading by this compound occured.Possibly serum lysosomal enzymes secretion was a
result of macrophage damage by GdCl$_3$ (Kupffer cells).

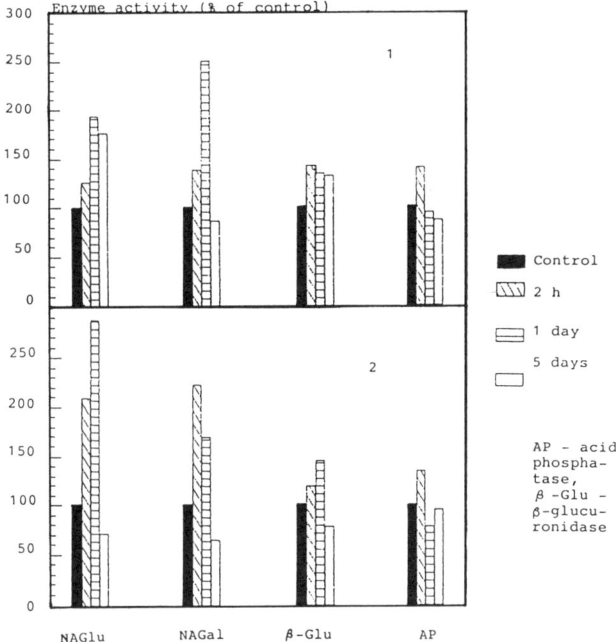

Figure 1. Serum secretion of lysosomal hydrolases after macrophage stimulation by zymosan (1) and macrophage depression by
gadolinium chloride ($GdCl_3$) (2)

Zymosan treatment was followed by the significant (3-fold at 5th
day) elevation of liver lysosomal hydrolases NAGlu and NAGal
(fig.2); the specific activity of acid phosphatase, β-glucosidase
β-galactosidase in liver was also increased (fig.2). $GdCl_3$ administration resulted in raising of β-galactosidase activity up to
170% only (fig.2) at 1st day after injection (period of MPS depression).The liver cysteine proteinases activity increased at the
5th day after zymosan using,reaching 143% for cathepsin B and
137% for cathepsin L comparatively to the control values (table 1).
There were no changes of cysteine proteinases studied in case of
MPS depression by $GdCl_3$ (table 1).
Zymosan induces migration of peripheral monocytes into liver, especially at 4-6th days after the treatment (1-3). The significant
increase of lysosomal hydrolases in liver and serum of zymosan-
treated mice can be explained as enzymes synthesis de novo (2).
It is known that macrophages enriched by cathepsin B and other
cysteine proteinases comparatively to hepatocytes (5,8). $GdCl_3$ ef-

Table 1.Effect of zymosan and GdCl$_3$ administration to mice
on liver cysteine proteinases activity

Group of animals, number	Cysteine proteinases specific activity (nmol/min per mg of protein)	
	Cathepsin B	Cathepsin L
Control (5)	0.25 ± 0.oo6 (100%)	0.79 ± 0.028 (100%)
Zymosan, 2h (6)	0.21 ± 0.008 (84%)	0.78 ± 0.046 (99%)
GdCl$_3$,2h (6)	0.22 ± 0.010 (88%)	0.74 ± 0.056 (94%)
Control (5)	0.19 ± 0.009 (100%)	n.d.
Zymosan,1 day (6)	0.17 ± 0.007 (91%)	n.d.
GdCl$_3$,1 day (6)	0.19 ± 0.010 (100%)	n.d.
Control (5)	0.14 ± 0.007 (100%)	0.51 ± 0.046 (100%)
Zymosan,5 days (6)	0.20 ± 0.006 (143%) p<0.01	0.70 ± 0.027 (137%) p<0.01
GdCl$_3$,5 days (6)	0.15 ± 0.005 (107%)	0.56 ± 0.038 (110%)

Control - mice with the injection of the same volume of
saline solution

fect can be related to its uptake by Kupffer cells followed by
releasing of macrophage marker lysosomal enzymes NAGlu and NAGal.
According to morphologic investigations the number of Kupffer
cells decreased sharply 1 day after GdCl$_3$ -induced suppression
of MPS.Until now the mechanism of action of GdCl$_3$ is unknown,so
the further studies are necessary.
Zymosan-induced model of inflammation was followed by increased
liver NAGlu and NAGal activity,elevation of these enzymes secretion into serum and increased level of cathepsin B and cathepsin L activity in liver.The prominent changes were noted during
granuloma formation in liver (at 5th day).

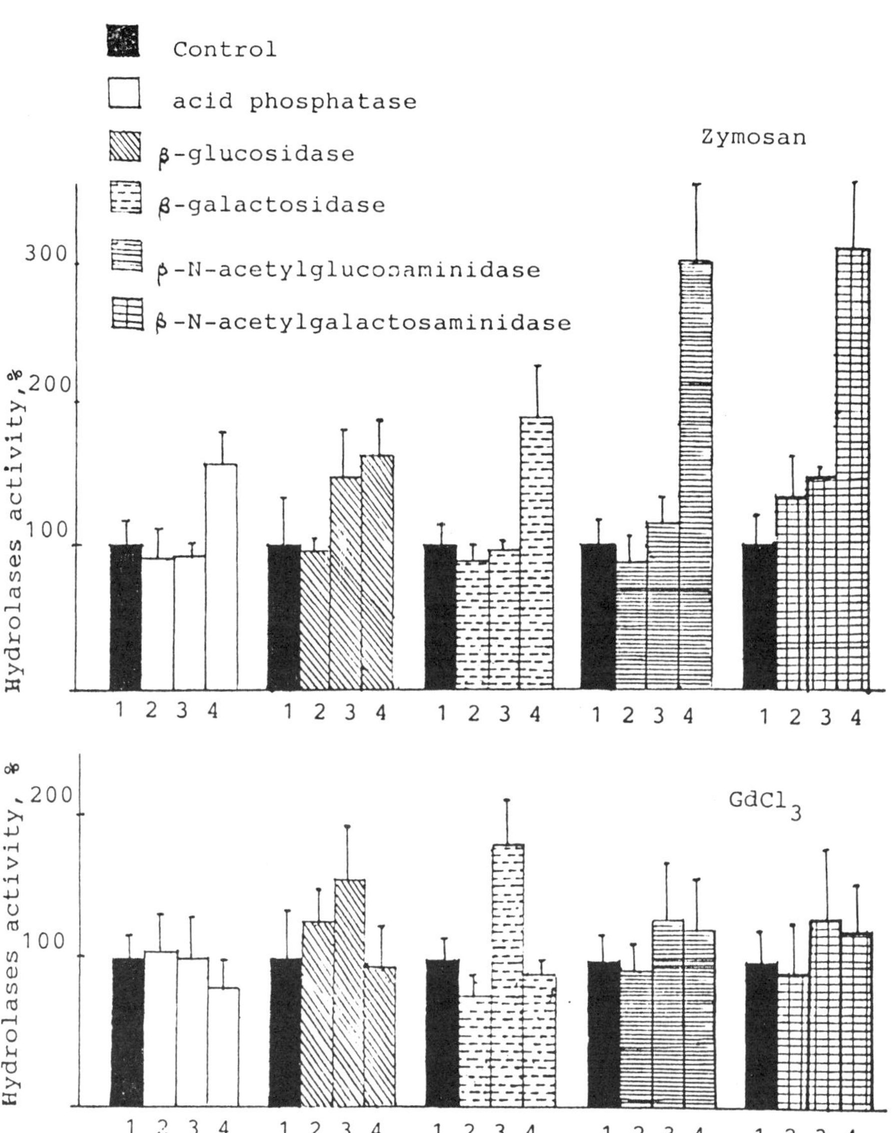

Figure 2. Effects of zymosan and GdCl₃ single administration to mice on liver specific acid hydrolases activity (as a percentage of the control).
All value are mean ± SD. Number of animals in each group = 10.
1 – 0 h; 2 – 2 h; 3 – 1 day later; 4 – 5 days later

It is necessary to note that increased level of liver cysteine proteinases activity was observed only in case of macrophage stimulation by zymosan; there was no change of cathepsins B and L during macrophage depression induced by $GdCl_3$.
In conclusion it can be said that zymosan-induced model of inflammation includes increased activity in liver tissue of marker macrophage enzymes - NAGlu and NAGal, cathepsin B and cathepsin L, serum secretion of acid glucosidases studied.Similar data (serum secretion) were obtained during macrophage depression induced by $GdCl_3$.

CONCLUSION

Zymosan-induced macrophage stimulation was used as a model for study of inflammation in vivo. The results were compared with the data obtained during macrophage depression by $GdCl_3$.Serum acid glucosidases secretion occured both after macrophage stimulation by zymosan and macrophage depression induced by $GdCl_3$.Zymosan treatment was followed by the increased activity in liver of marker macrophage enzymes as well as cysteine proteinases - cathepsin B and cathepsin L during granuloma formation in liver.

ACKNOWLEDGEMENTS

We thank Prof.Hardonk M.J. and Prof. Bouma J.M.W. (The Netherlands) for kind gift of gadolinium chloride, Dr.K.Hanada (Japan) for kind gift of Ep-475, Prof.Hasilik A. (Germany) for the kind gift of MUF-substrates for lysosomal enzymes.

REFERENCES

1. Tarayre JP,Delhon A,Aliaga M,Barbara M,Bruniquel F,Caillol V,
   Puech L, Consul N, Tisne-Versailles J. Pharmacological studies on zymosan inflammation in rats and mice. 1: Zymosan-induced paw oedema in rats and mice. Pharmacological Research
   1989; 21:375.

2. Bouwens L, Wisse E. Proliferation, kinetics and fate of monocyte in rat liver during a zymosan-induced inflammation. J Leukocyte Biol 1985; 37: 531.

3. Warren L. Stimulated secretion of lysosomal enzymes by cells in culture. J Biol Chem 1989; 264: 8835.

4. Jochum M, Dusurald K-H, Newmann S, Witte I, Fritz H, Seemuller U.Proteinases and their inhibitors in inflammation, basic concept and clinical implications. In: Proteinase inhibitors: medical and biological aspects. Katunuma N,Umezawa H, Holzer H, editors.Tokyo:Japan Scientific Societies Press, Berlin,Heidelberg,N.Y.,Tokyo:Springer-Verlag,1983:85-95

5. Assfalg-Machleidt, Jochum M, Joka T, Rothe G, Valet G, Zauner R, Scheuber H-P, Machleidt W. Cathepsin B - indicator for the release of lysosomal cysteine proteinases in severe trauma and inflammation. Biol Chem Hoppe-Seyler Suppl. 1990;371:211.

6. Bouma JMW, Smit MJ. Gadolinium chloride selectively blocks endocytosis by Kupffer cells. In:Kupffer Cell Foundation. Cells of the Hepatic Sinusoid 1989; 2:132.

7. Barrett AJ. Lysosomal enzymes. In: Lysosomes.A Laboratory Handbook. Dingle JT editor.Amsterdam,London:North-Holland Publ.Co. 1972; 46.

8. Barrett AJ, Kirschke H. Cathepsin B,cathepsin H and cathepsin L. In:Methods in Enzymology 1981;80: 535.

AAS 38/II
Recent Progress on Kinins
© 1992 Birkhäuser Verlag Basel

α_1-PROTEINASE INHIBITOR AND RESISTANCE TO ACUTE BLOOD LOSS DURING INJECTION OF β-1,3-CARBOXYMETHYLGLUCAN

E. Vereschagin, T. Korolenko and S. Arkhipov

Institute of Physiology, Siberian Branch of the Russian
Academy of Medical Sciences, Novosibirsk, Russia

SUMMARY: The present study was undertaken to evaluate the mechanism of protective effect of semisoluble β-1,3-carboxymethylglucan during massive acute hemorrhage. CBA mice were injected i.v. with glucan (25 mg/kg) 24 h prior to hemorrhage (50% of blood circulating volume). Survival data indicated that glucan increased survival compared with the control. However α_1-proteinase inhibitor activity in serum has been even decreased 24 h after glucan administration. Moreover enhancement of active oxygen form production and leakage of cytosolic and lysosomal enzymes after β-1,3-carboxymethylglucan application was noted.

INTRODUCTION

A close relationship between macrophage functions and resistance to circulatory shock have been shown (1). Increased tolerance to several types of shock was noted in animals pretreated with macrophage stimulator β-1,3-glucan (2). It was suggested that liberating proteinases (elastase, cathepsins) may overcome the inhibitory potential of their main antagonists and significantly aggravate the shock (3). Antiproteinase inhibitors, first of all α_1-proteinase inhibitor (α_1-PI), α_2-macroglobulin are known to be secreted by reticulo-endothelial system (RES). Lipopolysaccharides increased more than 8-fold secretion of α_1-PI by monocytes and macrophages in vitro (4). It is possible that protective effect of glucan during several types of shock was mediated partly by α_1-PI enhancement. The present study was undertaken to investigate the semisoluble β-1,3-carboxymethylglucan (CMG) effect during hemorrhage and to evaluate the role of α_1-PI.

MATERIALS AND METHODS

Experiment were carried out on male CBA mice (20 - 25 g). Animals were anesthetized by ether and calculated blood volume was removed from retroorbital venous sinus during 2 minutes (about 50% of blood circulating volume or 3.5% of body weight). Control animals were treated similarly except hemorrhage. CMG (Chemical Institute, Bratislava, Czecho-Slovakia) for RES stimulation was administered i.v. 24 h prior to hemorrhage in a dose of 25 mg/kg. The NBT test have been conducted on isolated peritoneal macrophages using nitroblue tetrazolium (Sigma, USA) (5). α_1-PI was assayed with the method, based on interaction of α_1-PI with tripsin in the system with low molecular substrate Nα -benzoyl-L-arginine (6). Lysosomal enzyme secretion was measured as increase of acid hydrolases level in serum; β -galactosidase activity was performed spectrofluorimetrically using methylumbelliferyl- β -D-galactopyranoside and acid phosphatase with β -glycerophosphate as was described (7). Activity of LDG and ALT in serum was estimated with help of standard test combination (Boehringer Mannheim, Germany). All data were statistically analyzed with Student t- test.

RESULTS AND DISCUSSION

CMG pretreatment increased the survival rate in shocked mice comparatively to the controls.In CMG-treated group only one from twenty mice died after hemorrhage, and in the control group five animals from twenty have died.The percentage of peritoneal macrophages reduced NBT was elevated from 33% (control) up to 53% after CMG application. Increased production of oxygen active forms showed that CMG had potent stimulatory effect on macrophages.Activity of LDG and acid phosphatase (but not ALT and β -galactosidase) in serum was enhanced 24 h after CMG administration (table 1). This effect of macrophage stimulators have been previously explained by the leakage of cytosolic and lysosomal enzymes due to the changes of cell membranes (8). So macrophage stimulation by CMG was accompanied by releasing of some "destructive potential" of RES. These factors (active oxygene forms, lysosomal enzymes) could lead to tissue injury, especially during shock. CMG pretrestment significantly reduced cytosolic and lysosomal enzymes leakage observed in hemorrhage (table 1).

Table 1. Serum lysosomal and cytosolic enzymes activity during hemorrhage after CMG administration to mice

Group of animals	LDG, U/l	ALT, U/l	Acid phosphatase,nmoles P_i min/l	β-Galactosidase,nmoles MUF/min/l
0 h prior to hemorrhage				
Control	296 ± 24	0.74 ± 0.03	4.4.± 0.25	0.27 ± 0.05
CMG	921 ± 35*	0.70 ± 0.04	6.0 ± 0.40*	0.23 ± 0.04
1 h after hemorrhage				
Control	643 ± 24*	1.62 ± 0.14*	9.3 ± 1.00*	0.45 ± 0.03*
CMG	813 ± 36*	1.10 ± 0.04*	6.9 ± 0.25*	0.24 ± 0.03

CMG was administered i.v. in a dose of 25 mg/kg b.w., 24 h before hemorrhage.N = 10 in each group.

* $p < 0.05$ compared to 0 h control value.

This fact shows that preliminary administration of CMG protected the tissues from injury during hemorrhage.One of the possible mechanisms of protection during shock may be the increase of α_1-PI in blood after CMG application. Surprisingly it was shown that CMG i.v. administration even decreased the α_1-PI level in serum.Comparatively to the control animals CMG administration was followed by decrease of α_1-PI in blood of mice 24 h after injection (figure 1). Both in the control and CMG groups α_1-PI level was decreased after hemorrhage (1 h). There was no difference in α_1-PI level between the control and CMG-treated groups. The possible mechanism of depletion of α_1-PI could be decrease

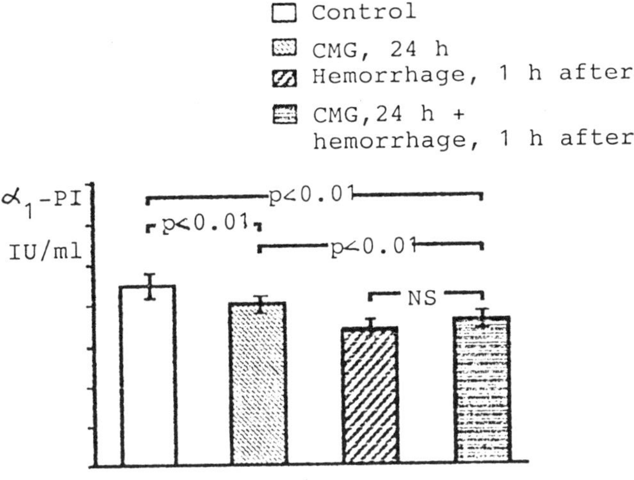

Figure 1. Effect of preliminary administration of β-1,3-carboxymethylglucan (25 mg/kg) on α_1-proteinase inhibitor after hemorrhage in mice. All values are mean ± SD, N= 10 in each group.

of proteinase inhibitory potential due to the enhanced proteolytic enzymes secretion and inactivation of α_1-PI by active forms of oxygen after glucan administration (9). The data obtained suggest that preliminary administration of semisoluble CMG has protective effect during acute massive hemorrhage in despite of initial enhancement of active oxygen form production and α_1-PI depletion after CMG injection.

CONCLUSION

Protective effect of semosoluble β-1,3-carboxymethylglucan during acute massive hemorrhage was shown. 24 h prior to hemorrhage (50% of blood circulating volume) glucan administration to CBA mice increased survival rate comparatively to the control. α_1-PI level in serum decreased 24 h after glucan administration; enhancement of active oxygen form production and leakage of cytosolic and lysosomal enzymes after CMG application was noted. CMG protective effect during acute blood loss was observed in despite of initial enhancement of active oxygen form production and α_1-PI depletion after CMG injection.

ACKNOWLEDGEMENTS

We thank Dr.J.Sandula for kind gift of β-1,3-carboxymethylglu-
can (Institute of Chemistry, Slovak Acad.Sci.,Bratislava, Czecho-
Slovakia),Prof.Hasilik A. (Germany) for the kind gift of MUF-
substrates for lysosomal enzymes.

REFERENCES

1. Altura BM.Reticuloendothelial system function and histamine
   release in shock and trauma:relationship to microcirculation.
   Klin Wochensch 1982; 60:882.

2. Di Luzio NR. Immunopharmacology of glucan: broad spectrum en-
   hancer of host defence mechanism Trend Pharmacol Sci 1983;
   4:344-347.

3. Jochum M,Witte J, Duswald KN, Inthorn D, Welter H,Fritz H.
   Pathobiochemistry of sepsis: role of proteinases,proteinase
   inhibitors and oxydizing agents. Behring Inst Mitt 1989;
   79: 121-130.

4. Barbey-Morel C, Pierce JA, Campbel EI. Lipopolysaccharide
   modulates the expression of α_1-proteinase inhibitor and
   other serine proteinase inhibitor in human monocytes and
   macrophages. J Exper Med 1987; 166: 1041-1048.

5. Herscowitz HB, Holden HT, Bellanti JA. Manual of macrophage
   methodology.Collection, characterization and function.
   Immunol Ser. Dekker M ed. N.Y and Basel, 1981.

6. van Wees J, Tegtmeyer F-K, Otte J, Wood WG, Braun J. Protei-
   nase-antiproteinase imbalance in meningitis: determination
   of α_1-proteinase inhibitor,elastase-α_1-proteinase inhibitor complex and elastase inhibition capacity in cerebrospi-
   nal fluid. Klin Wochenschr 1990; 68: 1054-1058.

7. Barrett AJ. In: Lysosomes: A Laboratory Handbook. Dingle JT
   editor.Amsterdam,London:North-Holland 1972; 46-135.

8. Decker K. Biologically active products of stimulated liver
   macrophages. Eur J Biochem 1990; 192: 245-261.

9. Travis J, Guzdek A, Potempa J, Watorek W. Serpins:structure
   and mechanism of action. J Biol Chem 1990; 371: 3-11.

PROTEIN PROTEINASE INHIBITOR THERAPY IN EXPERIMENTAL PANCREATITIS: PHARMACOLOGICAL CHARACTERIZATION OF THE INHIBITOR

T.A.Valueva[*], N.L.Matveev, V.V.Mosolov[*], V.A.Penin
[*]A.N.Bach Institute of Biochemistry, Russian Academy of Sciences, N.A.Semashko Medical Stomatologic Institute, Moscow, Russia

SUMMARY: The pharmacodynamical properties of the duck ovomucoid and its effect on the development of experimental pancreatitis in rats have been studied. It has been shown that after intravenous injection the ovomucoid initially accumulated in the liver, kidneys and blood, while after intraperitoneal injection - mainly in the pancreas and kidneys. The inhibitor is removed from circulation by renal filtration, one-half of the injected protein being removed for 4 hr. For the treatment of experimental pancreatitis two modes of ovomucoid administration were used: intravenous and combined (intravenous/intraperitoneal). The ovomucoid intravenous injection in a dose of 16,300 ATU/kg/ 24 hr resulted in decrease of both the trypsin-like activity and the level of the trypsinogen activation peptide in the blood to the level in intact rats and also in reduction of the primary pancreas destruction. The same effect observed in the case of the ovomucoid combined injection, but with a lower intravenous dose.

INTRODUCTION

During recent years an intensive search has been made for protein proteinase inhibitors suitable for the treatment of diseases accompanied by superactivation of proteolytic systems, including acute pancreatitis [1,2].

Aprotinin and trasylol used for the treatment of acute pancreatitis contain the basic pancreatic trypsin inhibitor (BPTI). BPTI is usually administered either intravenously or intraperitoneally in the case of surgical intervention [3]. However, BPTI is effectively adsorbed by the renal membrane and

fast removed from organism, 90% of the injected trasylol is detected in the kidney in 1 hr [4]. Besides BPTI does not inhibit
the leukocytic cathepsins and pancreatic elastase involved in
the pathogenesis of acute pancreatitis [5] and as a result fa-
ils to prevent the progressed distruction of the pancreas [6].

We have studied the effect of duck egg white ovomucoid on
the development of experimental pancreatitis in rats, as well
as its pharmacodynamical properties. Duck ovomucoid is a glycoprotein with M_r of about 31 kDa that efficiently inhibits the
activity of pancreatic enzymes (trypsin, chymotrypsin and elastase with K_i =10^{-7}-10^{-9}M) and some cellular enzymes (leukocytic
elastase and acrosin), as well as subtilisin and some other mi-
crobial proteinases [7]. The duck ovomucoid has three independent proteinase binding sites and is able to bind simultaneously
two trypsin and one chymotrypsin molecules [8].

MATERIALS AND METHODS

Bovine trypsin (type VIII), N,α-benzoyl-L-arginine p-nitroani-
lide (BAPNA), N-succinimidyl-3(-4-hydroxy-5-[^{125}]-iodophenyl)-
propionate (Botton-Hunter Reagent, 5 mCi/ml), were obtained
from Sigma Chemical Co., St. Louis, MO.

Ovomucoid with a specific activity of 1630 ATU/mg protein
was isolated from the duck egg white as described earlier [9].

The ^{125}I-labelled ovomucoid with the specific radioactivity of 46 mCi/mg protein was prepared by incubation with Botton-
Hunter Reagent for 20 hr followed by dialysis against 0.5 M
$NaHCO_3$ at 4°C for 48 hr [10].

The ^{125}I-labelled ovomucoid (5 mg/ml) in 0.9% NaCl was injected in a dose of 0.33 mg/kg animal weight into the lateral
tail vena of 44 Balb/c mice and intraperitoneally in the same
dose into 35 Balb/c mice. Mice were killed at intervals between
0 and 5 hr and in 24 hr after the injection. The heart, lungs,
spleen, kidneys, and liver were removed. Radioactivity was measured with a Wallac Compugamma 1282-032 gamma counter from LKB-
Produkter AB, Bromma, Sweden. The specific radioactivity was
calculated as the counts per minute for 1 g of the organ paren-

chyma (CPM/g) or 1 ml of the circulated blood (CPM/ml).

Experimental pancreatitis was provoked in 92 rats of the Vistar line by the method reported in [11]. The volume of the administered bile was 0.1 ml per 100 g weight of the animal. 48 rats were used as control animals (CA).

The ovomucoid (5 mg/ml) in 0.9% NaCl was injected in a dose of 16,300 ATU/kg in 2 hr after the development of acute pancreatitis. In another series of experiments (16 rats), the animals were subjected to relaparotomy followed by lavage of the abdomen with 0.9% NaCl, and then the ovomucoid solution was injected intravenously and intraperitoneally in doses of 8150 ATU/kg and 14,670 ATU/kg, respectively. No other treatment was provided.

The trypsin-like activity was determined by the procedure reported in [12] with some modification. The trypsin inhibitor activity was estimated by inhibition of the activity of trypsin after 5 min incubation of enzyme (50 µg) with 0.01 ml of the plasma. The concentration of the trypsinogen activation peptide was determined by competitive enzyme immunoassay with antibodies against the trypsinogen activation peptide [13]. The plasma was preliminary stabilized with EDTA.

Histological studies of the pancreas were performed after autopsy and fixation with 10% formol.

RESULTS

Figure 1A shows the distribution of the specific radioactivity in organs after the intravenous injection of the ^{125}I-labelled ovomucoid. The protein was found in the liver (125,388 CPM/g or 27% of the injected amount), kidneys (273,118 CPM/g or 15%), blood (141,866 CPM/ml or 34%), lungs (45,273 CPM/g or 1%), spleen (36,892 CPM/g or less than 1%) and less than 0,5% in the pancreas and heart in 2 min after the injection. The ovomucoid level in the blood decreased to 24,932 CPM/ml or 6% of the injected amount in 10 min. In the liver, kidneys and spleen the protein remained for 1 hr and its level decreased to 0.1% in 24 hr. Radioactivity was measured in the urine in 2 min after the

injection. The renal clearance was 0.0293±0.0047 ml/min. In all
cases ovomucoid was removed from circulation by renal filtration, one-half of the injected protein being removed for 4 hr.

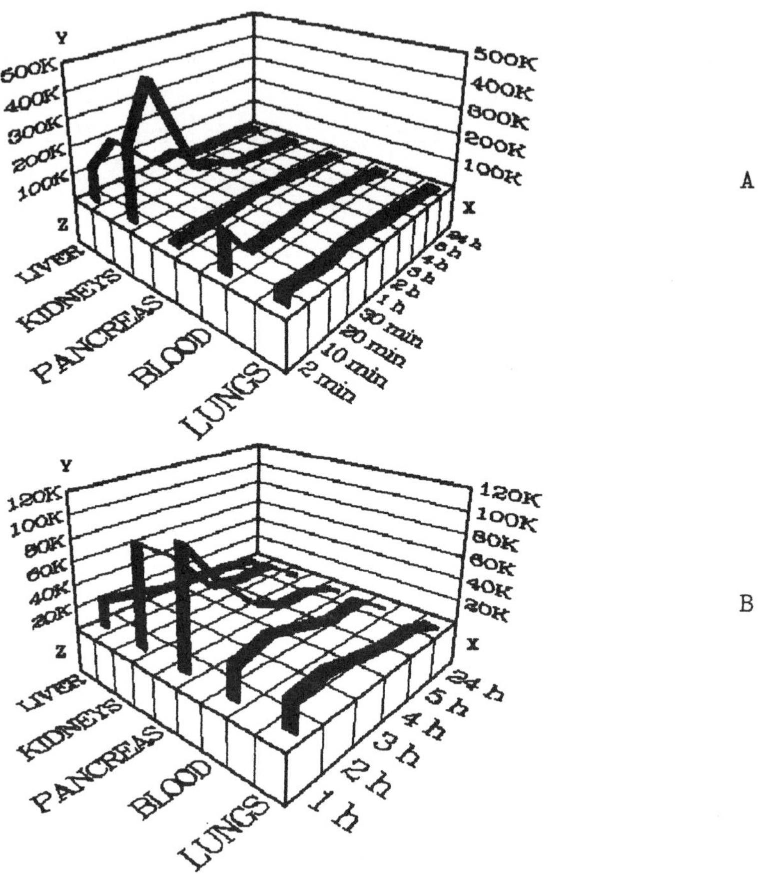

Figure 1. The level of the specific radioactivity (Y) in organs
(Z) vs time after the intravenous (A) or intraperitoneal (B)
injection (X) of the labelled duck ovomucoid. K = 1000.

Figure 1B shows the distribution of the specific radioactivity in organs after the intraperitoneal injection of the
^{125}I-labelled ovomucoid. One can see that the inhibitor is initially accumulated in the pancreas (181,858 CPM/g compared
with 6,937 CPM/g after intravenous injection) and kidneys

(88,583 CPM/g). Less than 3% of the injected inhibitor accumulated in the liver (23,998 CPM/g) and less than 1% in the lungs and spleen in 1 hr. The maximal level of the ^{125}I- labelled ovomucoid is observed in the blood in 2 hr.

Histological studies showed the development of the hemorrhagic component of necrosis and steatonecrosis in the pancreas of CA in 3 hr after the start of the experiment. The necrosis was progressing, and in 24 hr we observed thrombosis.

The first maxima of a trypsin-like activity and of the trypsinogen activation peptide concentration in the CA plasma were observed to the 3rd hr of the experiment, and to the 24th hr the pancreatitogenic increasing of the enzymatic activity was well-defined. The second maximum of the blood enzymatic activity was observed to the 6th hr of the experiment (Fig. 2). At the same time the trypsin inhibitor activity in the CA plasma was higher than in healthy animals and remained almost constant. 66.7% of CA died in the stage of enzyme toxemia (in 48 hr).

Ovomucoid was injected an hour before the development of the first maximum of the proteinase activity and the appearance of destructive changes in the pancreas, i.e. in 2 hr after simulation of pancreatitis. The plasma of test animals (TA) was analyzed at the 3rd hr of the experiment, when a maximal pancreatitogenic increase of the proteinase activity was observed in the plasma of CA (Fig. 2). The dose of the administered ovomucoid was equal to 16,300 ATU/kg animal weight.

One hour after the ovomucoid injection, the trypsin-like activity decreased to the level in intact animals (Fig. 2). Later this activity slightly increased, but it never reached the maximum observed in CA. The level of the trypsinogen activation peptide also significantly decreased, while the trypsin inhibitor activity authentically increased. In 4 hr after the injection (Fig. 2), the ovomucoid effect on the pancreatic enzymes in the blood plasma of TA remained, and the trypsin inhibitor activity even increased compared to that of CA. In 24 hr, the ratio of trypsin-like and trypsin inhibitor activities in the blood of TA remained normal, but the concentration of the trypsinogen activation peptide was somewhat higher.

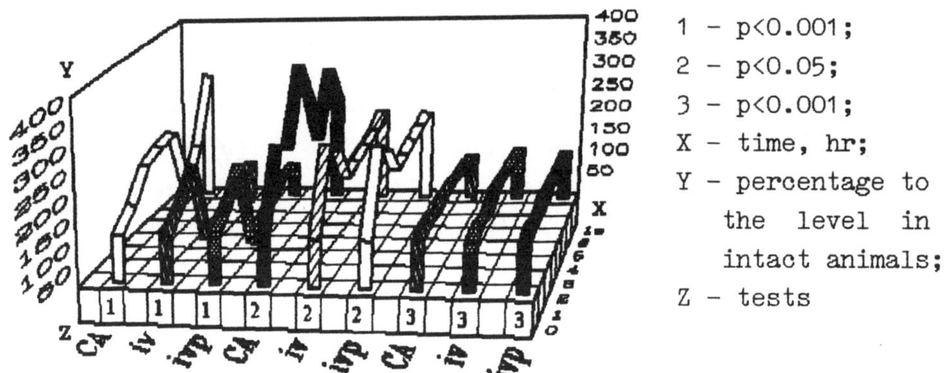

Figure 2. The effect of the duck ovomucoid intravenous (iv) and combined injection (ivp) on the trypsin-like enzymes (1), trypsin inhibitor (2) and the level of the trypsinogen activation peptide (3) in the rat plasma.

Histological studies of the TA pancreas one hour after the ovomucoid injection showed a regression of pancreonecrosis. In 24 hr, a distinct demarcation appeared around destruction foci, and the blood flow was restored in initially damaged vessels. To the 48th hr of the experiment 33.3% TA died.

In another series of tests, acute pancreatitis was treated by a combined injection of the ovomucoid (8150 ATU/kg intravenously and 14,670 ATU/kg intraperitoneally). However, the final ovomucoid concentration in the blood was somewhat higher due to the resorption of the inhibitor through the peritoneum.

A significant decrease in the trypsin-like activity and in the level of the trypsinogen activation peptide in the blood of TA was observed in an hour after the ovomucoid combined injection, while the trypsin inhibitor activity was rather low. In 4 and 24 hr, the parameters of enzymatic activity remained at the same level (Fig. 2).

DISCUSSION

It is shown that after the intravenous injection the ovomucoid has higher affinity for the liver tissue than for the renal tissue. The protein also accumulates in the lungs and spleen, while its level in the pancreas is very small. After intraperitoneal injection the ovomucoid concentration is 5 times higher in the pancreas than in the liver and 1.5 time higher than in the kidneys. The ovomucoid circulates in the organism 2 times longer than BPTI [4].

The chosen model of experimental pancreatitis is characterized by macrofocal progressing pancreonecrosis accompanied by hemorrhages and adiponecrosis, and by authentical increase of the blood proteinase activity that reached the first maximum to the 3rd hr of the experiment. The blood trypsin inhibitor activity is constantly below normal.

After the ovomucoid intravenous injection the trypsin-like activity and the concentration of the trypsinogen activation peptide decreased both to the 3rd and to the 24th hr of the experiment. At the same time no significant increase of the trypsin inhibitor activity was observed, which can be explained by recovery of the system of endogenous proteinases and their inhibitors. Morphological changes in the pancreas definitely correlate with changes in the plasma enzymatic activity, which indicates that duck ovomucoid has a curative effect on the pancreatic tissue. It is noteworthy that a single ovomucoid injection efficiently corrects the enzyme level in the blood. The ovomucoid combined injection gives the same results, but enables two-fold reduction of the dose of the intravenously injected ovomucoid. The slow resorption of the protein from the abdomen assures the prolonged effect.

Thus duck ovomucoid was found to be more efficient for the injection in a organism than BPTI that should be intravenously infused in significant doses [3] and can be used for the treatment of pancreonecrosis and other diseases accompanied by activation of proteolytic processes.

REFERENCES

1.   Corfield AP, Cooper MJ, Williamson RCN. Acute pancreatitis: a lethal disease of increasing incidence. Gut 1985; 26:724-729.

2.   Renner IG, Savage WT, Pantoja JL, Renner VJ. Death due to acute pancreatitis: a retrospective analysis of 405 autopsy cases. Dig Dis Sci 1985; 30:1005-1018.

3.   Fritz H, Wunderer G. Biochemistry and applications of aprotinin, the kallikrein inhibitor from bovine organs. Arzneim Forsch Drug Res 1983; 33:479-494.

4.   Balldin G, Lasson A, Ohlsson K. Aprotinin turn-over studies in dog and man acute pancreatitis. Z Physiol Chem 1984; 365: 1417-1425.

5.   Balldin G, Ohlsson K. Demonstration of pancreatic protease-antiprotease complex in the peritoneal fluid of pacients with acute pancreatitis. Surgery 1979; 85:451-456.

6.   Penin VA, Petrov BB, Titova GP, Mesentzev SS. Effect of endolymphatic injection of protease inhibitors on the morphology and function of the pancreas in the experimental acute pancreatitis. Pharmacologiya and Toxicologiya 1982; 45:83-87.

7.   Valueva TA, Vanchugova LV, Römashkin VI, Rosenfel'd MA, Valuev LI, Mosolov VV, Plate NA. The interaction of duck egg white ovomucoid with serine proteinases. Biochimiya 1988; 53:1455-1561.

8.   Vanchugova LV, Valueva TA, Rosenfel'd MA, Sinani VA, Mosolov VV, Valuev LI, Plate NA. Pecullarities of the interaction of a multisite proteinase inhibitir with serine proteinases. Doklady Akademii Nauk SSSR 1988; 300:635-638.

9.   Shul'gin MN, Valueva TA, Kestere AY, Mosolov VV. Properties of duck ovomucoid purified by affinity chromatography on trypsin-sepharose. Biochimiya 1981; 46:473-481.

10. Bolton AE, Hunter WM. The labelling of proteins to high-specific radioactivities by conjugation to a (125)I-containing acylating agent. Biochem J 1973; 133:529-539.

11. Aho HJ, Koskensalo SML, Nevalainen TJ. Experimental pancreatitis in the rat. Sodium-taurocholat - induced acute haemorrhagic pancreatitis. Scand J Gastroenterology 1980; 15: 411- 416.

12. Kakade ML, Simons N, Liener GE. The evalution of natural vs synthetic substrates for measuring the antitryptic activity of soybean samples. Cereal Chem 1969; 46:518-526.

13. Penin VA, Vinogradov SI, Matveev NL. The method of acute pancreatitis diagnostic. Avtorskoye svidetel'stvo SSSR N 1334078 1989.

AAS 38/II
Recent Progress on Kinins
© 1992 Birkhäuser Verlag Basel

VASOACTIVE EFFECTS OF APROTININ

Allan D Cumming, Graham R Nimmo, Kathrine J Craig, Alastair McGilchrist, Peter C Hayes

University Department of Medicine, Royal Infirmary, Edinburgh, EH3 9YW, UK

SUMMARY: The protease inhibitor aprotinin was given **a)** in experimental septic shock, and **b)** in patients with hepatic cirrhosis and ascites, since in both conditions, activation of the plasma kallikrein-kinin system is associated with pathological systemic vasodilatation, which may trigger reflex neuroendocrine activation and renal solute retention. Given early in experimental sepsis, aprotinin maintained the arterial pressure, systemic vascular resistance (SVR), creatinine clearance and sodium excretion, all of which fell in controls. Aprotinin also blocked increases in pulmonary artery pressure and plasma renin activity (PRA). Given late in sepsis, aprotinin caused a rapid rise in arterial pressure and SVR towards baseline levels. In cirrhosis, aprotinin increased SVR in patients with low baseline values, and improved glomerular filtration rate, renal plasma flow and sodium excretion in all subjects; PRA was suppressed by aprotinin.
Aprotinin reverses pathological systemic vasodilatation in these two conditions, and this is associated with a reduction in renin release and improved renal function.

INTRODUCTION

Aprotinin is a broad spectrum protease inhibitor, manufactured as a purified extract of bovine lung [1]. It has previously been studied in a wide range of experimental and clinical states, but apart from the recently discovered action to reduce peroperative blood loss in cardiac surgery, it has proved disappointing as a therapeutic agent [2]. Recent reassessment of the appropriate dose regime has prompted further evaluation of its use [3].

In high doses, aprotinin binds to and inhibits active plasma kallikrein, the key enzyme in the plasma kinin-generating pathway [1,4]. Kinins are potent vasodilator substances, and can antagonise the constrictor effect of Angiotensin II at equimolar concentrations [5]. We were therefore interested in studying the effect of aprotinin in two disease states characterised by pathological systemic vasodilatation, namely septic shock and decompensated hepatic cirrhosis.

Septic shock is an important cause of morbidity, mortality and renal failure. The plasma kallikrein-kinin system is known to be activated in endotoxaemia and sepsis [6]. Kinins could mediate several important features of clinical sepsis - hypotension, systemic vasodilatation, increased capillary permeability, pulmonary vasoconstriction [7]. We therefore studied the effect of aprotinin on systemic and pulmonary haemodynamics and renal function, in a previously established ovine model of septic shock due to intraperitoneal sepsis [8].

Vasodilator systems are also activated in hepatic cirrhosis, and it has been proposed that peripheral arterial vasodilatation is the key event in causing sodium retention and ascites, perhaps by reflex activation of renin-angiotensin-aldosterone [9]. Plasma prekallikrein is known to be activated in hepatic cirrhosis [10]. We therefore hypothesised that inhibition of the plasma kallikrein-kinin system by aprotinin would increase systemic vascular resistance (SVR), suppress plasma renin activity (PRA), and increase sodium excretion in these patients.

MATERIALS AND METHODS

Aprotinin in septic shock

In these studies, septic shock was induced in anaesthetised sheep by the caecal ligation/puncture method of Brigham and Demling, as previously described [8]. Systemic haemodynamics were assessed using an arterial cannula and a Swann Ganz pulmonary artery catheter. In **Study 1**, aprotinin (or placebo in controls), was infused intravenously (6000 units/kg/hr) commencing 30 minutes after surgical induction of sepsis; there were 6 animals in both the treatment and control groups. In **Study 2**, aprotinin infusion was commenced, in 5 animals, once they had developed hypotensive septic shock (fall in MAP >40 mm Hg), resistant to volume expansion. A bolus of 10^6 KIU was given over 10 minutes, followed by 10^6 KIU per hour.

Aprotinin in hepatic cirrhosis

We studied 8 cirrhotic subjects with ascites; patients were in hospital, on no diuretics and taking 40 mmol dietary sodium daily. A standard renal clearance protocol was employed, and a Swann Ganz catheter inserted for haemodynamic measurements. Measurements were made before and during intravenous infusion of aprotonin (1×10^6 KIU stat, 1×10^6 KIU/hr for 2 hours).

PRA was measured by radioimmunoassay, and urinary kallikrein by a chromogenic substrate assay [11]. Treatment effects were assessed using analysis of variance.

RESULTS

Aprotinin in septic shock

Study 1 (pre treatment): In control animals (n=6), there were significant falls in mean arterial pressure (MAP) and systemic vascular resistance (SVR), an early increase in pulmonary artery pressure (PAP), and a reduction in creatinine clearance and urinary sodium excretion (**Table 1**). None of these changes were observed in aprotinin-treated animals (n=6). Significant treatment effects (between groups) were seen for MAP, PAP, and sodium excretion (p<0.05). Other haemodynamic and renal function parameters were similar in the two groups. Aprotinin treatment was associated with low urinary kallikrein excretion; the increase in plasma renin activity seen in controls did not occur. There were no apparent adverse effects.

Study 2 (intervention study): Infusion of aprotinin in the late stage of septic shock produced an immediate and rapid increase in MAP and SVR, in some cases virtually to pre-sepsis levels, with no significant change in cardiac output. The pressor effect ceased rapidly after discontinuing the infusion. Representative examples are shown in **Figures 1 and 2**, and summary data in **Table 2**.

Table 1. Changes in haemodynamics and renal function in control and treatment groups

	CONTROLS		APROTININ	
	baseline	sepsis	baseline	sepsis
Cardiac index (l/min/m²)	5.77 ±0.44	6.49 ±0.53	6.32 ±0.23	7.96 ±1.0
Mean arterial pressure (mm Hg)	103.8 ±3.6	66.8 ±5.4*	107.2 ±7.6	94.4 ±2.8**
SVR (dyne/sec/cm⁻⁵)	1394 ±82	582 ±154*	1404 ±151	1035 ±78
Pulmonary artery pressure (mm Hg)	13.4 ±1.2	25.2 ±3.4*	15.0 ±2.1	17.0 ±1.7**
Creatinine clearance (ml/min)	77 ±18	22 ±7*	87 ±11	47 ±16
Urinary kallikrein (nkat x 10⁻³/min)	2.7 ±1.4	1.7 ±0.9	1.8 ±1.0	0.7 ±0.5
PRA (ng/ml/hr)	0.21 ±0.01	6.34 ±0.92*	0.20 ±0.01	1.78 ±0.7**

* $p < 0.05$ from baseline ** $p < 0.05$ from controls   Mean ± SEM

Table 2. Acute pressor effect of aprotinin given late in the course of septic shock

	Change in MAP (mm Hg)	Change in SVR (dyne/sec/cm⁻⁵)
Baseline	0	0
Pre-aprotinin	- 53.8 ± 4.6	- 714 ± 75
During aprotinin	- 12.6 ± 5.0 *	- 281 ± 36 *
Post aprotinin	- 49.8 ± 10.8 **	- 636 ± 180 **

* $p < 0.01$ vs pre-aprotinin   ** $p < 0.01$ vs aprotinin

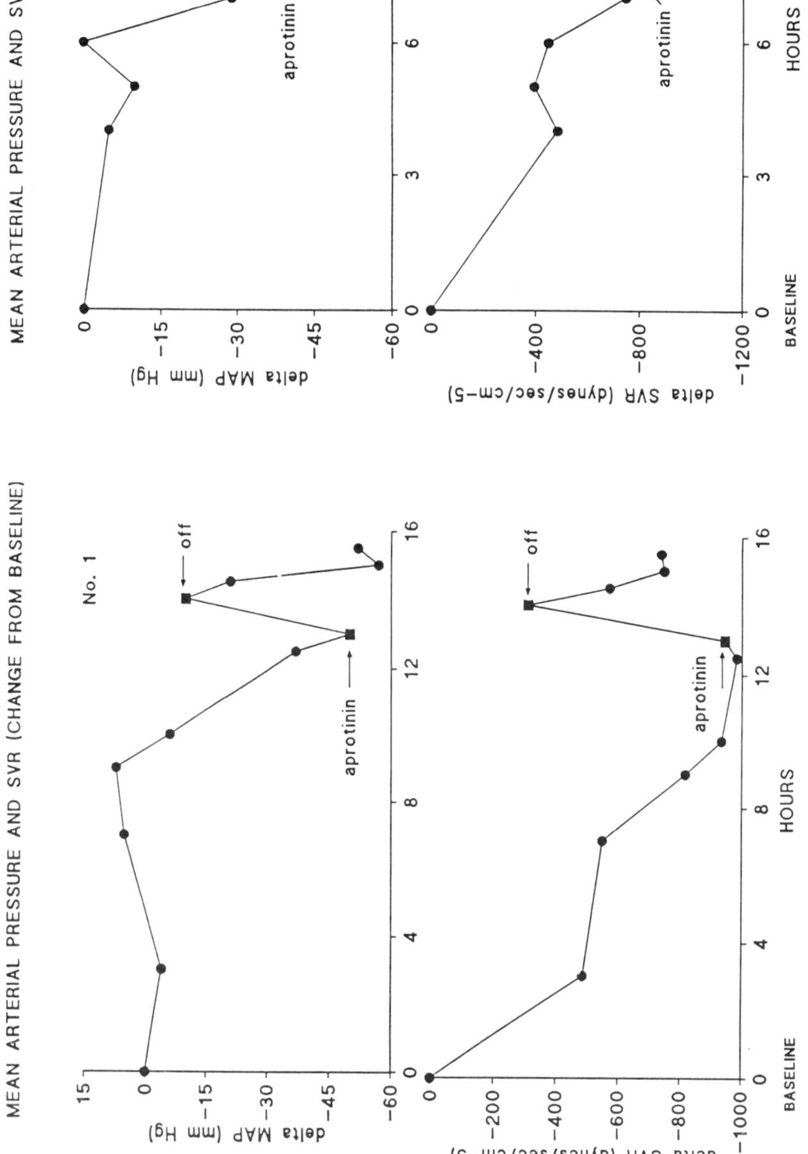

Figure 2. Change in mean arterial pressure and systemic vascular resistance during experimental septic shock.

Figure 1. Change in mean arterial pressure and systemic vascular resistance during experimental septic shock.

Aprotinin in hepatic cirrhosis

6 patients had low baseline SVR (<1200 dyne/sec/cm^{-5}). In 5 of these, SVR increased and cardiac output fell during aprotinin infusion (**Fig 3**). Renal plasma flow (PAH clearance) increased in all subjects (454 ± 54 to 663 ± 65 ml/min, $p<0.05$) and glomerular filtration rate (inulin clearance) increased (72 ± 10 to 121 ± 19 ml/min, $p<0.05$). Sodium excretion increased in 7 subjects, by a mean of 151% ($p<0.05$). PRA fell in all subjects (10.0 ± 2.9 to 5.9 ± 1.9 ng/ml/hr, $p<0.05$).

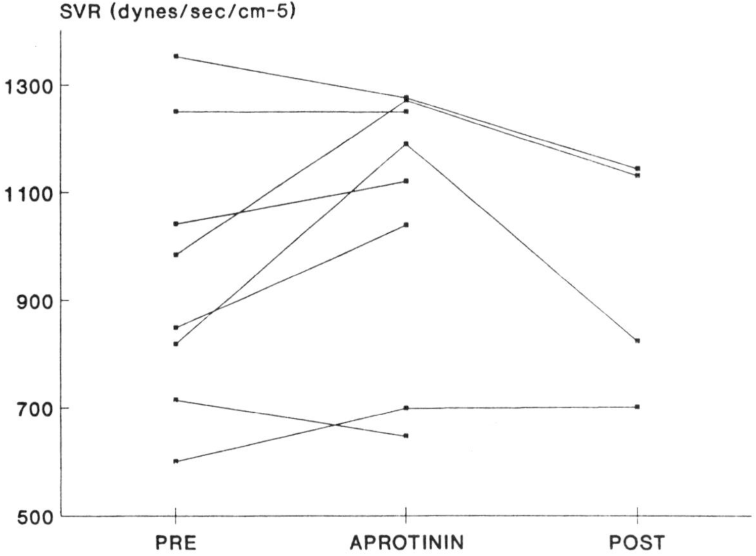

Figure 3. Change in systemic vascular resistance before, during and after aprotinin infusion in 8 patients with hepatic cirrhosis and ascites.

CONCLUSION

The results indicate that in two separate pathological states characterised by excessive systemic vasodilatation, aprotinin therapy is associated with an increase in systemic vascular resistance. In the experimental model which reproduces the important features of clinical **septic shock**, treatment with aprotinin shortly after the initiation of sepsis appeared to benefit systemic and pulmonary haemodynamics, renal function, and hormonal stimulation. In the sepsis intervention study, even more striking effects of aprotinin were observed, and the drug appeared to reverse almost completely the systemic haemodynamic changes of the fully-evolved sepsis syndrome. The observed haemodynamic improvement did not persist after the infusion was discontinued, suggesting that extremely high plasma levels are necessary for this effect; this is in keeping with the known pharmacokinetics of aprotinin [1, 3]. If reproduced in clinical practice, aprotinin could prove useful as a pressor agent, to allow time for conventional support therapy to take effect. It should be emphasised, however, that even the intervention study was carried out within 12 hours of the initiation of sepsis, and that to achieve comparability in clinical practice, aprotinin would have to be considered at an early stage, rather than as a treatment of last resort.

In **cirrhosis**, aprotinin infusion was associated with improved renal function, natriuresis, and suppression of PRA, with in most cases, detectable reduction in systemic vasodilatation. The findings suggest that in these patients, there is relative renal vasoconstriction, hypofiltration and sodium retention in response to the systemic haemodynamic changes. Overall the results are in keeping with the peripheral arterial vasodilatation theory of ascites formation as proposed by Schrier and others [9]. If this effect of aprotinin was sustained, then it could prove useful as an adjunctive therapy in cirrhotic patients who are frequently resistant to conventional diuretic treatment.

In both sets of studies, aprotinin was associated with a reduction in PRA. While this could reflect a reduction in vasodilatation-induced renin release, it is also possible that renal tissue kallikrein is involved in the activation of prorenin, and that this is inhibited by aprotinin [12]. It has been suggested that the renin-angiotensin system is important in the renal response to both sepsis [13] and cirrhosis [9], and the reduction in PRA could be partly responsible for the improved renal function observed in both studies.

Because of the broad inhibitory profile of aprotinin, it is not possible to ascribe the observed effects with certainty to any one enzyme system. However, both septic shock and hepatic cirrhosis have been clearly associated in previous studies with activation of the plasma kallikrein-kinin system [6, 10]. There is also striking similarity between the known biological effects of kallikrein-kinin activation and the clinical features seen in these conditions, which are reversed by aprotinin [5]. Similar results in experimental endotoxaemia in mice have recently been reported using a new selective kinin antagonist [14]. One can therefore speculate that at least some of the aprotinin effect is due to kallikrein inhibition. More potent inhibitors of plasma kallikrein are becoming available, and may prove even more effective in these conditions.

REFERENCES

1. Fritz H, Wunderer G: Biochemistry and applications of Aprotinin, the kallikrein inhibitor from bovine organs. Drug Research 1983; 33:479.

2. Traber DL, Adams T, Sziebert L et al: Failure of a protease inhibitor to affect the cardiopulmonary response to endotoxin when combined with a cycloxygenase inhibitor. Circ Shock 1984; 13:319.

3. Philipp E: Calculations and hypothetical considerations on the inhibition of plasmin and plasma kallikrein by Trasylol. In: Davidson JF, Rowan RM, Sanama MM, Desnoyers PC (eds): Progress in Chemical Fibrinolysis and Thrombolysis, Raven Press, New York, 1978, p 291.

4. Kaplan AP, Meier HL, Mandle RJ: The role of Hageman factor, prekallikrein and high molecular weight kininogen in the generation of bradykinin and the initiation of coagulation and fibrinolysis. Monographs in Allergy 1977; 12:120.

5. Regoli D, Barabe J: Pharmacology of bradykinin and related kinins. Pharmacol Rev 1980; 32:1.

6. O'Donnell TF, Clowes GHA, Talamo KC, et al: Kinin activation in the blood of patients with sepsis. Surg Gynaecol Obstet 1976; 143:539.

7. Robinson JA, Klodnycky ML, Loeb MS, et al: Endotoxin, prekallikrein, complement and systemic vascular resistance. Sequential measurements in man. Am J Med 1975; 59:61.

8. Cumming AD, Dreidger AA, McDonald JW, et al: Vasoactive hormones in the renal response to systemic sepsis. Am J Kidney Dis 1988; 11:23.

9. Schrier RW, Arroyo V, Bernardi M et al: Peripheral arterial vasodilation hypothesis: a proposal for the initiation of renal sodium and water retention in cirrhosis. Hepatology 1988; 8:1151.

10. Colman RW, Wong PY: Participation of Hageman factor dependent pathways in human disease states. Thromb Haemost 1977; 38:751.

11. Amundsen E, Putter J, Friberger P, et al: Methods for the determination of glandular kallikrein by means of a chromogenic tripeptide substrate. Adv Exp Med Biol 1979; 120A: 83.

12. Seto S, Kher V, Scicli AG, et al: The effect of aprotinin (a serine protease inhibitor) on renal function and renin release. Hypertension 1983; 5: 893.

13. Cumming AD, Kline R, Linton AL: Association between renal and sympathetic responses to non-hypotensive systemic sepsis. Crit Care Med 1988; 16:1132.

14. Noronha-Blob L, Prosser JC, Lowe VC et al: NPC17731 delays the onset of hypotension and reduces mortality in response to lethal doses of endotoxin in rats and mice. Abstracts, Kinin '91 Symposium, Munich, Germany, September 1991; p 365.

Coagulation and Fibrinolysis

THE CONTACT ACTIVATION PROTEINS: A STRUCTURE/FUNCTION OVERVIEW

Joost C. M. Meijers, Brad A. McMullen,[*] and Bonno N. Bouma

Dept. of Haematology, University Hospital Utrecht, the Netherlands and
[*]Dept. of Biochemistry, University of Washington, Seattle, Washington, U.S.A.

SUMMARY: In recent years, extensive knowledge has been obtained on the structure/function relationships of blood coagulation proteins. In this overview, we present recent developments on the structure/function relationships of the contact activation proteins: factor XII, high molecular weight kininogen, prekallikrein, and factor XI, with the emphasis on the localization of domains on these proteins that are involved in the interaction with activators, substrates and cofactors.

INTRODUCTION

Exposure of blood to negatively charged surfaces (collagen, kaolin, glass) results in the activation of the contact system of the intrinsic pathway of blood coagulation. The proteins involved in this contact reaction are: prekallikrein, factor XII, high molecular weight kininogen, and factor XI. The assembly of these components on a negatively charged surface leads to the activation of factor XI, thereby propagating the intrinsic coagulation pathway. Simultaneously, several other reactions occur such as the activation of factor VII and the initiation of the fibrinolytic system, the kinin-forming pathway, and the renin-angiotensin pathway.

The first step in the contact phase is the binding of factor XII to the negatively charged surface, which makes it highly susceptible for proteolysis by kallikrein (1-3). Prekallikrein is bound to high molecular weight kininogen in plasma. High molecular weight kininogen associates with a negatively charged surface, thereby localizing prekallikrein to this surface. Limited proteolysis by α-factor XIIa converts prekallikrein to kallikrein. Kallikrein can dissociate from the surface and act on surface-bound factor XII at distant sites, thereby propagating the reciprocal proteolytic cycle (4). Although there are other mechanisms for activation of either factor XII or prekallikrein, the reciprocal activation is the most important process under physiologic or pathophysiologic conditions.

Factor XI circulates in plasma in a complex with high molecular weight kininogen. High molecular weight kininogen links factor XI to a negatively charged surface. Factor XI is then activated by limited proteolysis by surface-bound α-factor XIIa.

<u>Alternative activation of factor XI</u>

Although the contact system is a powerful activator of factor XI *in vitro*, its role *in vivo* was doubted because of the lack of bleeding manifestations in patients deficient in either factor XII, prekallikrein or high molecular weight kininogen. Therefore, alternative activators of factor XI were thought to be present in plasma or provided by cells lining the vessel wall. Recently, two groups have shown that activation of factor XI by thrombin or by autoactivation by factor XIa can occur in the presence of appropriate negatively charged surfaces (5,6). However, the presence of high molecular weight kininogen was inhibitory for these reactions, and the surfaces used in these studies were non-physiological. Therefore, it remains unknown if a physiological surface for the activation of factor XI exists. The existence of a possible tissue activator for factor XI cannot be excluded.

STRUCTURE/FUNCTION OF CONTACT ACTIVATION PROTEINS

Over the last few years, considerable progress has been made in the elucidation of structure/function relationships of blood coagulation proteins. In this presentation, we would like to give an overview on the structure/function relationships of factor XI, factor XII, high molecular weight kininogen and prekallikrein as they have been obtained by protein and cDNA sequencing, monoclonal antibody studies and cDNA expression studies.

FACTOR XII

The structure of human factor XII has been established by amino acid sequence analysis and cDNA cloning (7-9). The mature protein consists of 596 amino acids, and consists of a number of different domains. Starting with the amino-terminal end of the protein, there is a fibronectin type II domain, a growth factor domain, a fibronectin type I domain, a second growth factor domain, a kringle domain, and a serine protease or catalytic domain (see Fig. 1). The cleavage site for the activation of factor XII by kallikrein was identified as an internal peptide bond between Arg-353 and Val-354. This results in the formation of a heavy chain (353 amino acids) and a light chain (243 amino acids), and these two chains are held together by a disulfide bond. The heavy chain is responsible for the binding of the protein to anionic surfaces during the contact activation reaction. With antibodies that block the binding of high molecular weight kininogen, and synthetic peptides, the putative surface-binding site on factor XII is located in the first 28 amino acids of the mature protein (10). Further cleavage of the heavy chain results in the formation of ß-factor XIIa. This consists of a nonapeptide (Asn-335 to Arg-343) disulfide linked to the light chain of factor XIIa.

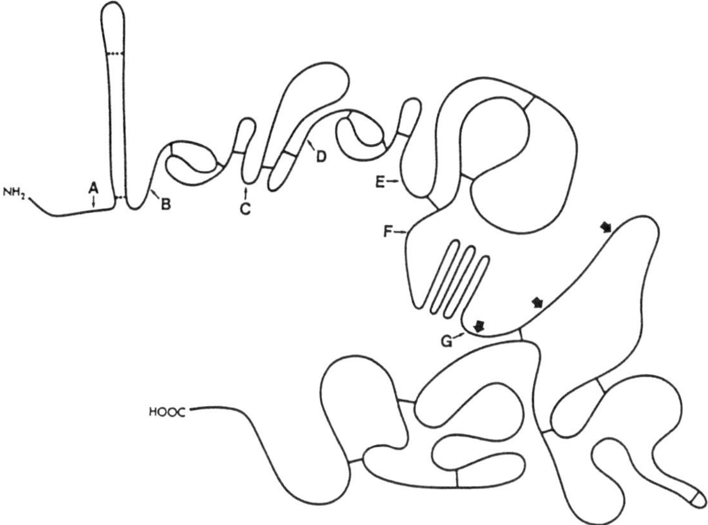

Figure 1. Structure of human factor XII. Thin arrows are drawn at positions of proposed structural domains. Region A-B represents a fibronectin type II homology; B-C and D-E are growth factor-like regions; C-D region is a fibronectin type I homology; region E-F is a kringle structure; F-G is a proline-rich region whose structure is undefined, and G-COOH represents the catalytic region. Kallikrein cleavage sites that give rise to ß-factor XIIa are indicated by the heavy arrows. Reprinted with permission from ref. 9.

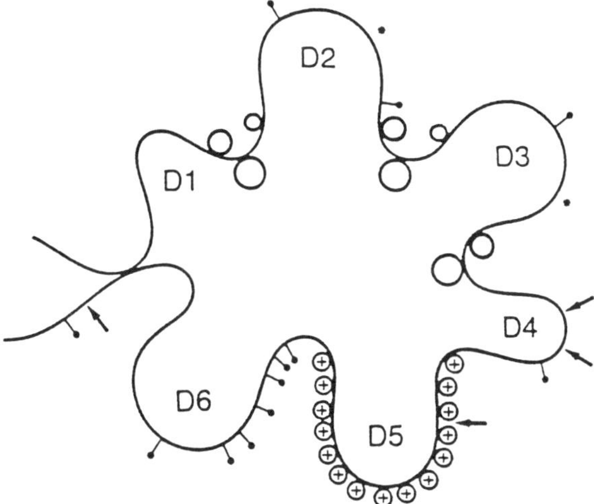

Figure 2. Structure of human high molecular weight kininogen. The domains are numbered D1-D6. The kallikrein cleavage sites are indicated by arrows. The putative reactive sites for cysteine proteinase inhibition are marked by asterisks. The D5-domain is rich in histidine, proline and lysine and is marked with +. Carbohydrate attachments sites are indicated by the ♀. Reprinted with permission from ref. 16.

The light chain of factor XIIa contains the catalytic portion of the enzyme, and shows considerable amino acid sequence homology with the catalytic domain of plasmin, tissue plasminogen activator, and urokinase (7). These findings suggest that factor XII may play a more significant role in fibrinolysis than in the coagulation cascade.

Inhibition of factor XIIa

The major inhibitor for both α- and ß-factor XIIa is C1 inhibitor. The inactivation of α-factor XIIa was studied by plasma inhibitors in a purified system and in plasma (11). C1 inhibitor was responsible for 91% of the inactivation of α-factor XIIa, with minor roles for α_2-antiplasmin, α_2-macroglobulin and antithrombin III.

Similarly, for the inhibition of ß-factor XIIa was C1 inhibitor the most efficient inhibitor. In plasma deficient in C1 inhibitor, the rate of inactivation of ß-factor XIIa was reduced to 13% compared to the inactivation of normal plasma (12).

HIGH MOLECULAR WEIGHT KININOGEN

The structure of high molecular weight kininogen was deduced by amino acid sequencing and cDNA sequence analysis (13-15). The mature protein consists of 626 amino acids. A complex domain structure has been proposed for high molecular weight kininogen (16, see Fig. 2), in which three domains (D1 to D3) constitute the heavy chain, and two of them (D2 and D3) form the structural units for cysteine protease inhibition (17,18). These domains are followed by a minidomain (D4) containing the kinin peptide, and two domains (D5 and D6) forming the high molecular weight kininogen light chain. Domain D5 is rich in histidine, proline, and lysine and anchors the protein to the negatively charged surface (19). The D6 domain is responsible for the interaction with prekallikrein and factor XI. The binding sites for prekallikrein and factor XI on high molecular weight kininogen were localized by fragmentation of high molecular weight kininogen, and sequence analysis of the peptides retaining affinity to prekallikrein (20). Both prekallikrein and factor XI bind to the same binding site, which was mapped to residues 565-595 (20,21). This binding site was confirmed by an elegant study by Vogel et al. (22), in which lambda-gt11 expression libraries were screened by a ligand assay. Recombinant fusion proteins of ß-galactosidase and high molecular weight kininogen were probed by unlabeled prekallikrein, followed by specific antibodies to prekallikrein. Synthetic peptides containing the binding site competed with the binding of prekallikrein and factor XI to high molecular weight kininogen. Also, a monoclonal antibody directed against a peptide of 27 residues covering the binding site interfered effectively with the binding of prekallikrein to high molecular weight kininogen. Furthermore, anti-idiotypic antibodies raised against this monoclonal antibody represented internal images of the prekallikrein-binding site of high molecular weight kininogen (22).

PREKALLIKREIN

The primary structure of prekallikrein was deduced by partial amino acid sequencing and cDNA sequence analysis (23, see Fig. 3). The amino acid sequence of prekallikrein shows 58% identity with factor XI. Prekallikrein consists of a mature polypeptide chain of 619 amino acids. The activation of prekallikrein to kallikrein by factor XIIa is due to the cleavage of the peptide bond following Arg-371. This generates kallikrein, an enzyme composed of a heavy chain (371 amino acids) and a light chain (248 amino acids), and these two chains are held together by a disulfide bond. The heavy chain of the molecule originates from the amino-terminal end of the zymogen and contains 4 tandem repeats of 90 or 91 amino acids. The disulfide structure of these repeats has recently been elucidated (24), and is identical to that of the repeats in factor XI. These repeats have been called apple domains. The functions of these domains in prekallikrein are not yet resolved. Van der Graaf et al. (25) localized the binding site for high molecular weight kininogen on the heavy chain of kallikrein. This was confirmed by studies with a monoclonal antibody to prekallikrein that blocked the interaction with high molecular weight kininogen (26). Page and Colman (27) have localized the binding sites of both high molecular weight kininogen and activated factor XII to a 28 kDa fragment of prekallikrein, encompassing amino acids 141-371. This fragment largely consists of the third and fourth apple domains. This is surprising, because the high molecular weight kininogen binding site on factor XI has been localized to the second half of the first apple domain (28). Further studies are necessary to define the binding sites of high molecular weight kininogen and factor XII on prekallikrein.

The light chain of kallikrein contains the three important amino acids (His-415, Asp-464, and Ser-559), that are directly involved in catalysis.

Inhibition of kallikrein

The inactivation of kallikrein was studied in normal plasma and plasmas deficient in inhibitors (29). In plasma deficient in C1 inhibitor the rate constant of the inactivation of kallikrein was only 10% of the rate constant in normal plasma, whereas the rate constant in α_2-macroglobulin deficient plasma was reduced to 63%. The absence of antithrombin III had little effect on the inactivation of kallikrein in plasma. Thus, C1 inhibitor and α_2-macroglobulin are the major inhibitors of kallikrein.

The kallikrein-inhibitor complexes in normal plasma and plasmas deficient in various inhibitors were analysed by SDS-polyacrylamide gel electrophoresis with ^{125}I-kallikrein (29). Calculation of the incorporation of radiolabeled kallikrein in the different complexes indicated that 35% of kallikrein formed a complex with α_2-macroglobulin, 52% with C1 inhibitor, and 13% with antithrombin III and an unidentified inhibitor in normal plasma (29), which is in agreement with the kinetic studies reported by Schapira et al. (30). The unidentified inhibitor was recently identified as protein C inhibitor (31). These data confirm that C1 inhibitor and α_2-macroglobulin are the major inhibitors of kallikrein in plasma.

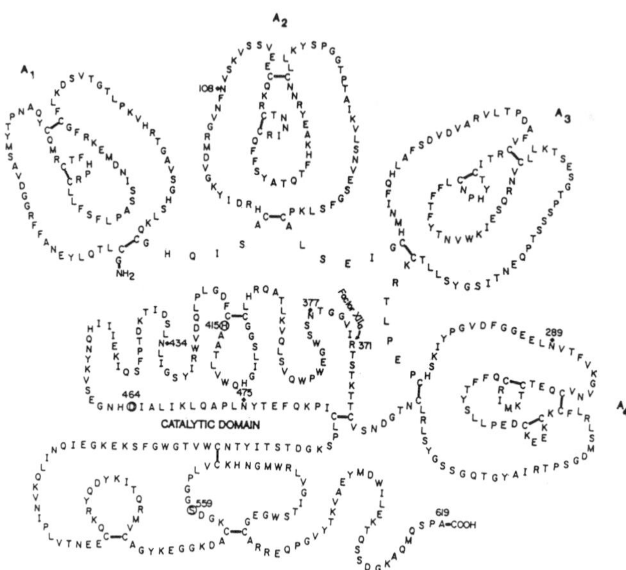

Figure 3. Structure of human plasma prekallikrein. The four apple domains in the amino-terminal portion of the molecule are labeled A_1, A_2, A_3, and A_4. The Arg-Ile bond that is cleaved by factor XIIa during the activation reaction is marked by a solid curved arrow. The circled residues (His-415, Asp-464, and Ser-559) are members of the catalytic triad characteristic of serine proteases. The Asn residues marked by solid diamonds (residues 108, 289, 377, 434, and 475) are attachment sites for carbohydrate chains. Reprinted with permission from ref. 24.

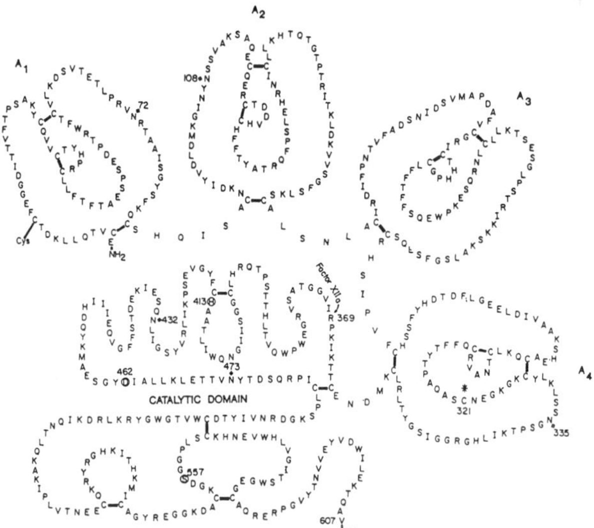

Figure 4. Structure of human factor XI. The four apple domains in the amino-terminal portion of the protein are labeled A_1, A_2, A_3, and A_4. The asterisk on Cys-321 in the fourth apple domain identifies the disulfide bond between two identical subunits. The Arg-Ile bond that is cleaved by factor XIIa or thrombin during the activation reaction is marked by a curved arrow. The circled residues (His-413, Asp-462, and Ser-557) are members of the catalytic triad typical of serine proteases. The solid diamonds on Asn residues at positions 72, 108, 432, and 473 indicate carbohydrate sites. The open diamond on Asn-335 indicates that this potential carbohydrate attachment site is not glycosylated. Reprinted with permission from ref. 33.

FACTOR XI

The primary structure of factor XI was deduced by partial amino acid sequencing and cDNA sequence analysis (32, see Fig. 4). The amino acid sequence of factor XI shows 58% identity with human plasma prekallikrein.

Factor XI consists of two identical polypeptide chains of 607 amino acids. The cleavage site for the activation of factor XI by factor XIIa (or thrombin) was identified as an internal peptide bond between Arg-369 and Ile-370 in each polypeptide chain. This results in the formation of two heavy chains and two light chains which are still held together by disulfide bonds. Each heavy chain of factor XIa (369 amino acids) was found to contain 4 tandem repeats of 90 (or 91) amino acids. Each of these repeats contain six cysteine residues that are linked in a typical 1-6, 2-5, 3-4 fashion (33). These domains have been called apple domains. Apple domains also occur in prekallikrein (24), but have not been identified in any other protein.

The light chains of factor XIa (each 238 amino acids) contain the catalytic portion of the enzyme with sequences that are typical of the trypsin family of serine proteases. Each molecule of factor XIa contains two active sites (34,35). Both active sites can be inhibited by inhibitors, such as antithrombin III (34,36), C1 inhibitor (37), and protein C inhibitor (31).

Dimerization of factor XI

The first and fourth apple domain of factor XI contain an extra Cys-residue, which were thought to be involved in the formation of the dimer (32). However, the Cys-residue in the first apple, Cys-11, was found to be linked to a single Cys-residue (33). The dimer was formed by linkage of the extra Cys-residue (Cys-321) of the fourth apple domain to a Cys-321 of another fourth apple domain (33). These results were confirmed by in vitro expression of the factor XI cDNA. Mutation of Cys-11 to Ser still resulted in the expression of a dimeric molecule, while mutation of Cys-321 to Ser resulted in the appearance of a monomeric factor XI on SDS-PAGE (38). However, this mutant exhibited dimeric properties in gel filtration studies, indicating a non-covalent association of the monomers of factor XI (38). The dimerization process appears to be an important step in the intracellular processing and secretion of the molecule. *In vitro* expression studies with naturally occurring factor XI mutants showed decreased or no secretion of the mutant molecule when the intracellular dimerization was partially or totally blocked (39,40). The physiological role of the disulfide link, or the reason for factor XI to be a dimer remain to be investigated.

Glycosylation of factor XI

Five potential Asn-linked carbohydrate attachment sites are present in the factor XI monomer.

Table I. Amino Acid Sequence of Peptides of factor XI Containing Potential Carbohydrate-Attachment Sites

CNB1-T2	V (N) R
CNB1-T5	K G I N Y (N) S S V A K
CNB1-T20-D/T3	L S S N G S P T K
CNB2-T16/22-6	V Y S G I L (N) Q S E I K E D
	D N E X T T K
CNB2-T10	
	L E T T V (N) Y T D S Q R P I X L P S K G D R

Peptides were obtained in a previous study (33). (N) denotes asparagine from published sequence, but was not detected. X is Cys as determined from the cDNA sequence (32)

These are located at residues 72, 108 and 335 of the heavy chain and 432 and 473 of the light chain. Glycosylation of these residues was demonstrated by protein sequencing of peptides obtained in a previous study (33). The sequence of each of these peptides was determined (Table I). Glycosylated asparagine residues were assigned to the positions indicated for the following reasons. First, the cDNA sequence as reported (32) agrees with the asparagine assignments. Second, in all cases, the potential attachment site was followed by the sequence of X-(T/S). Accordingly, four out of five potential Asn-linked carbohydrate attachment sites were identified to be glycosylated. Only Asn-335 in the heavy chain of factor XIa was not glycosylated. This amino acid is located in the fourth apple domain, the domain that is responsible for dimer formation (33,38).

Interaction of factor XI with high molecular weight kininogen

Factor XI in plasma is non-covalently bound to high molecular weight kininogen (41). Van der Graaf et al. (42) were able to locate the binding site for high molecular weight kininogen on the heavy chain of factor XIa. They isolated the active light chain of factor XIa by affinity-adsorption of heavy chain containing fragments on a resin to which high-molecular weight kininogen was coupled. Studies with monoclonal antibodies corroborated that the heavy chain of factor XIa is responsible for the binding of high molecular weight kininogen (43,44) Recent studies with peptides from factor XI showed the binding-site for high molecular weight kininogen to be on a region from Phe-56 through Ser-86 (28). This is the second part of the first apple domain in factor XI.

Interaction of factor XI with factor IX

Although the light chain of factor XIa contains the active site of the molecule, it was found that the heavy chain of factor XIa was required for activation of factor IX (42). This suggested the presence of a factor IX binding site on the heavy chain of factor XIa. This has been confirmed with monoclonal antibodies that blocked the activation of factor IX (44). Recently, a further localization of the factor IX binding site suggested that the second apple domain of factor XI, and in particular the region of Asn-145 to Ala-175, is important in the interaction of factor IX with factor XIa (46).

<u>Inhibition of factor XIa</u>

Regulation of the activity of factor XIa occurs by plasma proteinase inhibitors. Several inhibitors have been shown to inhibit the activity of factor XIa: C1 inhibitor (47), antithrombin III (48), α_1-antitrypsin (49), α_2-antiplasmin (50), and protein C inhibitor (31). In kinetic experiments, Scott et al. (51) found a predominant role for α_1-antitrypsin (68%), with minor roles for antithrombin III, C1 inhibitor and α_2-antiplasmin with 16, 8 and 8% of the factor XIa inhibition, respectively. Using inhibitor deficient plasmas, we have also studied the kinetics of inactivation of factor XIa. α_1-Antitrypsin was the major inhibitor accounting for 35% of the factor XIa inhibition, and C1 inhibitor and antithrombin III accounted for 24 and 15%, respectively (52).

Recently, Smith et al. (53) purified an inhibitor of factor XI from platelets, that was shown to be a truncated form of the Alzheimer amyloid precursor protein. Platelets also contain a low molecular weight inhibitor of factor XIa, PIXI (54). The role of these inhibitors, if any, in the regulation of factor XI is not yet known.

REFERENCES

1. Bagdasarian A, Talamo RC, Colman RW. Isolation of high-molecular weight activators of prekallikrein. J Biol Chem 1973; 248:3456-3463.

2. Cochrane CG, Revak SD, Wuepper KD. Activation of Hageman factor in solid and fluid phases. A critical role of kallikrein. J Exp Med 1973; 138:1564-1583.

3. Griffin JH. Role of surface in surface-dependent activation of Hageman factor (blood coagulation factor XII). Proc Natl Acad Sci USA 1978; 75:1998-2002.

4. Cochrane CG, Revak SD. Dissemination of contact activation in plasma by plasma kallikrein. J Exp Med 1980; 152:608-619.

5. Naito K, Fujikawa K. Activation of human blood coagulation factor XI independent of factor XII. Factor XI is activated by thrombin and factor XIa in the presence of negatively charged surfaces. J Biol Chem 1991; 266:7353-7358.

6. Gailani D, Broze Jr GJ. Factor XI activation in a revised model of blood coagulation. Science 1991; 253:909-912.

7. Fujikawa K, McMullen BA. Amino acid sequence of human ß-factor XIIa. J Biol Chem 1983; 258:10924-10933.

8. McMullen BA, Fujikawa K. Amino acid sequence of the heavy chain of human α-factor XIIa (activated Hageman factor) J Biol Chem 1985; 260:5328-5341.

9. Cool DE, Edgell CJS, Louie GV, Zolle MJ, Brayer GD, MacGillavray RTA. Characterization of human blood coagulation factor XII. Prediction of the primary structure of factor XII and the tertiary structure of ß-factor XIIa. J Biol Chem 1985; 260:13666-13676.

10. Clarke BJ, Cote HCF, Cool DE, Clark-Lewis I, Saito H, Pixley RA, Colman RW, MacGillivray RTA. Mapping of a putative surface-binding site of human coagulation factor XII. J Biol Chem 1989; 264:11497-11502.

11. Pixley RA, Schapira M, Colman RW. The regulation of human factor XIIa by plasma proteinase inhibitors. J Biol Chem 1985; 260:1723-1729.

12. De Agostini A, Lijnen HR, Pixley RA, Colman RW, Schapira M. Inactivation of factor XII active fragment in normal plasma. Predominant role of C1 inhibitor. J Clin Invest 1984; 73:1542-1549.

13. Takagaki Y, Kitamura N, Nakanishi S. Cloning and sequence analysis of cDNAs for human high molecular weight and low molecular weight prekininogens. Primary structure of two human prekininogens. J Biol Chem 1985; 260:8601-8609.

14. Lottspeich F, Kellerman J, Henschen A, Foertsch B, Müller-Esterl W. The amino acid sequence of the light chain of human high-molecular-mass kininogen. Eur J Biochem 1985; 152:307-314.

15. Kellerman J, Lottspeich F, Henschen A, Müller-Esterl W. Completion of the primary structure of human-high-molecular-mass kininogen. The amino acid sequence of the entire heavy chain and evidence for its evolution by gene triplication. Eur J Biochem 1986; 154:471-478.

16. Müller-Esterl W, Iwanaga S, Nakanishi S. Kininogens revisited. TIBS 1986; 11:336-339.

17. Salvesen G, Parkes C, Abrahamson M, Grubb A, Barrett AJ. Human low-Mr kininogen contains three copies of a cystatin sequence that are divergent in structure and in inhibitory activity for cysteine proteases. Biochem J 1986; 234:429-434.

18. Vogel R, Assfalg-Machleidt I, Esterl A, Machleidt W, Müller-Esterl W. Proteinase-sensitive regions in the heavy chain of low molecular weight kininogen map to the inter-domain junctions. J Biol Chem 1988; 263:12661-12668.

19. Iwanaga S, Kato H, Sugo T, Ikari N, Hashimoto N, Fujii S. In: Biological Functions of Proteinases. Holzer H, Tschesche H, editors. Berlin: Springer Verlag, 1979: 243-259.

20. Tait JF, Fujikawa K. Identification of the binding site for plasma prekallikrein in human high molecular weight kininogen. A region from residues 185 to 224 of the kininogen light chain retains full binding activity. J Biol Chem 1986; 261:15396-15401.

21. Tait JF, Fujikawa K. Primary structure requirements for the binding of human high molecular weight kininogen to plasma prekallikrein and factor XI. J Biol Chem 1987; 262:11651-11656.

22. Vogel R, Kaufman J, Chung DW, Kellerman J, Müller-Esterl W. Mapping of the prekallikrein-binding site of human H-kininogen by ligand screening of lambda-gt11 expression libraries. Mimicking of the predicted binding site by anti-idiotypic antibodies. J Biol Chem 1990; 265:12494-12502.

23. Chung DW, Fujikawa K, McMullen BA, Davie EW. Human plasma prekallikrein: A zymogen to a serine protease that contains four tandem repeats. Biochemistry 1986; 25:2410-2417.

24. McMullen BA, Fujikawa K, Davie EW. Location of the disulfide bonds in human plasma prekallikrein: The presence of four novel apple domains in the amino-terminal portion of the molecule. Biochemistry 1991; 30:2050-2056.

25.   Van der Graaf F, Tans G, Bouma BN, Griffin JH. Isolation and functional properties of the heavy and light chains of human plasma kallikrein. J Biol Chem 1982; 257:14300-14305.

26.   Hock J, Vogel R, Linke RP, Müller-Esterl W. High molecular weight kininogen-binding site of prekallikrein probed by monoclonal antibodies. J Biol Chem 1990; 265:12005-12011.

27.   Page JD, Colman RW. Localization of distinct functional domains on prekallikrein for interaction with both high molecular weight kininogen and activated factor XII in a 28-kDa fragment (amino acids 141-371). J Biol Chem 1991; 266:8143-8148.

28.   Baglia FA, Jameson BA, Walsh PN. Localization of the high molecular weight kininogen binding site in the heavy chain of human factor XI to amino acids phenylalanine 56 though serine 86. J Biol Chem 1990; 265:4149-4154.

29.   Van der Graaf F, Koedam JA, Bouma BN. Inactivation of kallikrein in human plasma. J Clin Invest 1983; 73:149-158.

30.   Schapira M, Scott CF, Colman RW. Contribution of plasma protease inhibitors to the inactivation of kallikrein in plasma. J Clin Invest 1982; 69:462-468.

31.   Meijers JCM, Kanters DHAJ, Vlooswijk RAA, van Erp HE, Hessing M, Bouma BN. Inactivation of human plasma kallikrein and factor XIa by protein C inhibitor. Biochemistry 1988; 27:4231-4237.

32.   Fujikawa K, Chung DW, Hendrickson LE, Davie EW. Amino acid sequence of human factor XI, a blood coagulation factor with four tandem repeats that are highly homologous with plasma prekallikrein. Biochemistry 1986; 25:2417-2424.

33.   McMullen BA, Fujikawa K, Davie EW. Location of the disulfide bonds in human coagulation factor XI: The presence of tandem apple domains. Biochemistry 1991; 30:2056-2060.

34.   Kurachi K, Davie EW. Activation of human factor XI (plasma thromboplastin antecedent) by factor XIIa (activated Hageman factor). Biochemistry 1977; 16:5831-5839.

35.   Bouma BN, Griffin JH. Human blood coagulation factor XI: Purification, properties, and mechanism of activation by activated factor XII. J Biol Chem 1977; 252:6432-6437.

36.   Soons H, Janssen-Claessen T, Tans G, Hemker HC. Inhibition of factor XIa by antithrombin III. Biochemistry 1987; 26:4624-4629.

37.   Meijers JCM, Vlooswijk RAA, Bouma BN. Inhibition of human blood coagulation factor XIa by C1 inhibitor. Biochemistry 1988; 27:959-963.

38.   Meijers JCM, Mulvihill ER, Davie EW, Chung DW. Apple four in human blood coagulation factor XI mediates dimer formation. Biochemistry 1992, in press.

39.   Meijers JCM, Davie EW, Chung DW. Expression of human blood coagulation factor XI: Characterization of the defect in factor XI type III deficiency. Blood 1992, in press.

40.   Asakai R, Meijers JCM, Davie EW, Chung DW. unpublished results.

41.   Thompson RE, Mandle Jr R, Kaplan AP. Association of factor XI and high molecular weight kininogen in human plasma. J Clin Invest 1977; 60:1376-1380.

42.   Van der Graaf F, Greengard JS, Bouma BN, Kerbiriou DM, Griffin JH. Isolation and functional characterization of the active light chain of activated human blood coagulation factor XI. J Biol Chem 1983; 258:9669-9675.

43.   Sinha D, Koshy A, Seaman FS, Walsh PN. Functional characterization of human blood coagulation factor XIa using hybridoma antibodies. J Biol Chem 1985; 260:10714-10719.

44.   Baglia FA, Sinha D, Walsh PN. Functional domains in the heavy-chain region of factor XI: A high molecular weight kininogen-binding site and a substrate-binding site for factor IX. Blood 1989; 74:244-251.

45.   Baglia FA, Jameson BA, Walsh PN. Identification and chemical synthesis of a substrate-binding site for factor IX on coagulation factor XIa. J Biol Chem 1991; 266:24190-24197.

46.   Forbes CD, Pensky J, Ratnoff OD. Inhibition of activated Hageman factor and activated plasma thromboplastin antecedent by purified C1 inactivator. J Lab Clin Med 1970; 76:809-815.

47.   Damus DS, Hicks M, Rosenberg RD. Anticoagulant activity of heparin. Nature (London) 1973; 246:355-357.

48.   Heck LW, Kaplan AP. Substrates of Hageman factor. I. Isolation and characterization of human factor XI (PTA) and inhibition of the activated enzyme by α1-antitrypsin. J Exp Med 1974; 140:1615-1630.

49.   Saito H, Goldsmith GH, Moroi M, Aoki N. Inhibitory spectrum of α2-plasmin inhibitor. Proc Natl Acad Sci USA 1979; 76:2013-2017.

50.   Scott CF, Schapira M, James HL, Cohen AB, Colman RW. Inactivation of factor XIa by plasma protease inhibitors. Predominant role of α1-protease inhibitor and protective effect of high molecular weight kininogen. J Clin Invest 1982; 69:844-852.

51.   Meijers JCM, Bouma BN. The relationship between the contact system and the protein C pathway. In: The Kallikrein-Kinin System in Health and Disease. Fritz H, Schmidt I, Dietze G, editors. Braunschweig: Limbach-Verlag, 1989: 277-288.

52.   Smith RP, Higuchi DA, Broze Jr GJ. Platelet coagulation factor XIa-inhibitor, a form of Alzheimer amyloid precursor protein. Science 1991; 248:1126-1128.

53.   Cronlund AL, Walsh PN. A low molecular weight platelet inhibitor of factor XIa: Purification, characterization and possible role in blood coagulation. Biochemistry 1992; 31: 1685-1694.

Factors Affecting the Rate of Contact Activation in Human Plasma

Tilo Brunnée, Gayle Coy, Sesha R. Reddigari and Michael Silverberg

Division of Allergy, Rheumatology and Clinical Immunology, Department of Medicine, Health Sciences Center, State University of New York at Stony Brook, Stony Brook, N.Y. 11794-8161, USA

Summary

The rate of high molecular weight kininogen cleavage in human plasma treated with dextran sulfate depends largely on the length of preincubation at 37°C and the sample size during preincubation. The longer the preincubation with aliquots < 100 µl, the more refractory to contact activation the plasma became. This effect is not due to prekallikrein or factor XII consumption/inhibition since both proteins are functional in clotting assays and detectable in immunoblots even after prolonged incubation times at 37°C.

Introduction

Contact activation of blood plasma is initiated when the plasma proteins Factor XII, prekallikrein, and high molecular weight kininogen interact with negatively charged solids like glass[1] or kaolin[2], colloids like ellagic acid/metal ion complexes[3] or soluble polyanions such as dextran sulfate (DS) or heparin[4]. Consequences of this process include the initiation of the intrinsic coagulation pathway and bradykinin generation. Dextran sulfate has become widely used in studies of contact activation since it is easily quantitated and the only true soluble contact activator known. The aim of this study was to find conditions under which contact activation in whole plasma gave reproducible kinetics. Since bradykinin in plasma has a very short halflife due to the action of kininases we monitored the cleavage of the substrate from which it is derived. The rate of appearance of cleaved high molecular weight kininogen, monitored by immunoblots[5], was used as a measure of the rate of kallikrein generation and compared with clotting assays for Prekallikrein and Factor XII.

Methods

Blood was drawn in Na_3-Citrate prefilled syringes (0.36 % final conc.), immediately centrifuged (3600 rpm, 15 min) and the plasma was stored in aliquots at –70°C. In order to minimize the exposure of plasma to warmth, aliquots of frozen plasma were thawed in ice water. All experiments were carried out in EDTA-washed polypropylene tubes to avoid contamination with metal ions. Before the addition of DS the samples were placed in a 37°C water bath; we determined with a needle temperature probe that fluid aliquots of 200 µl reached 30°C within 30 seconds and 37°C within 1 minute. Dextran sulfate (MW 500,000) was made 10 mg/ml in 10 mM EDTA, diluted 1:10 in H_2O, and then diluted further to the required concentration so that a 1/10 volume added to plasma gave the desired final concentrations. After various incubation times the DS treated plasma was added to boiling, non reducing, SDS buffer, and separated by SDS-PAGE. The proteins were transferred to nitrocellulose, immunoblotted with a mouse monoclonal antibody against the light chain of high molecular weight kininogen[5] or a rabbit polyclonal antibody against Factor XII with crossreactivity against Factor XIIa/XIIf. Clotting assays were performed with commercially available prekallikrein or factor XII deficient plasma.

Results

We have shown previously that plasma was more susceptible to activation by dextran sulfate at 0°C than at 37°C[6]. When we attempted to determine more precisely the effect of DS concentration on the rate of activation of plasma at 37°C we obtained results that were not at all reproducible. We investigated as many parameters of the reaction as we could identify. Finally, we discovered that two conditions had an unexpectedly strong influence on the rate of cleavage of HK. The first observation was that the longer plasma was incubated at 37°C before the addition of DS the more refractory to activation it became. The second factor was the sample size—the aformentioned phenomenon only occurred in small (50 µl or less) aliquots.

Effect of Preincubation Time

In order to control the time of exposure of the plasma to 37°C, aliquots of frozen plasma were thawed in ice water. The thawed plasma samples were then transferred to 37°C and incubated for measured preincubation times; under these conditions, the plasma reached 37°C within 1 minute. DS solution was then added to give the desired final concentration and samples taken for gel analysis at various times as shown below. DS at 15 µg/ml gave complete cleavage of HK in 5 minutes; less DS did not cause cleavage. This compares with our earlier result in which plasma treated with DS in the

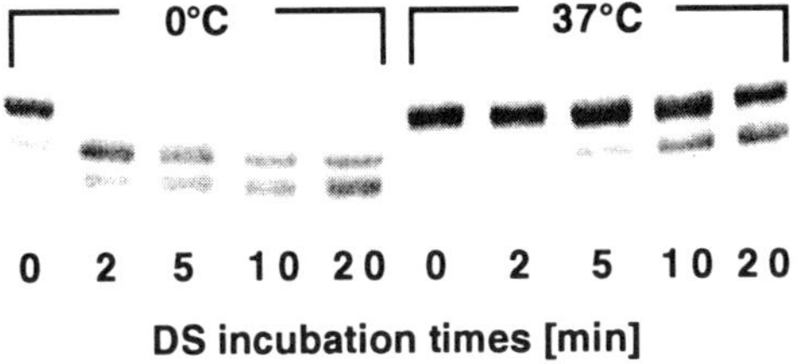

Figure 1: High molecular weight kininogen blot of normal human plasma, preincubated for 2 h 45 min at 0°C and 37°C, activation with 100 µg/ml dextran sulfate [MW 500,000] with varied incubation times at 37°C.

cold showed cleavage with only 5 µg/ml DS[6]. When the time of preincubation was prolonged, however, the results were different; much greater concentrations of DS and longer times were needed to induce HK cleavage.

Figure 1 is an immunoblot that shows the rate of HK cleavage in plasma samples treated with 100 µg/ml DS at 37°C after preincubation for 2 h 45 min at either 0°C or 37°C. While the plasma that was preincubated in the cold showed complete cleavage in 2 minutes, the plasma incubated at 37°C showed only partial cleavage after 30 minutes. We thought that this might be due to a loss of either factor XII or prekallikrein during the long preincubation but there was no significant diminution in the clotting activities of prekallikrein and factor XII in either sample (Table 1).

Table 1
Clotting assays of normal human plasma,
incubated for 2 h 45 min at 37 °C

n=6	U/ml (mean ± SD)
Factor XII	0.82 ± 0.19
Prekallikrein	0.87 ± 0.26

Immunoblots with a prekallikrein antibody did not show the creation of a kallikrein—C$\overline{\text{I}}$-INH complex. Blotting with a F XII/F XIIa polyclonal antibody showed no traces of F XIIa generation during prolonged preincubation times. Therefore, we concluded that the loss of activatability was not due to a significant loss of either zymogen. The loss of the ability to cleave HK did not require such long incubations, however, since this could be demonstrated after only 10–15 minutes of

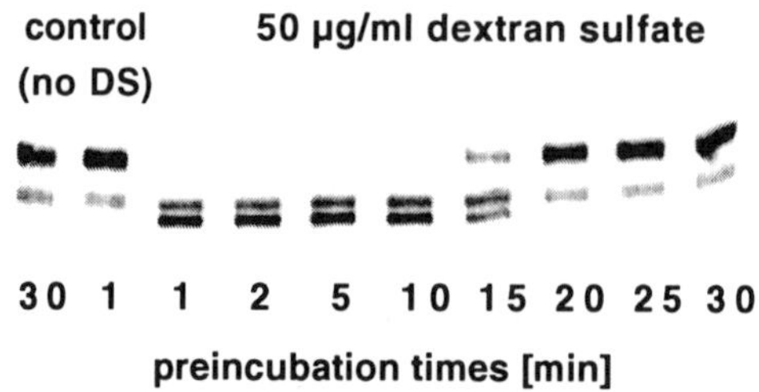

Figure 2: High molecular weight kininogen blot of normal human plasma, pre-incubated at 37°C for varied times, activation with 50 µg/ml dextran sulfate [MW 500,000] for 15 minutes at 37°C.

incubation at 37°C. There was a correlation between the time of the preincubation and the concentration of DS required to induce cleavage of HK; at any given [DS], the rate of activation was inversely correlated with the time of preincubation.

The extent of cleavage after a 15 minute incubation with 50 µg/ml DS following preincubation times varying from 1 to 30 minutes is shown in figure 2. It is clear that as the time of exposure to 37°C increases, less subsequent cleavage is seen. The time required for loss of activatability while quite short, is much longer than the time for the plasma to reach 37°C.

Effect of Sample Size

When we attempted to scale-up our initial experiments, we found that the phenomenon of increasing refractibility disappeared. The effect of sample size was reproducible. Experiments with small (≈50 µl) aliquots of plasma gave the results described above. Larger (>100 µl) aliquots incubated under the same conditions for over 2 hours retained their susceptibility to cleavage with DS.

Figure 3 shows two immunoblots combining the results from three aliquots, 40 µl preincubated at 0°C, 40µl preincubated at 37°C and 400 µl preincubated at 37°C. It is readily apparent that only the small sample incubated at 37 °C loses its susceptibility to activation. The effect of sample size is a function of the preincubation conditions because a 40 µl aliquot was removed for the reaction with DS in all samples. This phenomenon is not apparently due to the oxidation of some plasma component because small samples preincubated at 37°C under nitrogen were not cleaved upon subsequent activation with DS.

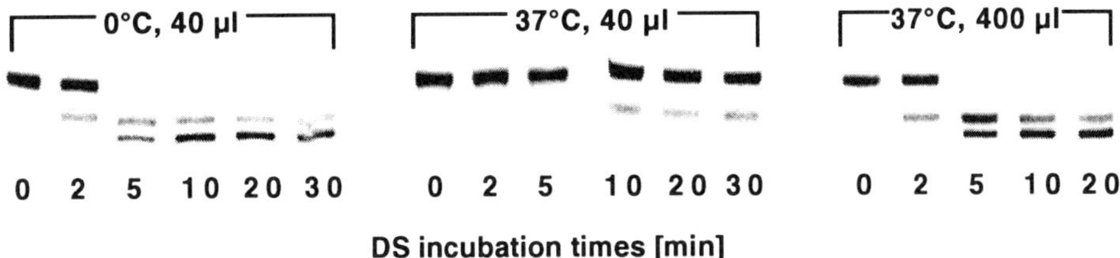

Figure 3: High molecular weight kininogen blot, different sizes of normal human plasma, preincubated for 2 h 15 min at 0°C and 37°C, activation with 100 µg/ml dextran sulfate [MW 500,000] with varied incubation times at 37°C.

Discussion

In order to investigate the kinetics of the contact activation system in whole plasma it is neccessary to find conditions in which the process occurs reproducibly. Although one must expect variability in a complex biological tissue such as blood plasma, we expected that the response of pooled normal human plasma to dextran sulfate would show only limited variability in terms of the concentration and time required to accomplish cleavage of HK. Our initial results, however, showed considerable variation, to the extent of being essentially non-reproducible. We would note that within any given experiment the results were totally rational, i.e the degree of cleavage increased as a function of time or DS concentration. It was only as we accummulated data from multiple experiments that we realized that the dependence of the rate of activation on these two parameters was not reproducible.

This induced us to attempt to find the sources of variation which we assumed to be artifacts of some kind. Our first suspicion was that the use of disposable plastic tubes direct from the box could potentially introduce heavy metal ion contamination. Accordingly, we boiled all of our tubes in EDTA and made the first DS stock solution in EDTA. This eliminated some of the variation, but we still found that the rate of cleavage could vary markedly from experiment to experiment. Finally, we identified the two phenomena described in this paper as having marked and unexpected effects on the rate of contact activation. The effect of temperature is a significant potential artifact because one's assumption is that plasma at 37°C is in a relatively "natural" state and therefore should be stable. When we first discovered that preincubation markedly decreased the rate of activation, we thought that a hysteretic effect of temperature on C$\overline{\text{I}}$ -INH was responsible for an increased susceptibility to activation in plasma that was newly warmed from 0°C and that the less-reactive plasma showed the natural susceptibility to activation. Fresh plasma however, without cooling, behaves like plasma freshly thawed on ice, and preincubated plasma recooled to 0°C does not regain its reactivity. We must conclude, therefore, that the incubation at 37°C results in some irreversible change from the original state of normal human plasma. The effect of the size of the sample on the effect suggests that it is a function of the ratio of surface area to volume. The ineffectiveness of a nitrogen atmosphere in preventing the effect would appear to rule out the oxidation of some plasma component as the cause. We are led to surmise, therefore, that the absorption of some plasma component to the walls of the tube is responsible for the loss of reactivity. There is no measurable loss of zymogen factor XII or prekallikrein, however, as measured by clotting assay and the immunoblot shows that the HK is not appreciably dimished.

Presently, therefore, we have not been able to establish the cause for these effects but by awareness of their existence it is possible to obtain reproducible activation kinetics for plasma treated with DS. The results of these experiments show that the concentrations of DS able to give rapid cleavage of HK at physiological temperatures are much lower than previously realized.

References

1. Margolis, J. Glass surface and blood coagulation, Nature 1956; 178: 805-806.
2. Proctor, RR & Rapaport, SJ. The partial thromboplastin time with kaolin: a simple screening test for first stage clotting deficiencies, Am J Clin Pathol 1961; 35: 212.
3. Bock, PE, Srinivasan, KR & Shore, JD. Activation of intrinsic blood coagulation by ellagic acid: insoluble ellagic acid metal ion complexes are the activating species, Biochemistry 1981; 20: 7258-7271.
4. Silverberg, M & Diehl, SV. The autoactivation of factor XII (Hageman factor) induced by low Mr heparin and dextran sulphate, Biochem. J. 1987; 248: 715-720.
5. Reddigari, SR & Kaplan, AP. Quantification of human high molecular weight kininogen by immunoblotting with a monoclonal anti-light chain antibody, J. Immunol. Meth. 1989; 19-25.
6. Cameron, CL, Fisslthaler, B, Sherman, A, Reddigari, S & Silverberg, M. Studies on contact activation: effects of surfaces and inhibitors, 1989; 15: 53-62.

ACTIVATION OF THE CONTACT SYSTEM IN ASCITES FROM PATIENTS WITH GASTROINTESTINAL CANCER

L. Buø[1], T.S. Karlsrud[3], H.T. Johansen[3] and A.O. Aasen[1,2]

[1]Institute for Surgical Research and [2]Department of Surgery B Rikshospitalet, Oslo, and [3]Department of Pharmacology, Institute of Pharmacy, University of Oslo, Norway

SUMMARY: Our observations indicates that the plasma contact system is activated in ascites from patients with gastrointestinal cancer: Factor XII is activated, plasma kallikrein is present in complex with the protease inhibitor α_2-macroglobulin, and the plasma kallikrein substrate high molecular weight kininogen, is highly degraded. Contact activation seems to take place in spite of a high level of inhibition. Activation of the contact system generates mediators, which may play a role in the accumulation of ascites.

INTRODUCTION

Gastrointestinal malignancies are often accompanied by accumulation of ascites (1,2). Increased fluid leakage from blood vessels, due to increased vascular permeability, and decreased reabsorption by lymphatics and blood vessels are probably implicated in this fluid accumulation (1,2). It has been proposed that factors secreted by tumor cells may be responsible for increases in macromolecular permeability (3,4), and that neovascularity induced by certain tumors is abnormally permeable to proteins (5). Involvement of the kinin-generating cascade in enhancement of vascular permeability has also been suggested (6). It has been demonstrated that kinins, which are known to enhance vascular permeability, are present in ascitic tumor fluid; and that kinins are generated via the kallikrein-dependent cascade in the ascitic tumor fluid (6). Lymphatic obstruction by tumor cells demonstrated histologically, is suggested to impair drainage of the peritoneal cavity (1).

The plasma contact activation system has the potensial to generate mediators which may contribute to increased vascular permeability and give accumulation of ascites (2,7). The four main proteins of the contact activation system are factor XII, prekallikrein, factor XI, and high molecular weight kininogen (8,9). C1-inhibitor and α_2-macroglobulin are the most important natural inhibitors of the contact activation system (9-11). Several defence mechanisms, such as blood coagulation, fibrinolysis, activation of complement, and the plasma kallikrein-kinin system, can be initiated by contact activation (12,9).

If the role of mediators and proteases in ascites accumulation could be described in greater detail, this could perhaps explain more about underlying mechanisms in ascites accumulation.

The present study characterizes the plasma contact system in ascites from patients with gastrointestinal malignancies.

MATERIALS AND METHODS

Materials: Glu-Pro-Arg-pNA (S-2366), H-D-Pro-Phe-Arg-pNA (S-2302), Plasma Prekallikrein Activator, Plasma Kallikrein, and α_2-Macroglobulin / α_1-Antitrypsin (α_1-protease inhibitor) Coa-Set were obtained from Kabi Vitrum AB, Stockholm, Sweden. C1-Esterase Inhibitor, Nycotest[R], was from Nycomed Diagnostica, Oslo, Norway. H-D-HHT-Gly-Arg-pNA/Pefabloc PK and Kalliplastin were purchased from Pentapharm Ltd., Basel, Switzerland. Factor XII Deficient Human Plasma was aquired from Baxter Merz & Dade AG, Düdingen, Switzerland. Corn inhibitor was from Channel Diagnostics, Walmer, Kent, England. Factor XI Deficient Human Plasma was obtained from George King Inc., Overland Park, KS, USA. Rabbit antiserum to human α_2-macroglobulin was aquired from Behring Diagnostica, Marburg, Germany. Chemicals for the casting of polyacrylamide gels, nitro-cellulose membrane, and Immunoblot Assay kit-Rabbit Anti-Goat Ig G (H+L) Alkaline Phosphatase Conjugate were products of Bio-Rad laboratories, Richmond, CA, USA. Kaolin and sodium dodecyl sulphate (SDS) were purchased from Sigma Chem. Co., St.Louis, MO., USA. Rainbow[R] Protein Molecular Weight Marker was from Amersham Laboratories, Buckinghamshire, England. Goat antiserum to human factor XII was aquired from ICN ImmunoBiologicals, Lisle, IL, USA. Factor XII was purified from human plasma as described by Laake and Østerud (13). All other reagents were obtained from commercial sources and were of analytical grade.

Patients: Ascites and plasma were collected from 9 patients (ages 47-83 years; mean 67; 3 female and 6 male) with advanced gastrointestinal cancer admitted to the Department of Surgery, Ullevaal University Hospital, Oslo, Norway. Plasma collected from 8 healthy blood donors (ages 27-53 years; mean 36; 4 female and 4 male) at the Ullevaal Hospital Bloodbank served as controls. Pool plasma, collected from 118 healthy blood donors at the Ullevaal Hospital Bloodbank, served as a reference for values determined in the patients and controls.

Sampling procedure: Ascites samples were drawn from the patients by percutaneous puncture. Blood samples were collected by venous puncture. Ascites and blood samples were mixed with 0,13 mol/l sodium citrate (1 volume of anticoagulant and 9 volumes of ascites or blood) in plastic tubes, centrifuged for 10 minutes at 1900 rpm (800 g), decanted and frozen at $\div 70°C$ until assayed en bloq.

Functional assays: Plasma kallikrein, prekallikrein and functional kallikrein inhibition were assayed with the chromogenic peptide substrate S-2302 as previously described (14,15). α_2-Macroglobulin, α_1-protease inhibitor and C1 inhibitor were determined using kits according to the procedure outlined by the manufacturers (Kabi Vitrum AB, Stockholm, Sweden and Nycomed Diagnostica, Oslo, Norway). Total proteins were determined by the method of Kingsley (16). Analyses of plasma kallikrein, prekallikrein, kallikrein inhibition, α_2-macroglobulin, α_1-protease inhibitor, C1 inhibitor, and total proteins were performed on an automated centrifugal enzyme analyzer (Cobas Bio, Hoffman La Roche, Basel, Switzerland) as previously reported (17). Factor XII was assayed with the chromogenic peptide substrate H-D-HHT-Gly-Arg-pNA according to the method of Stürzebecher et al. (18). Factor XI was determined with the chromogenic peptide substrate S-2366 by the method of Scott & Colman (19). The analyses of factor XII and factor XI were performed on a microplate reader (Model 3550 EIA Reader and software Kinetic Collector, Bio-Rad Corp., Richmond, CA). Plasma kallikrein-, factor XII-, and factor XI-like activities were determined by the same methods as used for the determination of prekallikrein, factor XII and factor XI respectively, but without the addition of any activators of the proenzymes.

Gel filtration was performed at room temperature and a flow rate of 0.3 ml per min on a Pharmacia Superose 12 column connected to a Pharmacia FPLC system. The column was equilibrated with 0.1 M tris pH 8.0 containing 0.02% Na-azid. 200 μl ascites was applied to the column via a sample loop. The eluent was photometrically monitored at 280 nm and fractions of 400 μl were collected. Molecular weight standards were dissolved in column buffer and applied to the column in the same manner as the ascites. A standard curve was established based on the eluation volumes of the different standards, and molecular weights corresponding to the separate fractions were determined. Enzyme activity of the fractions was assayed with the kallikrein susceptible chromogenic peptide substrate S-2302 using the microplate reader as outlined by De La Cadena et al. (20). The fractions were also tested for functional α_2-macroglobulin activity using a kit according to the procedure outlined by the manufacturer (Kabi Vitrum AB, Stockholm, Sweden).

Rocket immunoelectrophoresis was carried out according to Laurell (21), on the ascites and gel filtration fractions. Antiserum (produced in rabbits against α_2-macroglobulin) was mixed with agarose solution (13.5 ml 1% agarose in tris-barbital buffer pH 8.6, 2% PEG (M_r 6000)) at 54-56°C. Sample aliquots of 5 μl were applied in wells. Electrophoresis was carried out for at least 18 hours (3 V/cm, 10°C), in a flat bed apparatus (FBE-3000, Pharmacia AB, Uppsala, Sweden). After extensive washing the plates were stained with 1% Coomassie blue R-250. Rocket heights were compared to dilution curves established from pool plasma.

Immunoblotting: Proteins were separated by electrophoresis in a homogeneous SDS polyacrylamide gel (T=10%, C=2,7%), according to the method of Laemmli (22), using the Mighty Small II Dual Slab Gel Electrophoresis Unit (Hoefer Scientific Instruments, San Francisco, CA). The proteins were then electrotransferred onto a nitrocellulose membrane essentially according to Towbin et al. (23), using the Trans-Blot SD Semi-Dry Transfer Cell (Bio-Rad Laboratories, Richmond, CA) according to the manufacturers instructions. The nitrocellulose sheet was washed and quenched and then incubated with goat antiserum spesific to human factor XII. Immunodetection was carried out with alkaline phosphatase conjugated rabbit antibodies against goat IgG. Relative molecular weight was determined by the use of molecular weight standards.

Statistical methods: Median and range values are given. Statistical significance was determined by the Rank sum test (Wilcoxon). Values of $p < 0.05$ were considered significant.

RESULTS

Contact factors: Factor XII was present in ascites with a median enzyme activity of 53% of the activity found in pool plasma (Fig.1). In plasma obtained from the cancer patients factor XII values were significantly reduced when compared to controls and pool plasma values (Fig.1). In most of the ascites samples a considerable amount of factor XII-like activity was present (Table 1).

Immunoblotting of factor XII under nonreducing conditions, showed one protein band which could be identified as factor XII (Fig.2). Its relative molecular weight was calculated to be about 80 kilodaltons, which is in accordance with previous reports on the molecular weight of factor XII (24). The identity of this protein band as factor XII, was verified by the presence of a similar band in a purified factor XII preparation, and its absence in plasma congenitally deficient of factor XII (Fig.2).

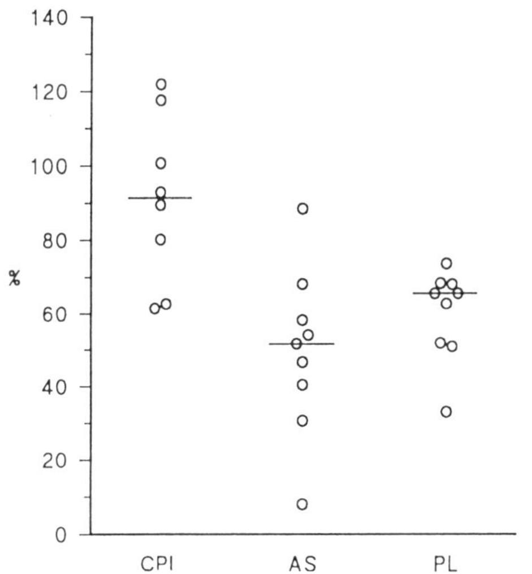

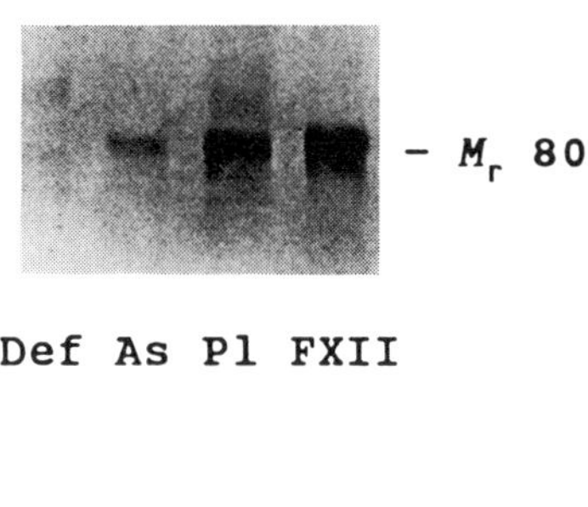

Figure 1. Factor XII activity in ascites (AS) and plasma (PL) from patients with GI cancer, and in control plasma (CPL), given as % of activity in pool plasma. Median values are indicated by horizontal lines.

Figure 2. SDS-PAGE immunoblot of factor XII deficient plasma (Def), ascites (As) and plasma (Pl) from patient with GI cancer, and a purified factor XII preparation (FXII). Relative M_r (kD) is given.

Table 1. Enzyme activity in ascites and plasma from 9 patients with GI cancer compared with control plasma from 8 healthy persons.

	Ascites	Plasma	Controls
FXII-like activity[a]	1.3[c] (0-2.7)	0.2 (0-0.8)	0.5 (0-0.6)
FXI-like activity[a]	0.3[c] (0-1.0)	0.2 (0-0.7)	0.1 (0-0.4)
Kallikrein-like activity[b]	34 (1-133)	5 (1- 20)	16 (4- 36)

Activities were determined spectrophotometrically with chromogenic peptide substrates. Median (range) values are given as: [a] ΔmOD/min; [b] U/l. [c] Patient values significantly different from controls.

Factor XI activity in ascites showed a median value of 63% of the activity in pool plasma (Fig.3). The factor XI values varied greatly in both ascites and plasma obtained from the patients. In the patient plasma, factor XI values were both higher and lower than values found in controls (Fig.3). Very little factor XI-like activity was found in both ascites and plasma (Table 1).

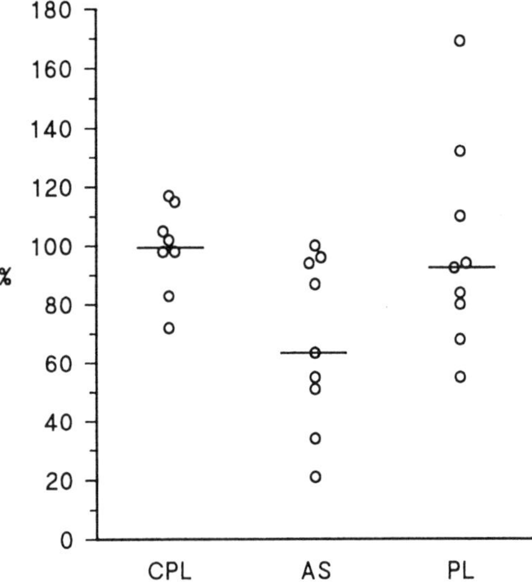

Figure 3. Factor XI activity in ascites (AS) and plasma (PL) from patients with GI cancer, and in control plasma (CPL), as % of activity in pool plasma. Median values are indicated by horizontal lines.

Plasma prekallikrein values in ascites were 39% of the pool plasma values (Fig.4). Prekallikrein values were also significantly lower in plasma from patients when compared to healthy persons (Fig.4). Determination of plasma kallikrein-like activity yielded remarkable high values in some of the ascites samples (Table 1). This was not found in the patient plasma samples (Table 1).

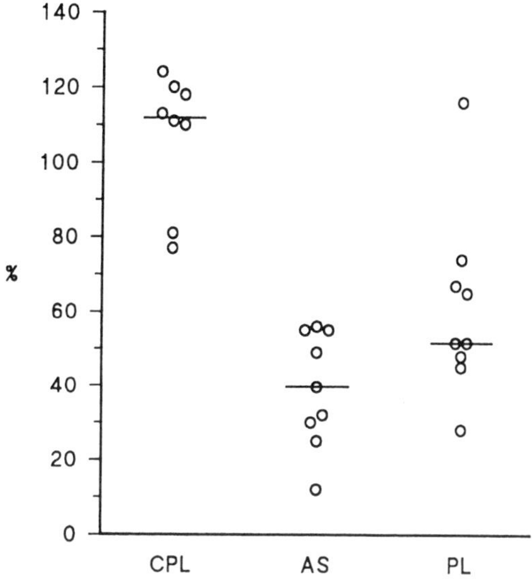

Figure 4. Prekallikrein activity in ascites (AS) and plasma (PL) from patients with GI cancer, and in control plasma (CPL), given as % of activity in pool plasma. Median values are indicated by horizontal lines.

Gel filtration of ascites followed by assay of enzyme activity revealed amidolytic activity towards the plasma kallikrein susceptible substrate S-2302 in the fractions corresponding to a high M_r (>660.000) (Fig.5). In these fractions α_2-macroglobulin was detected by both immunological (Fig.5) and functional tehniques. Enzyme activity towards S-2302 was also detected in fractions corresponding to a lower M_r-range (<40.000).

Inhibition studies: In the ascites functional plasma kallikrein inhibition, C1 inhibitor, α_2-macroglobulin, and α_1-protease inhibitor values were 66%, 82%, 45% and 156% respectively, of the values in pool plasma (Table 2). Compared to values in the controls, the plasma inhibition values of functional kallikrein inhibition, C1 inhibitor, and α_1-protease inhibitor, in the patient plasma, were significantly higher (Table 2).

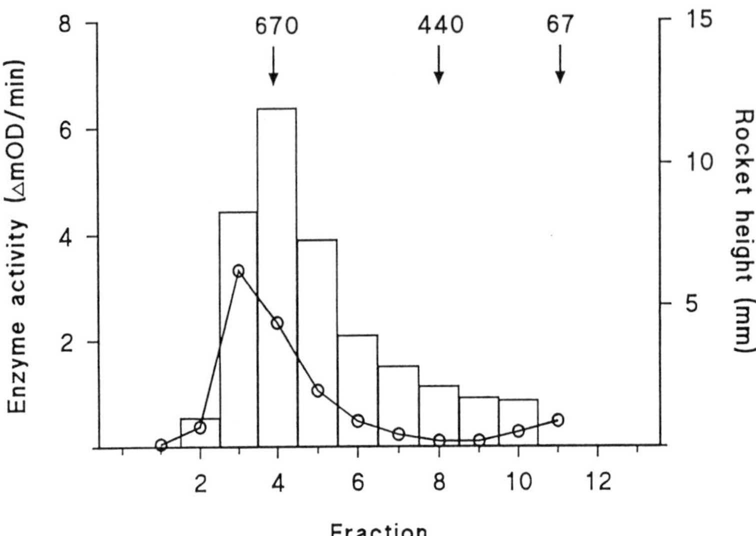

Figure 5. Gel filtration of ascites on a Superose 12 column. Enzyme activity of fractions is given as ΔmOD/min. α_2-macroglobulin in fractions was determined by rocket immuno-electrophoresis (vertical bars). Vertical arrows indicate relative elution volume of standard proteins. Molecular weight (kD) is given above each arrow.

Table 2. Functional activity of plasma inhibitors in ascites and plasma from 9 patients with gastrointestinal cancer compared with control plasma from 8 healthy persons.

	Ascites	Plasma	Controls
Kallikrein inhibition	66[a] (48- 82)	110[a] (87-123)	99 (77-105)
C1 inhibitor	82[a] (42-103)	142[a] (114-182)	99 (74-126)
α_2-Macroglobulin	45[a] (16- 85)	104 (66-137)	78 (66-135)
α_1-Protease inhibitor	156[a] (47-233)	193[a] (139-266)	106 (96-121)

Activities were determined spectrophotometrically with chromogenic peptide substrates. Median (range) values are given as % of the activity in pool plasma. [a]Patient values significantly different from controls.

Total proteins in the patients were 74 (58-88)% in ascites and 89 (74-108)% in plasma when compared to pool plasma. In the controls total proteins were 98 (95-105)%. The protein content in ascites was significantly lower than in plasma from both patients and healthy persons.

DISCUSSION

Our study demonstrates the presence of plasma contact factors in ascites from patients with gastrointestinal cancer. Factor XII, factor XI, and prekallikrein values were calculated to 53, 63, and 39% respectively, of the values in normal pool plasma, when determined by functional techniques. Immunoblotting verified the presence of factor XII in ascites. The present study also revealed decreased functional factor XII and prekallikrein values in plasma obtained from the cancer patients when compared to plasma from healthy persons.

Decreased values of contact factors in patients could be due to reduced synthesis by the liver. When compared to healthy persons, our cancer patients have a decreased level of total proteins. However, this study does not reveal any statistically significant differences in total protein content between patients with and those without liver metastasis. A larger group of patients would possibly be needed in order to obtain such differences.

C1 inhibitor, α_2-macroglobulin and α_1-protease inhibitor, which are the main inhibitors of the contact system (8,10), were all found in the ascites. In view of the low level of contact factors, functional inhibition values in both ascites and plasma obtained from the cancer patients were unexpected high, as activation of contact factors would be expected to result in a consumption of inhibitors. The findings are, however, in accordance with our previous studies on cancer patients (25). Increased values of α_1-protease inhibitor in ascitic fluid of patients with malignancy has also recently been demonstrated by others, and is suggested to be a valuable parameter in the differential diagnosis of ascites (26). The high inhibition values observed in patient plasma may be a secondary response to the disease, as protease inhibitors are able to act as acute phase reactants (27).

Plasma kallikrein-like activity in ascites far exceeded this activity in plasma. Evidence of the presence of kallikrein (M_r 85.000 and 88.000 (28)) in ascites, in complex with the high molecular weight inhibitor α_2-macroglobulin (M_r 718.000 (29)), (8-11), was provided by the results of gel filtration studies followed by immunological and functional assays. At the present time we do not know the identity of the enzyme activity detected in fractions corresponding to the lower M_r-range (< 40.000). The presence of other enzymes than plasma kallikrein, capable of splitting the chromogenic peptide substrate S-2302, should be considered. Recent studies by our group indicate that high molecular weight kininogen is adsorbed to the Superose 12 column (Karlsrud TS et al., unpublished data). High molecular weight kininogen contains binding sites for plasma prekallikrein and kallikrein (9). Binding to high molecular weight kininogen could lead to a delayed elution of plasma kallikrein indicating that the enzyme activity of fractions corresponding to the lower M_r-range also may be caused by plasma kallikrein.

Plasma kallikrein generates the potent vasoactive peptide bradykinin from high molecular weight kininogen by proteolytic cleavage. Bradykinin has a strong permeability increasing capasity (2,7) which may contribute to the accumulation of malignant acites. The relevance of this mechanism is also emphasized in recent studies by our group which showed a pronounced proteolyic breakdown of high molecular weight kininogen in malignant ascites (30). This also emphasize that the active enzyme plasma kallikrein has been generated as a result of contact activation, and that kallikrein has attacked its natural substrate high molecular weight kininogen. Contact activation seems to take place in spite of a high level of inhibition.

ACKNOWLEDGEMENTS

The authors thank Grethe Dyrhaug, Brit Engebretsen, Elisabeth Fahlstrøm, and Adam Babinski for providing technical assistance. Laila Buø is a Fellow of the Norwegian Cancer Society - Den Norske Kreftforening.

REFERENCES

1. Holm-Nielsen P. Pathogenesis of ascites in peritoneal carcinomatosis. Acta Path Microbiol Scand 1953; 33:10-21.
2. White MJ, Miller FN, Heuser LS, Pietsch CG. Human malignant ascites and histamin-induced protein leakage from the normal microcirculation. Microvasc Res 1988; 35:63-72.
3. Senger DR, Galli SJ, Dvorak AM, Perruzzi CA, Harvey VS, Dvorak HF. Tumor cells secrete a vascular permeability factor that promotes accumulation of ascites fluid. Science 1983; 219:983-985.
4. Stein WR. A permeability-enhancing factor produced by tumor. The genesis of malignant efflusions. J Cancer Res Clin Oncol 1980; 97:315-320.
5. Heuser LS, Miller FN. Differential macromolecular leakage from the vasculature of tumors. Cancer 1986; 57:461-464.
6. Matsumura Y, Kimura M, Yamamoto T, Maeda H. Involvement of the kinin-generating cascade in enhanced vascular permeability in tumor tissue. Jpn J Cancer Res 1988; 79:1327-1334.

7. Erdös EG. Commentary. The kinins. A status report. Biochem Pharmacol 1976; 25:1563-1569.

8. Colman RW. Surface-mediated defence reactions. The plasma contact activation system. J Clin Invest 1984; 73:1249-1253.

9. Colman RW, Schmaier AH. The contact activation system: Biochemistry and interactions of these surface-mediated defense reactions. CRC Crit Rev Oncol Hematol 1986; 5:57-85.

10. Schapira M. Major inhibitors of the contact phase coagulation factors. Semin Thromb Hemost 1987; 13:69-78.

11. Schapira M, Scott CF, Colman RW. Contribution of plasma protease inhibitors to the inactivation of kallikrein in plasma. J Clin Invest 1982; 69:462-468.

12. Kluft C, Dooijewaard G, Emeis JJ. Role of the contact system in fibrinolysis. Semin Thromb Hemost 1987; 13:50-68.

13. Laake K, Østerud B. Activation of purified plasma factor VII by human plasmin, plasma kallikrein and activated components of the human intrinsic blood coagulation system. Thromb Res 1974; 5:759-772.

14. Amundsen E, Gallimore MJ, Aasen AO, Larsbraaten M, Lyngaas K. Activation of human plasma prekallikrein: Influence of activators, activation time and temperatur and inhibitors. Thromb Res 1978; 13:625-636.

15. Aasen AO, Smith Erichsen N, Gallimore MJ, Amundsen E. Studies on components of the plasma kallikrein-kinin system in plasma samples from normal individuals and patients with septic shock. In: Adv. in Shock Res. Schumer W, Spitzer JJ, Marshall BE, editors. New York: A.R. Liss. Inc., 1980; 4:1-11.

16. Kingsley GR. The determination of serum total protein, albumin, and globulin by the biuret reaction. J Biol Chem 1939; 131:197-200.

17. Aasen AO, Kierulf P, Strømme J. Methodological considerations on chromogenic peptide substrate assays and application on automated analyzers. Acta Chir Scand Suppl 1982; 509:17-22.

18. Stürzebecher J, Svendsen L, Eichenberger R, Markwardt F. A new assay for the determination of factor XII in plasma using a chromogenic substrate and a selective inhibitor of plasma kallikrein. Thromb Res 1989; 55: 709-715.

19. Scott CF, Colman RW. A simple and accurate microplate assay for the determination of factor XI in plasma. J Lab Clin Med 1988; 111:708-714.

20. De La Cadena RA, Scott CF, Colman RW. Evaluation of a microassay for human plasma prekallikrein. J Lab Clin Med 1987; 109:601-607.

21. Laurell CB. Quantitative estimation of proteins by electrophoresis in agarose gel containing antibodies. Anal Biochem 1966; 15:45-52.

22. Laemmli UK. Cleavage of structural proteins during the assembly of the head of bacteriophage T4. Nature 1970; 227:680-685.

23. Towbin H, Staehelin T, Gordon J. Electrophoretic transfer of proteins from polyacrylamide gels to nitrocellulose sheets: Procedure and some applications. Proc Natl Acad Sci USA 1979; 76:4350-4354.

24. Chan JYC, Movat HZ. Purification of factor XII (Hageman factor) from human plasma. Thromb Res 1976; 8:337-349.

25. Røise O, Sivertsen S, Ruud TE, Bouma BN, Stadaas JO, Aasen AO. Studies on components of the contact phase system in patients with advanced gastrointestinal cancer. Cancer 1990; 65:1355-1359.

26. Villamil FG, Sorroche PB, Aziz HF, Lopez PM, Oyhamburu JM. Ascitic fluid α_1-antitrypsin. Dig Dis Sci 1990; 35:1105-1109.
27. Kluft C, Verheijen JH, Jie AHF, Rijken DC, Preston FE, Sue-Ling HM, Jespersen J, Aasen AO. The postoperative fibrinolytic shutdown: a rapidly reverting acute phase pattern for the fast-acting inhibitor of tissue-type plasminogen activator after trauma. Scand J Lab Invest 1985; 45:605-610.
28. Mandle RJ, Kaplan AP. Hageman factor substrates. Human plasma prekallikrein: Mechanism of activation by Hageman factor and participation in Hageman factor-dependent fibrinolysis. J Biol Chem 1977; 252:6097-6104.
29. Hall PK, Roberts RC. Physical and chemical properties of human plasma α_2-macroglobulin. Biochem J 1978; 173:27-38.
30. Karlsrud TS, Buø L, Aasen AO, Johansen HT. Characterization of kininogens in human malignant ascites. Thromb Res 1991; 63:641-650.

PURIFICATION OF FACTOR XI AND SOME PROPERTIES OF ACTIVATED
FACTOR XI FROM PORCINE PLASMA

H. Mashiko and H. Takahashi

Meiji College of Pharmacy, 1-35-23 Nozawa, Setagaya-ku, Tokyo
154, JAPAN

SUMMARY: Porcine Factor (F.) XI was purified by following three
succesive chromatographies. By this procedure, about 5.5 mg of F.
XI was obtained from 500 ml of the plasma. The F. XI forms dimer,
and is heterogeneous molecule, judging from SDS-polyacrylamide
gel electrophoresis. The properties of isolated porcine F. XIa
are great similar with those of bovine F. XIa.

INTRODUCTION

F. XI (plasma thromboplastin antecedent) is a plasma protein,
which participates in intrinsic blood coagulation (1). F. XI is
present in zymogen form and purified from human (2,3), bovine
(4) and rabbit (5) plasmas, and characterized. Human and bovine
F. XI formed dimer, two identical monomer is connected by disulfide bond (2-4), however, rabbit F. XI formed a monomer (5).
The F. XI is converted to an active form (F. XIa), receiving a
proteolytic cleavage of each monomer by activated F. XII (2,6).
And F. XIa composed of heavy (H)-chain and light (L)-chain. Each
H-chain bears two functionally important domains. The one is high
molecular weight (HMW) kininogen binding site, and the other is
F. IX binding site under the presence of Ca ion (7). Therefore,
F. XI circulates in plasma as a complex with HMW kininogen (8)
as like as plasma prekallikrein (9).

   Disordor of F. XI results in the excessive bleeding after
injury and minor surgery. Thus, F. XI is an important protein,
however, the purification of F. XI is very difficult, because of

its low concentration in plasma and also its high susceptibility
to proteolytic enzyme, F. XIIa.

   To study the initial reaction of intrinsic blood coagulation
system, we already purified the factors, such as plasma prekallikrein (10), HMW kininogen (11) and F. XII (12) from porcine
plasma. As a course of the study, we tried to purify F. XI from
porcine plasma. During the purification of F. XI, F. XIa was also
isolated from the plasma. This paper describes the purification
and some properties of F. XI and F. XIa.

MATERIALS AND METHODS

Fresh porcine blood containing 3.8% sodium citrate was collected
in polyethylene bottles at a slaughterhouse, and centrifuged at
3000 rpm for 30 min at 20°C. The plasma obtained was supplemented
with Polybrene at a final concentration of 0.5 g/liter, and
benzamidine at a final concentration of 5 mM. The plasma was
stocked at -80°C until use. Porcine HMW kininogen was prepared
by our method (11). Q-Sepharose Fast Flow and Protein A Superose
HR 10/2 were obtained from Pharmacia LKB Biotechnology, Japan.
Formyl-Cellulofine was obtained from Seikagaku Kogyo Co., Ltd.,
Japan. All of the clotting factor-deficient human plasmas were
obtained from George King Bio-Medical, U.S.A. Bovine serum
albumin, rabbit cephaline, soybean trypsin inhibitor (SBTI), egg
white trypsin inhibitor (EWTI) and a kit of standard protein
markers (MW-SDS-200) were purchased from Sigma Chemicals Co.,
U.S.A. The sources of other materials were as follows: diiso-
propylfluorophosphate (DFP) from Katayama Kagaku Kogyo Co., Ltd.,
Japan; Trasylol from Bayer, Germany; lima bean trypsin inhibitor
(LBTI) from Worthington Biochemical Corp., U.S.A.; various
fluorogenic peptide substrates and 7-amino-4-methylcoumarin (AMC)
from the Peptide Institute Inc., Japan; a silver staining kit
from Kanto Chemical Co., Inc., Japan and Polybrene from Aldrich
Chemicals Co., U.S.A.

   Assay of F. XI was carried out by a kaolin-activated partial

thromboplastin time (APTT) method using human F. XI-deficient
plasma (2). One unit is defined as the amount of activity which
is present in 1.0 ml of porcine plasma. In the case of F. XIa
assay, 0.15 M NaCl solution was used as substitution for kaolin
suspension. Assay of plasma prekallikrein, HMW kininogen or F.
XII was also carried out by a kaolin-APTT method. using pre-
kallikrein-, HMW kininogen- or F. XII-deficient human plasma,
respectively.

The purified porcine HMW kininogen (9.2 mg) was immobilized
to Formyl-Cellulofine (26.5 g) according to the instruction
manual. Free formyl residue was blocked by 0.2 M Tris-HCl buffer,
pH 7.2.

SDS-polyacrylamide gel electrophoresis (SDS-PAGE) was performed on 10% gels according to the method of Laemmli (13).
Protein was visualized with silver stain using a silver stain
kit.

Substrate specificity of porcine F. XIa against various
fluorogenic peptide substrates was examined in 0.1 M Tris-HCl
buffer, pH 8.0, containing 0.15 M NaCl according to the method
of Morita et al. (14) with minor modification.

Porcine F. XIa solution (0.1 ml) was mixed with 0.1 ml of
various proteinase inhibitor solutions in a total volume of 1 ml.
After 10 min-incubation at 37°C, 0.1 ml of 1 mM tert-butoxy-
carbonyl (Boc)-Phe-Ser-Arg-4-methylcoumaryl-7-amide (MCA) was
added, and the mixture was further incubated for 1 hr at 37°C.
The remaining amidase activity of F. XIa was determined as
described above.

Protein concentrations were determined by measurements of
the absorbance at 280 nm, assuming that an absorption value of
1.0 equals 1 mg/ml.

RESULTS AND DISCUSSION

Purification of F. XI from porcine plasma

All purification procedures were performed in a cold room. The
columns were silicon-coated before use, and polyethylene test

tubes were used. To each elution buffer or dialysed buffer, Polybrene and benzamidine were added at a final concentration of 0.5
g/liter, and 5 mM, respectively, during the chromatographies.

It was reported that plasma prekallikrein binds to HMW
kininogen with higher affinity than F. XI (3,15). Therefore, it
is necessary to separate F. XI from prekallikrein prior to the
use of HMW kininogen-Cellulofine. To achieve the purpose, the
plasma was chromatographed on a Q-Sepharose Fast Flow column (7.5
x 17 cm). Prekallikrein did not adsorb the column, while F. XI
adsorbed the column, and eluted by NaCl linear gradient in the
equilibration buffer. By this chromatography, F. XI was perfectly
separated from prekallikrein. The F. XI fraction was pooled and
dialysed. One-third of the dialysate was applied to the HMW
kininogen-Cellulofine column (3.5 x 3.5 cm) equilibrated with the
dialysed buffer. After washing the column with the equilibration
buffer containing 3 M NaCl, proteins were eluted with the buffer
containing 3 M NaSCN. F. XI adhered to the resin and only eluted
by the buffer containing 3 M NaSCN, however, was not eluted by
the buffer containing 1 M NaCl that is the elution condition of
human F. XI from human HMW kininogen-Sepharose column (16), or
3 M NaCl. So, the affinity of porcine F. XI to porcine HMW kininogen is stronger than that of human F. XI to human HMW kininogen.
When F. XI preparation was subjected to SDS-PAGE, the bands of
other protein in addition to F. XI were detected. From the
mobility of other protein on SDS-PAGE under the reducing or nonreducing condition, this protein may be a immunoglobulin. In
fact, it was reported that purified human F. XI preparation
contains IgG at a concentration from 5% to 25% (2). To remove
IgG from F. XI fraction, Protein A Superose HR 10/2 column
chromatography was done.

After remaining two-third of F. XI fraction was chromatographed on a HMW kininogen-Cellulofine column, F. XI fraction was
pooled and dialysed. The fraction was applied on a column (1 x 2
cm) of Protein A Superose equilibrated with the dialysed buffer.

Table 1. Summary of purification procedures for F. XI from
porcine plasma

Procedure	Total protein (mg)	Total activity (units)	Specific activity (units/mg)
Porcine plasma	42,100	500	0.01
Q-Sepharose Fast Flow	6,740	388	0.06
HMW kininogen-Cellulofine	18	315	17.5
Protein A Superose	5.5	225	40.9

After washing the column with the equilibration buffer, protein
was eluted with the equilibration buffer containing 3 M NaSCN.
Coagulant activity of F. XI was only detected in breakthrough
fraction.

By this procedure, about 5.5 mg of F. XI was obtained from
500 ml of the plasma (Table 1). Specific activity of porcine F.
XI was 40.9 units/mg of protein, and this value was lower than
that of human, bovine or rabbit F. XI. Specific activity of F. XI
from human, bovine, and rabbit plasmas, was 202 (2), 494 (4),
and 83 (5), respectively.

When final F. XI preparation was subjected to SDS-PAGE,
porcine F. XI showed minor microheterogeneity under reduced or
non-reduced condition (Fig. 1). Namely, reduced F. XI showed
two bands, and the major band was 90 Kd and the minor band was
85 Kd. On non-reduced condition, F. XI also showed adjacent two
bands, and the major and the minor bands were about 180 Kd. But,
the separation of these two bands is not sufficient, so, it is
difficult to confirm it from this figure. Microheterogeneity of
porcine F. XI appeared in both cases at reduced and non-reduced
conditions, so, microheterogeneity of F. XI may be derived from
amino-terminal or carboxyl-terminal portion in the molecule.
Such heterogeneity was also observed in bovine F. XI (6).
Considering bovine F. XI, this heterogeneity of porcine F. XI
may depend on the fragmentation in carboxyl-terminal portion of
the molecule. Moreover, it is indicated that porcine F. XI also
forms dimer linked with disulfide bond as like as bovine and

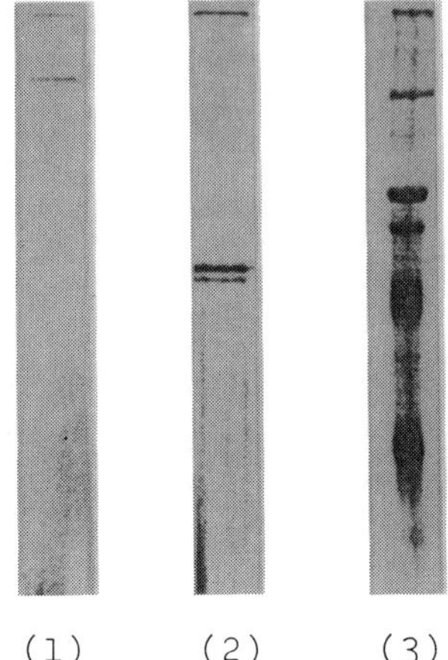

(1) Non-reduced F. XI
(2) Reduced F. XI
(3) Marker proteins

Figure 1. SDS-PAGE of purified porcine F. XI

human F. XI (2,3), but, is not a monomer as rabbit F. XI (5).

   The F. XI preparation shortened only the abnormal clotting
time of F. XI-deficient plasma, and did not affect against F.
XII-, HMW kininogen- or prekallikrein-deficient plasma. These
results indicate that the preparation is functionally pure. And
the preparation shortened the abnormal clotting time of F. XI-
deficient plasma only in the presence of kaolin. This result
also indicates that F. XI thus obtained is a precursor form.

Some properties of spontaneously activated porcine F. XIa

Spontaneously activated F. XIa was also isolated according to the
same method as described above. Using this preparation, properties of F. XIa were studied as compared with those of bovine F.
XIa.

   Substrate specificity of porcine F. XIa was examined using
various synthetic fluorogenic peptide substrates and compared
with that of bovine F. XIa (17). As shown in Table 2, porcine
F. XIa showed a similar substrate specificity with bovine F. XIa.
Among these substrates, porcine F. XIa hydrolysed Boc-Val-Pro-

Table 2. Hydrolysis of various synthetic fluorogenic peptide substrates with porcine or bovine F. XIa

Substrates	Relative activity (%)	
	Porcine F. XIa	Bovine F. XIa[17]
Boc-Phe-Ser-Arg-MCA	100	100
Boc-Val-Pro-Arg-MCA	115	86
Boc-Leu-Thr-Arg-MCA	83	182
Boc-Leu-Gly-Arg-MCA	57	51
Boc-Glu(OBzl)-Gly-Arg-MCA	56	52
Boc-Leu-Ser-Thr-Arg-MCA	35	56
Boc-Ile-Glu-Gly-Arg-MCA	30	32

Arg-MCA best, while, bovine F. XIa hydrolysed Boc-Leu-Thr-Arg-MCA best. This activity of porcine F. XIa was perfectly inhibited by DFP and partially inhibited by LBTI, SBTI and Trasylol, but, was not inhibited by EWTI at all.

REFERENCES

1. Davie EW, Fujikawa K. Basic mechanism in blood coagulation. Ann Rev Biochem 1975; 44: 799.

2. Bouma BN, Griffin JH. Human blood coagulation Factor XI. Purification, properties and mechanism of activation by activated Factor XII. J Biol Chem 1977; 252: 6432.

3. Bouma BN, Vlooswijk RAA, Griffin JH. Immunological studies of human coagulation Factor XI and its complex with high molecular weight kininogen. Blood 1983; 62: 1123.

4. Koide T, Kato H, Davie EW. Characterization of bovine Factor XI (plasma thromboplastin antecedent). Biochemistry 1977; 16: 2279.

5. Wiggins RC, Cochrane CG, Griffin JH. Rabbit blood coagulation Factor XI. Purification and properties. Thromb Res 1979; 15: 475.

6. Kurachi K, Fujikawa K, Davie EW. Mechanism of activation of bovine Factor XI by Factor XII and Factor XIIa. Biochemistry 1980; 19: 1330.

7. van der Graaf F, Greengard JS, Bouma BN, Kerbiriou DM, Griffin JH. Isolation and functional characterization of the active light chain of activated human blood coagulation Factor XI. J Biol Chem 1983; 258: 9669.

8. Thompson RE, Mandle Jr R, Kaplan AP. Association of Factor XI and high molecular weight kininogen in human plasma. J Clin Invest 1977; 60: 1376.

9. Mandle RJ, Colman RW, Kaplan AP. Identification of prekallikrein and high-molecular-weight kininogen as a complex in human plasma. Proc Natl Acad Sci USA 1976; 73: 4179.

10. Kikuno Y, Takahashi H, Suzuki T. Purification of prekallikrein from porcine plasma and its conversion to active kallikrein. J Biochem (Tokyo) 1983; 93: 235.

11. Miyamoto K, Mashiko H, Fujii K, Kohashi N, Takahashi H. High molecular weight kininogen in porcine plasma-Improved method for purification and fragmentation of the kininogen by tissue kallikrein-. Abstract at 108th Annual Meeting of the Pharmaceutical Society of Japan 1988; p. 436.

12. Kato K, Mashiko H, Fujii K, Shiina K, Miyamoto K, Kohashi N, Takahashi H. Purification of Factor XII from porcine plasma and its activation by porcine plasma kallikrein. In: Advances in Experimental Medicine and Biology; Vol. 247B. Abe K, Moriya H, Fujii S. editors. New York: Plenum Press, 1989: 243-248.

13. Laemmli UK. Cleavage of structural proteins during the assembly of the head of bacteriophage T4. Nature 1970; 227: 680.

14. Morita T, Kato H, Iwanaga S, Takada K, Kimura T, Sakakibara S. New fluorogenic substrates for α-thrombin, Factor Xa, kallikreins and urokinase. J Biochem (Tokyo) 1977; 82: 1495.

15. Tait JF, Fujikawa K. Primary structure requirements for the binding of human high molecular weight kininogen to plasma prekallikrein and Factor XI. J Biol Chem 1987; 262: 11651.

16. Fujikawa K, Chung DW, Hendrickson LE, Davie EW. Amino acid sequence of human Factor XI, a blood coagulation Factor with four tandem repeats that are highly homologous with plasma prekallikrein. Biochemistry 1986; 25: 2417.

17. Iwanaga S, Morita T, Kato H, Harada T, Adachi N, Sugo T, Maruyama I, Takada K, Kimura T, Sakakibara S. Fluorogenic peptide substrates for proteinases in blood coagulation, kallikrein-kinin and fibrinolysis system. In: Advances in Experimental Medicine and Biology; Vol. 120A, Fujii S, Moriya H, Suzuki T. editors. New York: Plenum Press, 1979: 147-163.

THE EFFECTS OF FRACTIONATED AND UNFRACTIONATED HEPARINS WITH AND WITHOUT APROTININ ON PLASMA INHIBITION OF ALPHA AND BETA FX11a

M.J. Gallimore, G. Fuhrer, W. Heller and H.-E. Hoffmeister

Department of Thoracic, Heart and Cardiovascular Surgery, University
of Tuebingen, D-7400 Tuebingen, Germany

SUMMARY: Chromogenic peptide substrate assays were used to compare the effects of fractionated and unfractionated heparins on plasma inhibition of alpha and beta FX11a, with and without various concentrations of aprotinin. All of the heparins reduced beta FX11a inhibition at 1 or 2U/ml. Four heparins increased alpha FX11a inhibition. Aprotinin counteracted the reduction in beta FX11a inhibition and augmented the heparin potentiation of alpha FX11a inhibition.

INTRODUCTION

We have previously reported (1) that the plasma kallikrein-kinin system becomes activated during cardiopulmonary bypass (CPB) with increasing activities of kallikrein bound to alpha-2-macroglobulin (kallikrein like activity) and falls in prekallikrein and kallikrein inhibition. We also reported that unfractionated heparin at doses equivalent to those used in CPB reduced the inhibition of beta FX11a by both plasma and C1-esterase inhibitor (2).

We have recently shown that that aprotinin reverses the effect of heparin on beta FX11a inhibition to some extent and have suggested that this effect contributes to the reduction of blood loss observed in high dose aprotinin therapy in CPB (3).

Chromogenic substrate assay kits for determining inhibitors of alpha FX11a and beta FX11a are now available and we have used these in a study to compare the effects of 3 un-fractionated and 3 fractionated heparins on plasma inhibition of alpha and beta FX11a. We have also compared the effects of aprotinin on alpha and beta FX11a inhibition in the presence or absence of the various heparins.

MATERIALS AND METHODS

Plasma from citrated blood (1 part blood plus 9 parts 0.11M trisodium citrate) was used. A standard plasma pool was prepared as described elsewhere (4) and used for all studies.

Unfractionated heparins were obtained from Medac, Germany, Hoffman LaRoche (Liquamine), Germany, and Braun, Germany. Fractionated heparins were obtained from Kabi (Fragmin), Sweden, Sandoz, (Mono Embolex) Germany and Rhone Poulanc (Enoxaparin), France.

Heparin levels were determined as anti FXa activity using assay kits from KabiDiagnostica, Munich, Germany.

Aprotinin was obtained from Bayer, Leverkusen, Germany.

Inhibition of alpha and beta FX11a was determined by reacting plasma, plasma plus heparin, or plasma plus aprotinin plus heparin with alpha or beta FX11a at 37 C and determining residual enzyme activities with a chromogenic peptide substrate for alpha and beta FX11a. Kits for these assays are available from Unicorn Diagnostics Ltd, 22 Gordon Road, London E18 1DN and full details of the methods are supplied with the kits. Typical standard curves for plasma inhibition of alpha and beta FX11a are shown in figures 1 and 2.

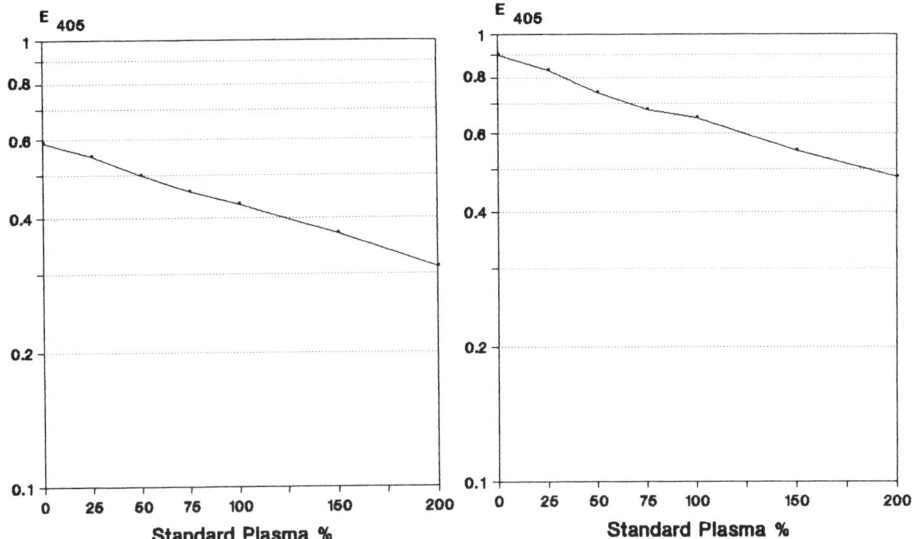

Figures 1 and 2. Standard curves for alpha (left) and beta FX11a inhibition (right). End point assays.

RESULTS

1. Effect of Heparins on Alpha and Beta FX11a Inhibition by Plasma

Unfractionated or fractionated heparins were added to plasma at final anti FXa activities of 0, 1, 2, 3 and 4 units/ml. The plasma samples were then assayed for inhibition of alpha or beta FX11a and the percentage inhibition calculated from standard curves for each parameter. The results were expressed in percent making the values without heparin 100%.

The results are shown in figures 3, 4, 5, and 6.

All three unfractionated heparins increased alpha FX11a inhibition by plasma (Fig. 3). Liquemin gave most enhanced inhibition. With the three fractionated heparins Fragmin and Enoxiparin gave reduced inhibition whilst Mono Embolex gave reduced inhibition at 1 u/ml and increased inhibition at higher heparin levels (Fig. 4).

All three unfractionated heparins reduced beta FX11a inhibition at all heparin concentrations with the exception of Liqemin which gave slightly elevated inhibition at 4 u/ml (Fig. 5). With the fractionated heparins pronounced reductions in plasma inhibition of beta FX11a were seen with Fragmin and Enoxaparin at all heparin concentrations whilst Mono Embolex gave reduced inhibition at 1 and 2 U/ml and slightly elevated inhibition at 4 U/ml (Fig. 6).

2. Effect of Aprotinin on Plasma Inhibition of Alpha And Beta FX11a in the Presence and Absence of Heparins

Aprotinin (0, 100, 200, and 400 KIU/ml) was added to plasma followed by unfractionated or fractionated heparins (final anti FXa activities 0, 1, 2, 3 and 4 units/ml) and after mixing the plasmas were assayed for inhibition of alpha and beta FX11a. The results are shown in Table 1.

Aprotinin produced small concentration dependent increases in alpha FX11a inhibition in the absence of heparins With beta FX11a inhibition very small changes were seen with aprotinin in the absence of heparins. When added together with unfractionated heparins aprotinin potentiated the heparin induced increases in alpha FX11a inhibition at all concentrations. With the fractionated heparins aprotinin potentiated alpha FX11a inhibition values whether the heparins had increased or decreased inhibition. With beta FX11a inhibition, at the heparin concentrations where beta FX11a inhibition was reduced aprotinin reversed this effect to some extent. Where beta FX11a inhibition was elevated aprotinin produced further dose-dependent increases in inhibition.

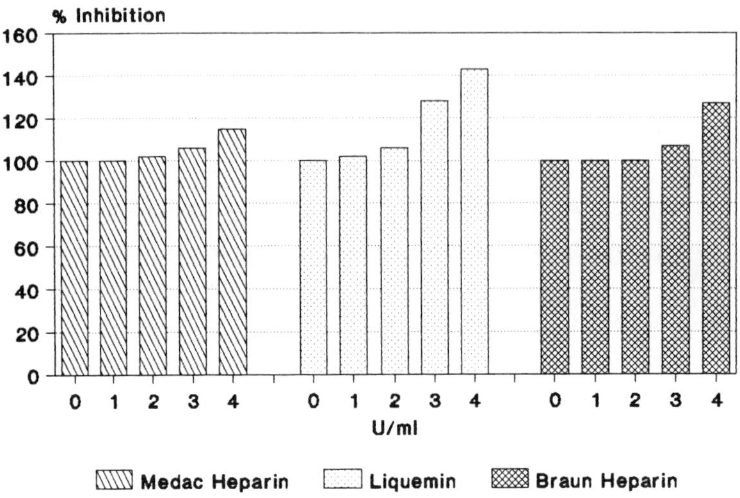

Fig. 3   Effect of Unfractionated Heparins on Alpha FXIIa Inhibition
by Plasma

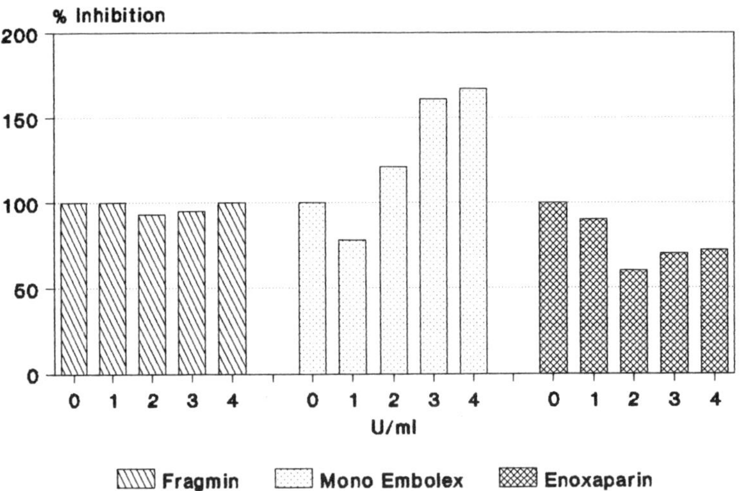

Fig. 4   Effect of Fractionated Heparins on Alpha FXIIa Inhibition
by Plasma

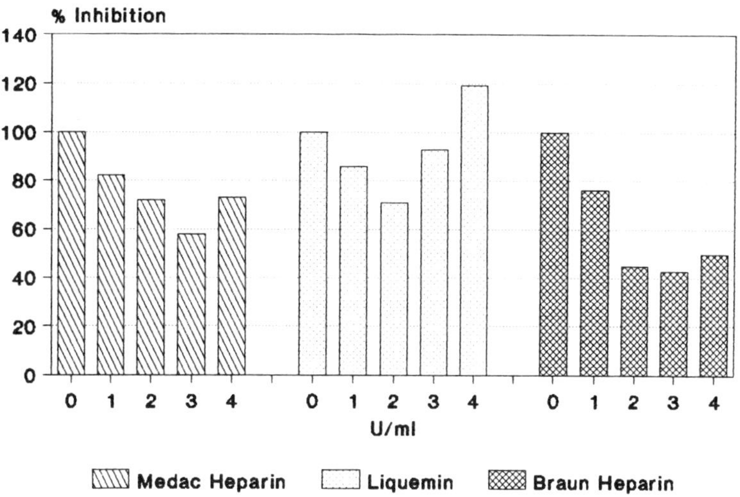

Fig. 5 Effect of Unfractionated Heparins on Beta FXII Inhibition by Plasma

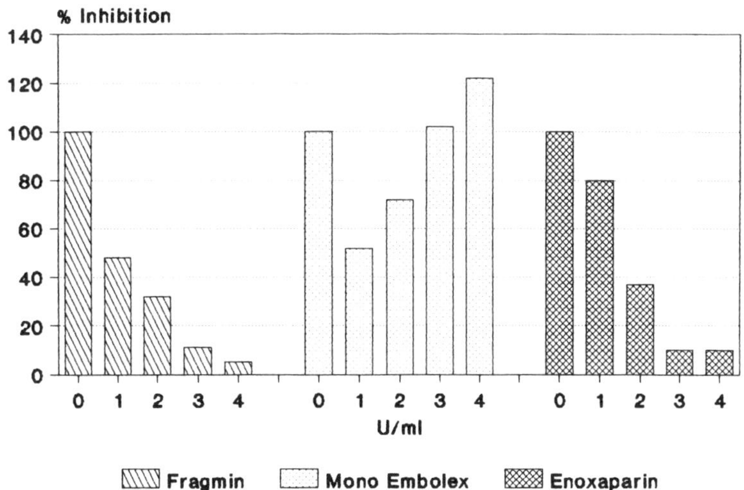

Fig. 6 Effect of Fractionated Heparins on Beta FXIIa Inhibition by Plasma

Table 1. Effect of aprotinin and heparin on alpha and beta FX11a inhibition by plasma

			Alpha FX11a Inhibition								
		Unfractionated (U/ml)						Fractionated (U/ml)				
Aprotinin (KIU/ml)		0	1	2	3	4	Aprotinin (KIU/ml)	0	1	2	3	4
Medac	0	100	100	102	106	115	Fragmin 0	100	100	93	95	100
	100	102	102	104	113	123	100	102	102	99	99	102
	200	104	104	106	118	131	200	104	104	100	100	107
	400	105	106	109	121	136	400	106	107	102	104	109
Lique-	0	100	102	106	128	143	Mono- 0	100	78	121	161	167
min	100	101	104	110	134	149	Embolex 100	102	90	134	170	189
	200	110	111	116	140	155	200	106	93	139	178	195
	400	116	118	120	148	161	400	109	101	148	184	198
Braun	0	100	100	100	107	127	Enoxa- 0	100	90	60	70	72
	100	103	104	108	120	135	parin 100	102	91	62	73	75
	200	106	106	110	123	148	200	104	92	67	77	77
	400	110	110	115	127	156	400	107	94	69	80	79
				Beta FX11a Inhibition								
Medac	0	100	82	72	58	73	Fragmin 0	100	48	32	11	5
	100	100	81	74	60	83	100	101	51	35	12	11
	200	100	82	75	65	90	200	98	60	38	14	14
	400	100	89	76	66	98	400	100	66	41	23	17
Lique-	0	100	86	71	93	119	Mono 0	100	52	72	102	122
min	100	101	88	82	97	128	Embolex 100	100	53	73	106	125
	200	104	89	83	100	130	200	100	55	78	107	128
	400	105	91	86	102	135	400	102	61	92	112	138
Braun	0	100	76	45	43	50	Enoxa- 0	100	80	37	10	10
	100	100	80	49	49	54	parin 100	97	82	42	15	10
	200	100	81	50	50	56	200	97	83	44	15	10
	400	102	83	50	51	56	400	100	85	48	18	10

Aprotinin KIU/ml = Kallikrein inhibitor units per ml.

DISCUSSION

It is widely accepted that the FX11-related blood contact systems (coagulation, fibrinolysis, kallikrein-kinin and complement) are activated during CPB. Unfractionated heparins are used in high doses in CPB and we have suggested that heparins contribute to enhanced contact phase activation in CPB (5). In the present study we have confirmed our previous observation that heparins reduce inhibition of beta FX11a by plasma (Figs 5 and 6) with this effect being particularly pronounced with two fractionated heparins (Fragmin and Enoxaparin Fig. 6).This effect was partly overcome by aprotinin. With alpha FX11a inhibition by plasma the unfractionated heparins gave increased inhibition (Fig. 3) whilst with the fractionated heparins Fragmin slightly reduced alpha FX11a inhibition, Mono Embolex increased inhibition at 2 -4 units per ml and Enoxaparin reduced inhibition. With Aprotinin alpha FX11a inhibition was potentiated with all of the heparins in a dose-dependent manner with inhibition values of over 150% of normal obtained with the highest concentrations of aprotinin and Liquemin, Braun and Mono Embolex (Table. 1).

Our results show that at similar anti FXa concentrations various heparins have different effects on the inhibition of alpha and beta FX11a with most of them increasing alpha FX11a inhibition and all decreasing beta FX11a inhibition at one or more concentrations. They also show that aprotinin increases plasma inhibition of alpha and beta FX11a in the majority of heparinised plasmas. These results suggest that some heparins would be preferred in CPB. Possible roles for aprotinin in CPB as well as inhibition of plasmin and plasma kallikrein, are the antagonisation of the reduction in beta FX11a inhibition by heparin and increase in alpha FX11a inhibition. These effects lead to reduced activation of the blood contact systems and the effects on cells by activated enzymes from these systems. These effects undoubtedly contribute to the clinical benefits of high dose aprotinin therapy in CPB (3,6).

REFERENCES

1. Fuhrer G, Gallimore MJ, Heller W. Hoffmeister H.E. Studies on components of the plasma kallikrein-kinin system in patients undergoing cardiopulmonary bypass. In: KININS 1V Advances in Experimental Medicine and Biology. Greenbaum LW, Margolis HS, editors. New York: Plenum Press, 1986: 198B:385-391.

2. Fuhrer G, Gallimore MJ, Heller W. Hoffmeister H.-E.Studies on the inhibition of plasma kallikrein, C1-esterase and beta FX11a in the presence and absence of heparins. In: KININS V. Avances in Experimental Medicine and Biology. Abe K, Moriya H, Fujii S, editors. New York: Plenum Press, 1989: 247B:61-66.

3. Fuhrer G, Gallimore MJ, Heller W. Hoffmeister H.-E. Aprotinin in cardiopulmonary bypass-Effects on the Hageman factor (FX11) - kallikrein system and blood loss. Blood Coagulation and Fibrinolysis. In Press.

4. Gallimore MJ. and Friberger P. Simple chromogenic peptide substrate assays for determining prekallikrein, kallikrein inhibition and kallikrein like activity in human plasma. Thromb Res 1982; 25:293-298.

5. Fuhrer G, Gallimore MJ, Heller W,. Hoffmeister H.-E. FX11. Blut 1990; 61:258-266.

6. Hunt BJ. Jacoub M. Aprotinin and cardiac surgery. Brit Med J 1991; 303:660-661.

HUMAN PLASMA KALLIKREIN PROCESSING: PROTEOLYSIS AS AN ALTERNATIVE CONTROL

Motta G, Fink* E, Sampaio MU and Sampaio CAM

Depto. Bioquímica, Escola Paulista de Medicina, S. Paulo, SP, Brazil, and *Dept. Clinical Chemistry and Clinical Biochemistry, University of Munich, Munich, Germany

SUMMARY

Human plasma kallikrein (HuPK) was detected in normal non-activated and dilution-activated plasma by immunoblotting, using polyclonal antibodies. In non-activated plasma, the predominatly detected protein corresponds to prokallikrein (Mr 80,000-90,000). Activated plasma, besides kallikrein, contains larger proteins (Mr > 130,000) that possibly represent complexes between kallikrein and proteinase inhibitors. Plasma also contains species (Mr 43,000) which corresponds to kallikrein heavy chain. In activated plasma, monoclonal antibodies against kallikrein heavy chain detected, besides these same bands described above, two additional bands (Mr 30,000 and 20,000) possibly correspondent to fragments of kallikrein heavy chain.

INTRODUCTION

Human plasma kallikrein is a serine proteinase present in plasma as prokallikrein, a glycoprotein zymogen synthesized by liver as a single polypeptide chain with 619 aminoacid residues. The activation of prokallikrein to kallikrein requires the cleavage of the peptide bond Arg^{371}-Ile^{372} in the single chain, forming a molecule with a heavy chain (371 residues) and a light chain (248 residues) held together by disulfide bridges (1).

Prokallikrein circulates in plasma complexed with high molecular weight kininogen as a bimolecular complex 1:1 (2), being the heavy chain of prokallikrein bound to the light chain of high molecular weight kininogen (3).

Prokallikrein is activated in blood by activated factor XII (4). Kallikrein itself activates factor XII at the early phase of intrinsic blood coagulation (5), and hydrolyzes high molecular weight kininogen liberating the hypotensive peptide bradykinin (6). Plasma kallikrein also participates in some reactions of fibrinolysis (7) and complement systems (8), and promotes the aggregation of platelets (9) and leucocytes (10).

Plasma kallikrein can be found in two different molecular weight species (Mr 88,000 and 85,000) (11). The NH_2-terminal heavy chain (43,000) is important for the specific activity of kallikrein and is similar to the heavy chain of factor XI (12); the COOH-terminal light chain (Mr 36,000-33,000) lodges the catalytic site of kallikrein, and is similar to trypsin (1).

Kallikrein is inactivated either by plasma inhibitors such as C1-inhibitor, alpha 2-macroglobulin, antithrombin III (13) and protein C inhibitor (14), or by the liver, where it is recognized by its alpha-galactose residues (15).

In this report, we studied the proteolysis of human plasma kallikrein in activated human plasma, as an alternative control of plasma kallikrein metabolization.

MATERIAL AND METHODS

Human plasma kallikrein (HuPK) was isolated from Cohn's fraction IV (16) or fresh plasma (17). The materials were submitted to SBTI-Sepharose chromatography (0.02 M tris-HCl, 0.3 M NaCl, pH 8.0 buffer) and the adsorbed kallikrein was eluted by benzamidine 1.0 M. The protein concentration was calculated according to the mesurement of the extinction coefficient (E_{280},$^{1\%}$=10.6), determined by Nagase and Barrett (18). The heavy and light chains of plasma kallikrein were isolated by reduction with dithiothreitol, alkylation with iodoacetamide (19) and separated on SBTI-Sepharose.

Polyclonal antibodies against HuPK were raised in rabbits. The antiserum was purified on HuPK-Sepharose (0.05 M tris-HCl, 0.15 M NaCl, pH 8.0 buffer), and the bound antibodies were eluted with 0.2 M glycine-HCl, pH 2.0 buffer, and the pH of the collected samples was kept at 8.0 by addition of 1.0 M tris. Antibody against rabbit IgG (second antibody) was raised in goats, and anti-serum was purified on anti-HuPK-Sepharose, by the same procedure.

Monoclonal antibodies (PK 9) against heavy chain of HuPK, kindly provided by Prof. Dr. Werner Muller-Esterl (University of Mainz-Germany), were precipitated from ascitic fluids with saturated ammonium sulfate solution, pH 7.0 (11:9, v/v). The solution was kept at 4°C during 60 minutes and centrifuged at 3,500 x g at 4°C for 30 minutes. The pellet was ressuspended in 50% ammonium sulfate solution and recentrifuged, under the same conditions. This pellet was ressuspended in 0.01 M tris-HCl, pH 7.5 buffer and dialyzed against the same buffer, overnight at room temperature. The antibodies were cromatographed on a column (100 ml) of DEAE-Sepharose CL 6B (0.01 M tris-HCl, pH 7.5 buffer), and eluted with a sodium chloride gradient from 0 to 0.25 M. The PK9 antibodies were eluted with 0.14 M sodium chloride.

Antibodies were labelled with iodine-125 using as oxidant reagents either Iodo-beads (Pierce) or Chloramine T (20). The specific activity of the polyclonal or monoclonal antibodies was 10-20 uCi/ug, and in each experiment 2×10^6 cpm (100 ng of protein) were used.

Human normal blood was collected directely into plastic tubes mixed with sodium citrate solution 3.8%, 9:1 (v/v). The sample was centrifuged at 1,500 x g,   during 15 minutes at 4°C, and the separeted plasma was aliquoted and kept frozen at -20°C.

For activation, plasma samples (2 ul) were thawed, diluted in water in a final volume of 200 ul, and incubated at 37°C during 15 minutes. The activation reaction was stopped by freezing, and the samples were submitted to electrophoresis. Control samples of non activated plasma (2 ul) were thawed and diluted directly in electrophoresis buffer.

Sodium dodecyl sulfate polyacrylamide gel electrophoresis (SDS-PAGE) was performed in slab gels from 5% to 15%, according to the method of Laemmli (21), with 3% stacking gels. Apparent molecular weights were determined by running standard proteins of known molecular weights (range 14,000 to 200,000) on the gel.

Immunoblotting was performed according to the modification described by Burnette et al. (22) or according to Kyhse-Andersen (23). The immunodetection of the antigen was achieved by a double antibody reaction: the nitrocellulose membranes were incubated with anti-HuPK antibody (20 ug/ml) and the complexes were developed with ^{125}I-second antibody (2 x 10^6 cpm per assay). Alternatively, the immunodetection of the antigens was achieved by reaction with the monoclonal antibody against heavy chain ^{125}I-PK9 (2 x 10^6 cpm per assay).

RESULTS

Human plasma kallikrein was purified by a described procedure (16, 17) and the two known forms, alpha and beta, were prepared; both preparations resulted in single bands on non reduced gel electrophoresis (Figure 1a).

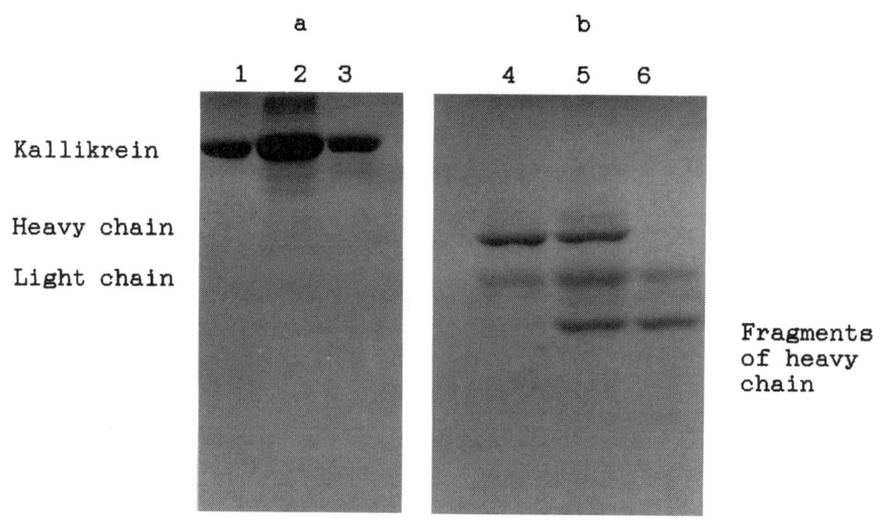

FIGURE 1: SDS-polyacrylamide electrophoresis of kallikrein (HuPK) forms.
a. Non reduced gel
1. alpha-HuPK (15 ug)
2. alpha-HuPK and beta-HuPK (20 ug)
3. beta-HuPK (10 ug)

b. Reduced gel
4. alpha-HuPK (15 ug)
5. alpha-HuPK and beta-HuPK (20 ug)
6. beta-HuPK (10 ug)

After reduction with DTT, alpha-HuPK presents a heavy chain (Mr 45,000) and a light chain (Mr 36,000 and 33,000); beta-HuPK has its heavy chain hydrolyzed into two bands (Mr 30,000 and 20,000), and a light chain (Mr 36,000 and 33,000).

On an immunoblotting using anti-HuPK and ^{125}I-second antibodies, in non-activated plasma (figure 2a) prokallikrein gives a strong band (Mr 80,000) and also weak (Mr > 150,000) bands. The 100-fold diluted plasma (figure 2b) presents the same prokallikrein-kallikrein band (Mr 80,000), and the high molecular bands (Mr > 130,000), that represent kallikrein-inhibitor complexes. The activated plasma also exhibits a band (Mr 43,000) that corresponds to the purified heavy-chain of the enzyme used as marker in the experiment (figure 2d); this band does not coincide with IgG fragments which may contaminate kallkrein preparations (figure 2c).

The same experiment indicated in figure 2 was performed with a monoclonal antibody against heavy chain (PK9). Diluted human plasma (1:100) was incubated with purified HuPK or its isolated heavy chain and the antigens were immunoprecipitated with ^{125}I-PK9 (figure 3).

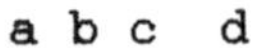

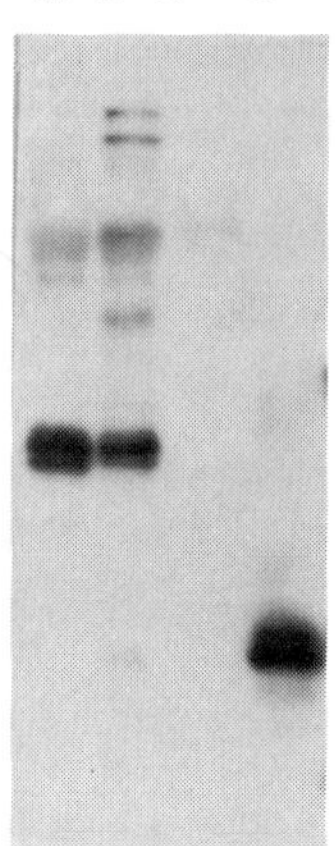

FIGURE 2: Activation of human normal plasma by dilution (1:100).

a. human plasma (2 ul)
b. human plasma (2 ul) diluted 1:100
c. human IgG (6.5 ug)
d. isolated heavy chain of HuPK (1.0 ug)
Immunoprecipitation: anti-HuPK
Development: ^{125}I-second antibodies

In activated plasma the monoclonal antibodies (PK9) identified kallikrein (Mr 80,000) and larger proteins (Mr > 130,000); in this case, the higher molecular weight complexes correspond to kallikrein-inhibitors complexes, and not to eventual complexes between free light chain of HuPK and inhibitors, because the monoclonal PK9 used to develop the blotting does not react with light chain (24).

The addition of isolated kallikrein heavy chain to activated plasma causes a strong enhancement of the weak protein band (Mr 43,000), showing that the band corresponds to heavy chain.

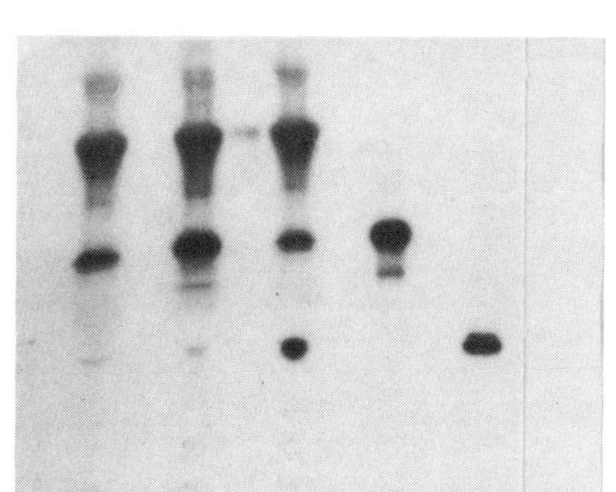

FIGURE 3: Diluted human plasma (1:100) incubated with purified
kallikrein and kallikrein heavy chain.

1. human normal plasma (2 ul)
2. human normal plasma (2 ul) and HuPK (0.5 ug)
3. human normal plasma (2 ul) and isolated heavy chain (0.3 ug)
4. HuPK (0.5 ug)
5. isolated heavy chain (0.3 ug)

Development: ^{125}I-PK9

Plasma (2 ul) was diluted (1:100) and incubated with
increasing quantities of purified HuPK, and the antigens were
immunoprecipitated with ^{125}I-PK9 (figure 4). The increasing
quantities of purified kallikrein added to activated plasma
causes a strong enhancement of the kallikrein-inhibitors
complexes bands (Mr > 130,000), as well as the heavy chain band
(Mr 43,000), and also the appearance of smaller proteins bands
(Mr 30,000 and 20,000). These results are the first indication
of the hydrolysis of kallikrein heavy chain, in plasma.

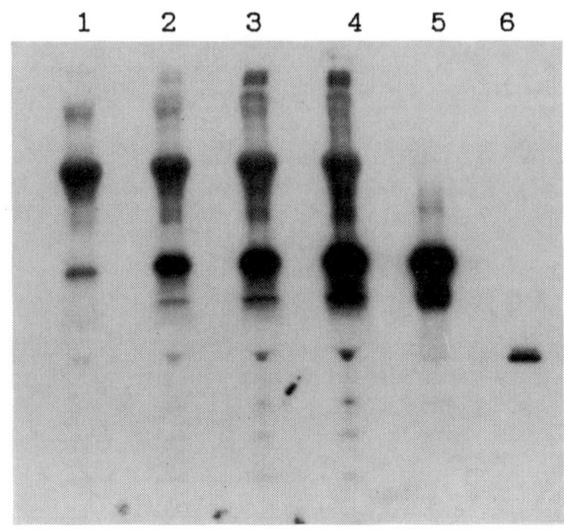

FIGURE 4: Diluted human plasma (1:100) incubated with different quantities of HuPK.

1. human plasma (2 ul)
2. human plasma (2 ul) and HuPK (0.5 ug)
3. human plasma (2 ul) and HuPK (1.0 ug)
4. human plasma (2 ul) and HuPK (2.5 ug)
5. HuPK (2.5 ug)
6. HC (0.2 ug)

Development: ^{125}I-PK9

DISCUSSION

Beta-HuPK derives from a clevage in the heavy chain of the alpha-HuPK, and one possibility for this modification is to occur to keep pure kallikrein solutions at room temperature. The beta form has the same activity on synthetic substrates, but alpha-kallikrein cleaves high molecular weight kininogen (HMWKgn) releasing braykinin, faster than the beta form (25).

Contact of plasma with negatively charged surfaces, such as glass or kaolin, causes the activation of the intrinsic pathway of blood clotting, by bringing together kallikrein, kininogen and factor XII on the surface. However, dilution induces activation by decreasing the inhibitor concentration in plasma and thus promoting activation of the key clotting enzymes. In our experiments the activation was confirmed by the formation of complexes, equivalent to those formed by incubation of kallikrein and purified inhibitors (13).

Only in the activated plasma the protein band corresponding to the heavy chain (Mr 43,000) was detected by both polyclonal and monoclonal antibodies (26). The addition of large quantities of active kallikrein in activated plasma brings evidences that the transformation of alpha to beta-kallikrein proceeds in the plasma, as it was observed for purified samples of kallikrein. The larger protein bands (Mr > 130,000) probably correspond to complexes of kallikrein and plasma proteinase inhibitors. The polypeptide chains with Mr < 43,000 may indicate that kallikrein or its heavy chain is being processed in activated plasma, resulting in shorter fragments.

No corresponding free light chain is found in activated plasma containing free heavy chain. One possible explanation for this finding is an extensive hydrolysis of the light chain, and no immunnodetectable fragments would be available for reaction with polyclonal antibodies. Or, alternatively, the formation of light chain-inhibitors complexes might occur but difficult to resolve from the HuPK-inibitor complexes.

Thus, the control of kallikrein activity, especially in the blood clotting cascade, might also be exerted by a proteolytic degradation of its molecule. The resulting free heavy chain might alter the surface binding ability of high molecular weight kininogen, and the whole activity of the contact phase would be lowered. Proteolysis of the heavy chain itself might also be taken as part of this control mechanism, that would not depend on inhibition and liver clearance alone.

REFERENCE

1. Chung DW, Fujikawa K, McMullen BA and Davie EW (1986).
   Biochemistry 25: 2410-2417.
2. Mandle RJr, Colman RW and Kaplan AP (1976). Proc. Nat. Acad.
   Sci. USA 73: 4179-4183.
3. Vogel R, Kaufmann J, Chung DW, Kellermann J and Muller-Esterl
   W (1990). J. Biol. Chem. 265: 12494-12502.
4. Kaplan AP and Austen KF (1970). J. Immunol. 105: 802-811.
5. Meier HL, Pierce JV, Colman RW and Kaplan AP (1977). J. Clin.
   Invest. 60: 18-31.
6. Habermann E (1970). Handb. Exper. Pharmacol. 25: 250-288.
7. Ichinose A, Fujikawa K and Suyama T (1986). J. Biol. Chem.
   261: 3486-3489.
8. Hiemstra PS, Daha MR and Bouma BN (1985). Thrombos. Res. 38:
   491-503.
9. Cassaro CMF, Sampaio MU, Maeda NY, Chamone DF and Sampaio CAM
   (1987). Thrombos. Res. 48: 81-87.
10. Schapira M., Despland E., Scott CF, Boxer LA and Colman RW
    (1982). J. Clin. Invest. 69: 1199-1202.
11. Mandle RJr and Kaplan AP (1977). J. Biol. Chem. 252: 6097-
    6104.

12. Fujikawa K, Chung DW, Hendrickson LE and Davie EW (1986). _Biochemistry_ 25: 2417-2424.
13. Graaf F van der, Koedam JA and Bouma BN (1983). _J. Clin. Invest._ 71: 149-158.
14. Espana F, Berrettini M. and Griffin JH (1989). _Thrombos. Res._ 55: 369-384.
15. Borges DR, Gordon AH, Guimarães JA and Prado JL (1982). _Agents and Actions Suppl._ 9: 46-51.
16. Sampaio C, Wong S-C and Shaw E (1974). _Arch. Biochem. Biophys._ 165: 133-139.
17. Oliva MLV, Grisolia D, Sampaio MU and Sampaio CAM (1982). _Agents and Actions_ 9: 52-57.
18. Nagase H and Barrett AJ (1981). _Biochem. J._ 193: 187-192.
19. Graaf F van der, Tans G, Bouma BN and Griffin JH (1982). _J. Biol. Chem._ 257: 14300-14305.
20. Greenwood FC, Hunter WM and Glover JS (1963). _Biochem. J._ 89: 114-123.
21. Laemli UK (1970). _Nature_ 227: 680-685.
22. Burnette WN (1981). _Analy. Biochem._ 112: 195-203.
23. Kyhse-Andersen J (1984). _J. Biochem. Biophys. Methods_ 10: 203-209.
24. Hock J, Vogel R, Limke RP and Müller-Esterl W (1990). _J. Biol. Chem._ 265: 12005-12011.
25. Motta G, Sampaio MU and Sampaio CAM (1989). _Adv. Exp. Med. Biol._ 247B: 239-242.
26. Veloso D, Tseng SY, Graig AR and Colman RW (1989). _Adv. Exp. Med. Biol._ 247A: 499-505.
27. Tans G, Rosing J, Berretini M, Lammle B and Griffin JH (1987). _J. Biol. Chem._ 262: 11308-11314.

AAS 38/II
Recent Progress on Kinins
© 1992 Birkhäuser Verlag Basel

CHLORAMINE T IMPAIRS THE RECEPTOR-MEDIATED ENDOCYTOSIS OF PLASMA KALLIKREIN BY THE LIVER

D.R. Borges[*] and M. Kouyoumdjian

Departments of Medicine[*] and Biochemistry, Escola Paulista de Medicina, 04023 - Sao Paulo, Brasil

SUMMARY: Treatment of rat plasma-kallikrein with chloramine T (which does not affect neither its amidolytic activity nor its Mr) impairs the hepatic clearance of the enzyme in a dose-related manner. Preperfusion of the liver with chloramine T before the addition of plasma-kallikrein also diminishes the hepatic clearance of the enzyme.

INTRODUCTION

The liver is the main organ to clear plasma as well as tissue kallikreins from circulation (1). Previous studies with two native tissue kallikreins, horse urinary and pig pancreatic, showed that their removal from circulation through hepatic receptor-mediated endocytosis is calcium-dependent; their receptors were characterized as galactosyl and mannosyl-specific lectins, respectively (2). Borges and co-workers (3) showed that rat plasma-kallikrein (RPK) is efficiently cleared by exsanguinated and perfused rat liver through an endocytosis mechanism. The binding site to hepatocytes is latent on prokallikren and located on its heavy chain (4). The labelling of RPK with ^{125}I, when performed following the method of Greenwood et al (5), is easily and efficiently achieved but the enzyme loses its capacity to be recognized by liver cells (6). We now report further results on the effects of chloramine T on the liver clearance of RPK.

MATERIALS AND METHODS

Male adult Wistar outbred albino rats from the colony EPM-1 were from the "Biotério Central da Escola Paulista de Medicina". Bovine serum albumin (BSA) was from Sigma Chemical Co. Inc. Milwaukee, USA. Na-^{131}I was from the Comissão Nacional de Energia Nuclear, São Paulo, Brasil; Na-^{125}I and ^{3}H-water were obtained from New England Nuclear, Boston, USA. Benzoyl-ProPheArg-para-nitroanilide (BzPPApNA) was synthesized and given by L. Juliano, Department of Byophysics, Escola Paulista de Medicina, São Paulo, Brasil.

Rat plasma-kallikrein (RPK): we prepared the Ê (integral, 84-87 kDa) form of RPK as described (7). In each rat liver perfusion 300 pmoles was used.

Preparation of ^{125}I-RPK and ^{131}I-BSA: RPK (36 ug) and BSA (100 ug) were labelled with iodine, ^{125}I and ^{131}I respectively, as described by Greenwood et al. (5). The reactions were carried out in 0.05 M NaPB pH 7.0 using a fresh solution of chloramine T (0.9 mM). After 1 minute sodium metabisulphite (3 mM) was added and the labelled protein separated from free iodine on a 5 ml Sephadex G-25 column. Specific radioactivities of 2 and 3.2 uCi/ug of protein were obtained for ^{125}I-RPK and ^{131}I-BSA, respectively.

RPK treatment with chloramine T: some aliquots (20 ug) of RPK were incubated at room temperature with different concentrations of chloramine T (0.4, 0.9 and 18 mM). The incubations of RPK with 0.4 and 0.9 mM chloramine T were interrupted after 1 minute with 3 mM sodium metabisulphite and immediately gel filtered in a Sephadex G-25 column. The incubation with 18 mM chloramine T was interrupted with 20 mM sodium metabisulphite; 20 ul of 0.12 M Tris-HCl pH 6.8 containing 1% SDS, 20% glycerol and 0.05% bromophenol blue was added and the sample introduced on SDS-PAGE.

Liver perfusion in situ: The livers of 280-320 g rats were perfused through the portal vein as described previously (3). The clearance rate of RPK was calculated from the residual RPK amidolytic activity (on BzPPApNA, 0.4 mM) in the perfusion fluid.

Pulse-labelling experiments: Three pulse experiments were performed with a mixture of ^{125}I-RPK (0.18 uCi), ^{131}I-BSA (0.17 uCi) and ^{3}H-water (10 uCi). After injection in the portal vein (within 0.5 second employing a mycroseringe) the effluent perfusate was collected over a period of 90 seconds with fractions of 0.5-2 seconds. The radioactivity of the perfusate aliquots were measured in a three channel spectrometer Beckman LS 6800 (8).

RESULTS AND DISCUSSION

The effect of the treatment of RPK with different concentrations of chloramine T prior to liver perfusion was studied. The treatment with 18 mM chloramine T had no effect, either in the amidolytic activity or on SDS-PAGE. On the other hand the incubation of RPK with 0.4 mM chloramine T decreased the clearance rate by rat liver whereas with 0.9 mM completely abolished this clearance (Table 1).

Table 1. Effect of chloramine T treatment of RPK on its enzymatic activity, Mr and hepatic clearance

Chloramine T (mM) [a]	Amidolytic activity [b] (%)	Mr [c]	Liver clearance (%)
0	100	84-87 kDa	100
0.4	100	ND [d]	53
0.9	100	ND	0
18.0	100	84-87 kDa	ND

[a] **in vitro** incubation of RPK with chloramine T
[b] determined as described by Kouyoumdjian et al (6)
[c] SDS-PAGE, without reduction
[d] ND: not determined

The damage caused to some proteins by chloramine T, used in iodination procedures, was described as early as 1966 by McConahey and Dixon (9). Parathyroid hormone and calcitonin are regularly altered during iodination whereas other substances may have their integral structure disrupted (10). Chloramine T oxidation has no affect upon the enzymatic activity of RPK or its behaviour on SDS-PAGE but the liver clearance was reduced or even abolished, depending on the chloramine T concentration used. The hepatic clearance was also lowered after sodium periodate or iodoacetate (5 mM) treatment (data not shown). These substances disturb the hepatic clearance of RPK most probably by oxidizing terminal sugars and/or by destabilizing its native conformation which may be important for RPK binding to liver cells. They do not affect the catalytic light chain in so far as it concerns small substrates. Paquin et al reported that RPK labelling (Tyr-iodinated) interferes with its recognition by specific antibody (11).

A mixture of ^{131}I-BSA, ^{3}H-water and ^{125}I-RPK was injected into the portal vein of rat and the outflow profile analyzed. Figure 1 shows the results of 3 pulse experiments and reveals that ^{125}I-RPK (iodinated using 0.9 mM chloramine T) did not exchange with the intracellular space (^{3}H-water marker) since its outflow profile was similar to ^{131}I-BSA, an extracellular marker.

During a single passage through the liver some substances will be distorted according to the events inside the organ; ^{131}I-albumin, which do not exchange significantly with the cellular space, will have an outflow profile with the least distortion whereas others, like ^{3}H-H$_2$O, which exchange very rapidly with the intracellular spaces, will have an outflow profile greatly distorted (8). The behaviour of ^{125}I-RPK in the experiment was identical to ^{131}I-albumin confirming that exposing RPK to chloramine T during iodination resulted in the failure for the enzyme to bind to the hepatic receptor.

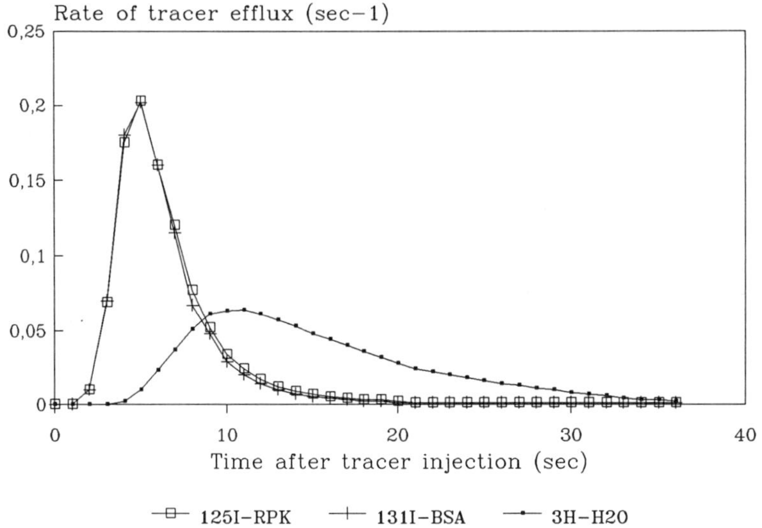

Figure 1. Outflow profile of ^{125}I-rat plasma-kallikrein.
The pulse-labelling experiments were performed in isolated livers; a mixture of 0.18 uCi ^{125}I-RPK, 0.17 uCi ^{131}I-albumin and 10 uCi ^{3}H-H$_2$O was injected and the effluent perfusate (second fractions) plotted versus the time following injection. Each point represents the mean of three experiments.

To study the effect of chloramine T upon the plasma-kallikrein liver receptor the oxidant was previously perfused through the liver for 10 minutes after which the perfusion medium was exchanged (now without chloramine T) and the RPK added in the perfusion system. In this manner RPK did not got in contact with chloramine T. A considerable reduction on RPK clearance (approximately 65%) was observed (Table 2, mean ± SEM).

Table 2. Effect of preperfusion of chloramine T on the hepatic clearance of RPK

		RPK clearance (pmol/g liver)		
		5	10	15
Perfusion	N	(perfusion time, minutes)		
control	3	8.9±0.6	12.1±0.9	14.4±1.4
chloramine T [a]	4	2.8±0.8	4.0±1.2	6.1±0.9
"t" test		p<0.01	p<0.01	p<0.01

[a] Prior to the addition of RPK to the perfusion fluid the liver was perfused with 0.18 mM chloramine T for 10 minutes.

Thus chloramine T has also an effect on the RPK-receptor. RPK endocytosis by liver cells is probably mediated by an S-type lectin (4). Although S-type lectins may be inactivated under oxidizing conditions (12) we cannot exclude, at present, the possibility that the diminished uptake following liver treatment with chloramine T may be due to effects on other steps of endocytosis besides binding.

In conclusion one must be aware that labelling process may affect irreversibly functional sites on the regulatory chain of plasma-kallikrein.

ACKNOWLEDGEMENTS: We thank Dr. Adelar Bracht (Dept. Bioquimica, Universidade Estadual de Maringá) for the pulse experiments and Miss Hercilia Mares Molina for technical assistance.

REFERENCES

1. Borges DR, Sampaio CAM, Llosa P de La and Prado JL. The liver is the main organ to clear plasma and tissue kallikreins from plasma **in vivo**. Adv Exp Biol Med 1986; 198A:229-233.

2. Kouyoumdjian M, Borges DR, Prado ES and Prado JL. Identification of receptors in the liver that mediate endocytosis of circulating tissue kallikreins. Biochim Biophys Acta. 1989; 980:299-304.

3. Borges DR, Gordon AH, Guimarães JA and Prado JL. Rat plasma kallikrein clearance by perfused rat liver. Brazilian J Med Biol Res 1985; 18:187-194.

4. Borges DR and Kouyoumdjian M. The recognition site for hepatic clearance of plasma-kallikrein is on its heavy chain and is latent on prokallikrein. J Hepatol (in press)

5. Greenwood FC, Hunter WM and Glover JS. The preparation of 131I-labelled human growth hormone of high specific radioactivity. Biochem J 1963; 89:114-123.

6. Kouyoumdjian M, Borges DR and Prado JL. Rat plasma kallikrein: enzymatic activity and liver clearance following iodination. Arq Biol Tecnol 1986; 29:193.

7. Kouyoumdjian M, Borges DR, Michelacci YM, Guimarães JA, Sampaio CAM and Prado JL. Purification and characterization of the alpha form of rat plasma kallikrein. Brazilian J Med Biol Res 1987; 20:549-552.

8. Ishii EL, Schwab AJ and Bracht A. Inhibition of monossacharide transport in the intact rat liver by stevioside. Biochem Pharmacol 1987; 361417-1433.

9. McConahey PJ and Dixon FJ. A method of trace iodination of proteins for immunologic studies. Int Arch Allergy 1966; 29:185-189.

10. Buckle RM and Potts JT. Assessment of damage to I-131-labelled parathyroid hormone by chromatoelectrophoresis and adsortion onto dextran-charcoal. J Lab Clin Med 1970; 76:46-53.

11. Paquin J, Benjannet S, Sawyer N, Lazure C, Chrétien M and Seidah NG. Rat plasma kallikrein: purification, NH_2-terminal sequencing and development of a specific radioimmunoassay. Biochim Biophys Acta 1989; 999:103-110.

12. Drickamer K. Two distinct classes of carbohydrate-recognition domains in animal lectins. J Biol Chem 1988; 263:9557-9560.

ON THE ROLE OF BRADYKININ IN SECRETION
FROM VASCULAR ENDOTHELIAL CELLS

J.J. Emeis and N. Tranquille

Gaubius Laboratory IVVO-TNO, P.O. Box 430,
2300 AK Leiden, the Netherlands

SUMMARY: Bradykinin will induce, in perfused rat hindlegs, the acute release from endothelial cells of tissue-type plasminogen activator and of von Willebrand factor. This release is mediated by B_2-receptors, requires the influx of extracellular calcium, and is modulated by cyclic nucleotides. A possible role of bradykinin in the physiological regulation of plasma levels of tissue-type plasminogen activator is discussed.

INTRODUCTION

The fibrinolytic and thrombolytic enzyme tissue-type plasminogen activator (t-PA) is very rapidly cleared from the circulation by the liver: its intravascular half-life varies from one minute in rodents to four minutes in man (1). In order to maintain a stable blood level, the protein must thus continuously be released into the circulation (2). It is likely that vascular endothelial cells are responsible for said continuous secretion of t-PA, as t-PA is synthetized and stored mainly by these cells. Which secretory mechanism is employed by endothelial cells to perform this function is still not definitively established (3). Of the two secretion mechanisms that might be involved -- constitutive (continuous) secretion and regulated (stimulated) secretion -- the latter possibility, stimulated or regulated secretion, here called acute release, is supported by the in vivo evidence, as tissues contain large, stable stores of t-PA (4) and as plasma levels of t-PA and acute release of t-PA remain virtually unchanged for many hours in rats in vivo after protein synthesis has been inhibited (5,6). Continuing stimulated secretion requires continuing stimulation, and bradykinin might be one of the compounds responsible for this stimulation. In the present paper we will discuss evidence regarding the acute induction of t-PA release from endothelial cells by bradykinin. At the same time we will discuss the induction of the release of von Willebrand factor, an other endothelial secretory product that is released in parallel with t-PA (7).

MATERIALS AND METHODS

The induction of acute release of t-PA and von Willebrand factor (vWF) from endothelial cells was studies using the perfused rat hindleg system described previously (5,8,9). In brief: rat hindlegs (male Wistar rats) were perfused via the aorta, at a constant flow rate of 10 ml/min, with oxygenated Tyrode's balanced salt solution containing bovine serum albumin (Tyrode/BSA) at 37°C. After a 30-min wash-out period, the hindlegs were perfused for five minutes with Tyrode/BSA containing bradykinin (routinely 0.8 μM, this fairly high concentration possibly being required because of the large capacity of rat vascular beds to degrade bradykinin; see ref 10). Samples were collected at one-minute intervals from an outflow cannula in the vena cava. In the effluent fractions we determined t-PA activity using a spectrophotometric assay (11), and vWF antigen using an enzyme-linked immunosorbent assay (12). Inhibitors were present, where indicated, in the Tyrode/BSA solution for the last 10 (or 20) minutes of the wash-out period, as well as during stimulation of release by bradykinin.

RESULTS

Bradykinin dose-dependently (8) induced the release of t-PA. Release of both t-PA and vWF was rapid, maximal release being observed at one to two min after the beginning of stimulation, and short-lived, as the concentration of both proteins had effectively returned to base-line values after five min of stimulation (figure 1). Stimulation of acute release by bradykinin showed tachyphylaxis (8). As desArg^9-bradykinin did not induce any release, the secretion from perfused rat hindlegs was presumably due to activation by bradykinin of the B$_2$-receptor (data not shown). Release was strictly calcium-dependent; no secretion of either t-PA or vWF was found during stimulation with bradykinin in the absence of calcium (9).

This requirement for extracellular calcium presumably reflected a requirement for calcium influx into the cell via receptor-operated calcium channels, as bradykinin-induced release of t-PA (though surprisingly not the release of vWF) was blocked by lanthanum chloride (table 1). In support of this conclusion, verapamil and diltiazem, antagonists of voltage-dependent calcium channels, did not affect release, while the calcium channel agonist Bay K-8644 even reduced release (compare ref 13). The acute release of t-PA and vWF was also inhibited by the calmodulin antagonists calmidazolium and trifluoroperazine, as well as by TMB-8, suggesting a role for calmodulin in endothelial release processes (table 1) (9).

As we have shown elsewhere (14), products of the phospholipase pathway are also necessary for induction of t-PA release by bradykinin to occur. These products are most likely epoxyeicosatrienoic acids, formed in endothelial cells by cytochrome P450-dependent mono-

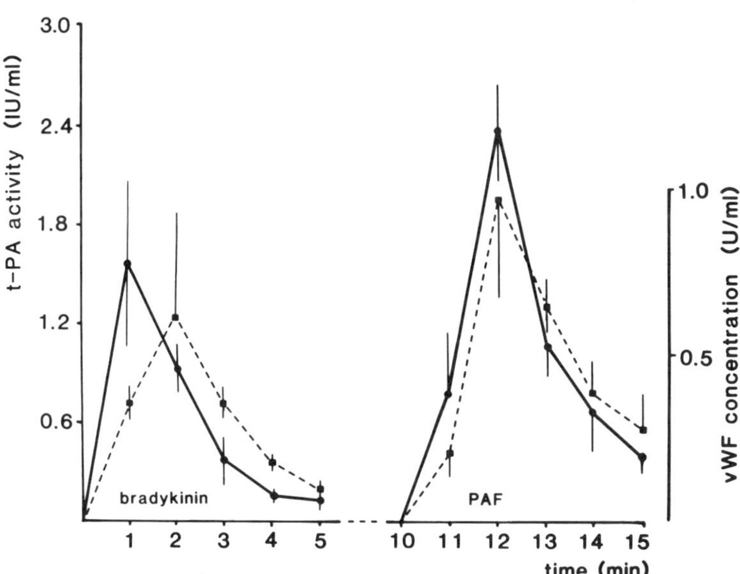

FIGURE 1. Time course of release of tissue-type plasminogen activator (t-PA; ●) and of von Willebrand factor (vWF; ■) from perfused rat hindlegs during a 5-min period of stimulation with bradykinin (0.8 μM), followed -- after a 5-min wash-out -- by a 5-min period of stimulation with platelet-activating factor (5 nM).

TABLE 1.   CALCIUM AND THE RELEASE OF t-PA AND vWF BY BRADYKININ

Inhibitor (concentration)	t-PA released (U/ml)	vWF released (U/ml)	n=
Controls	1.68 ± 0.27[*]	1.38 ± 0.57	7
No calcium	<0.03 [**]	<0.1 [**]	4
LaCl$_3$ (200 μM)	0.40 ± 0.11[**]	1.54 ± 0.21	4
Verapamil (10 μM)	1.24 ± 0.39	1.48 ± 0.54	4
Diltiazem (20 μM)	1.73 ± 0.46	2.35 ± 0.27	3
BAY K-8644 (1 μM)	1.19 ± 0.38[**]	0.70 ± 0.09[**]	4
Calmidazolium (10 μM)	0.89 ± 0.22[**]	1.62 ± 0.12	4
Trifluoroperazine (50 μM)	0.29 ± 0.07[**]	0.55 ± 0.26[**]	3
TMB-8 (70 μM)	1.51 ± 0.53	0.98 ± 0.35	6

[*] Data shown are means $\pm$ SD of maximal concentrations obtained during a 5-min stimulation with 0.8 μM bradykinin

[**] Significantly different from controls

TABLE 2.   CYCLIC NUCLEOTIDES AND THE RELEASE OF t-PA AND vWF BY BRADYKININ

Modulator (concentration)	t-PA released (U/ml)	vWF released (U/ml)	n=
Controls	1.66 ± 0.38[*]	1.00 ± 0.23	30
Nitroprusside (1 mM)	1.14 ± 0.40[**]	0.16 ± 0.10[**]	4
A.N.F. (20 nM)[†]	1.12 ± 0.20[**]	0.60 ± 0.16[**]	4
8-bromo-cyclic GMP (1 mM)	1.84 ± 0.30	1.15 ± 0.46	4
Forskolin (10 μM)	1.60 ± 0.25	1.02 ± 0.25	10
8-bromo-cyclic AMP (1 mM)	2.00 ± 0.31	1.72 ± 0.54[**]	4

[*] Data shown are means $\pm$ SD of maximal concentrations obtained during a 5-min stimulation with 0.8 μM bradykinin

[**] Significantly different from controls

[†] A.N.F.: atrial natriuretic peptide

-oxygenase(s). A third system that might be involved in bradykinin-induced release of t-PA and vWF is the cyclic nucleotide system. As shown in table 2, sodiumnitroprusside and atrial natriuretic factor (activators of soluble and particulate guanylate cyclase) both reduced bradykinin-induced release of t-PA and vWF. Surprisingly, the cell-permeant compound 8-bromo-cyclic GMP had no such effect. Forskolin, an inducer of adenylate cyclase activity, had no effect on bradykinin-induced release, though 8-bromo-cyclic AMP enhanced it (table 2). Concomitant treatment with N^G-nitro-L-arginine methyl ester, an inhibitor of nitric oxide formation (15), had no effect on release by bradykinin (not shown). None of the inhibitors or modulators mentioned was able to induce release by itself in the absence of bradykinin. Together these data suggest that bradykinin-induced release of t-PA and vWF from vascular endothelial cells involves a (B_2-receptor dependent) influx of extracellular calcium, which influx is followed by activation of phospholipase(s) and mono-oxygenase(s), while the release reaction is modulated by cyclic nucleotides.

DISCUSSION

We have shown that bradykinin will induce an acute, transient release of tissue-type plasminogen activator and von Willebrand factor from endothelial cells in perfused rat hindlegs. Similar results have been shown for perfused vascular systems of dogs and pigs (16,17). Induction of t-PA release by bradykinin also occurs **in vivo**, as has been shown in rats (8,18), dogs (19), pigs (20), monkeys (21) and men (22,23) (see ref 24 for details). The fact that bradykinin can induce the release of t-PA (and vWF) does not necessarily entail that it is involved in the physiological regulation of release in vivo. At present no data are available that show this to be the case. It is to be expected that the availability of potent and long-acting bradykinin receptor antagonists and of inhibitors of bradykinin degradation will, in the near future, help to solve this question.

Stimulation of endothelial cells by bradykinin will not only result in release of t-PA and vWF, but will also (see e.g. refs 25,26) increase the synthesis of prostaglandins, including prostacyclin, increase the synthesis of endothelium derived relaxing factor, and possibly also induce the release of endothelin, itself another inducer of t-PA and vWF release (27). The capacity of endothelial cells to produce and release bradykinin themselves (26) opens new and exciting possibilities for the autocrine or paracrine regulation of these processes.

REFERENCES

1. Mordenti J, Chen SA, Moore JA, Ferraiolo BL, Green JD. Interspecies scaling of clearance and volume of distribution data for five therapeutic proteins. Pharm Res 1991; **8**:1351-9.
2. Emeis JJ. Regulation of the acute release of tissue-type plasminogen activator from the endothelium by coagulation activation products. Ann N Y Acad Sci 1992; in press.
3. Emeis JJ. Mechanisms involved in short-term changes in blood levels of t-PA. In: Tissue-type plasminogen activator: physiological and clinical aspects. Kluft C, editor. Boca Raton, Florida: CRC Press, 1988; **2**:21-35.
4. Padró T, van den Hoogen CM, Emeis JJ. Distribution of tissue-type plasminogen activator (activity and antigen) in rat tissues. Blood Coagulation Fibrinolysis 1990: **1**:601-8.
5. Tranquille N, Emeis JJ. Protein synthesis inhibition by cycloheximide does not affect the acute release of tissue-type plasminogen activator. Thromb Haemostas 1989; **61**:442-7.
6. Emeis JJ, Padró T, van den Hoogen CM. The effect of protein synthesis inhibition on plasma fibrinolytic activity in rats. Fibrinolysis 1990; **4**,supplement 3:129.
7. Tranquille N, Emeis JJ. The simultaneous acute release of tissue-type plasminogen activator and von Willebrand factor in the perfused rat hindleg region. Thromb Haemostas 1990; **63**: 454-8.
8. Emeis JJ. Perfused rat hindlegs. A model to study plasminogen activator release. Thromb Res 1983; **30**:195-203.
9. Tranquille N, Emeis JJ. On the role of calcium in the acute release of tissue-type plasminogen activator and von Willebrand factor from the rat perfused hindleg region. Thromb Haemostas 1991; **66**:479-83.
10. Chen X, Orfanos SE, Ryan JW, Chung AYK, Hess DC, Catravas JD. Species variation in pulmonary endothelial aminopeptidase P activity. J Pharmacol Exp Ther 1991; **259**:1301-7.
11. Verheijen JH, Mullaart E, Chang GTG, Kluft C, Wijngaards G. A simple, sensitive spectrophotometic assay for extrinsic (tissue-type) plasminogen activator applicable to measurements in plasma. Thromb Haemostas 1982; **48**:266-9.
12. Ingerslev J. A sensitive ELISA for von Willebrand factor (vWF:Ag). Scand J Clin Lab Invest 1987; **47**:143-9.
13. Schilling WP, Ritchie AK, Navarro LT, Eskin SG. Bradykinin-stimulated calcium influx in cultured bovine aortic endothelial cells. Am J Physiol 1988; **255**:H219-27.
14. Tranquille N, Emeis JJ. The involvement of products of the phospholipase pathway in the acute release of tissue-type plasminogen activator from perfused rat hindlegs. Eur J Pharmacol 1992; in press.
15. Moore PK, al-Swayeh OA, Chong NWS, Evans RA, Gibson A. L-N^G-nitro arginine (L-NOARG), a novel, L-arginine-reversible inhibitor of endothelium-dependent vasodilatation in vitro. Br J Pharmacol 1990; **99**:408-12.
16. Klöcking H-P. Pharmakologische Beeinflussung der Freisetzung von t-PA aus dem Gefässendothel. Hämostaseologie 1991; **11**:76-88.
17. Kitaguchi H, Hijikata A, Hirata M. Effect of thrombin on plasminogen activator release from isolated perfused dog leg. Thromb Res 1979; **16**:407-20.
18. Smith D, Gilbert M, Owen WG. Tissue plasminogen activator release in vivo in response to vasoactive agents. Blood 1985; **66**:835-9.
19. Holemans R. Enhancement of fibrinolysis in the dog by injection of vasoactive drugs. Am J Physiol 1965; **208**:511-20.

20. Egberg N, Gallimore M, Green K, Jakobsson J, Vesterqvist O, Wiman B. Effects of plasma kallikrein and bradykinin infusions into pigs on plasma fibrinolytic variables and urinary excretion of tromboxane and prostacyclin metabolites. Fibrinolysis 1988; 2:101-6.

21. Holemans R, Mlynarczyk EJ, Silver MJ. Enhancement of fibrinolysis and blood clotting: role of microvascular changes. Med Exp 1968; 18:299-307.

22. Neri Serneri GG, Rossi Ferrini PL, Paoletti P, Panti A, D'Ayala Valva G. Effects of bradykinin on coagulation and fibrinolysis, study in vitro and in vivo. Thromb Diathes Haemorrh 1965; 14:508-18.

23. Tesi M, Caramelli L. Influence of the autonomic nervous system on fibrinolytic activity caused by bradykinin. In: Vasopeptides. Back N, Sicuteri F, editors. New York: Plenum Press, 1972: 209-20.

24. Kluft C, Dooijewaard G, Emeis JJ. Role of the contact system in fibrinolysis. Sem Thromb Haemostas 1987; 13:50-68.

25. Vanhoutte PM, Auch-Schwelk W, Biondi ML, Lorenz RR, Schini VB. Why are converting enzyme inhibitors vasodilators? Br J Clin Pharmac 1989; 28:95S-104S.

26. Wiemer G, Schölkens BA, Becker RHA, Busse R. Ramiprilat enhances endothelial autacoid formation by inhibiting breakdown of endothelium-derived bradykinin. Hypertension 1991; 18:558-63.

27. Pruis J, Emeis JJ. Endothelin-1 and -3 induce the release of tissue-type plasminogen activator and von Willebrand factor from endothelial cells. Eur J Pharmacol 1990; 187:105-12.

AAS 38/II
Recent Progress on Kinins
© 1992 Birkhäuser Verlag Basel

CONTACT SYSTEM DEPENDENT FIBRINOLYTIC ACTIVITY IN VIVO: OBSERVATIONS IN HEALTHY SUBJECTS AND FACTOR XII DEFICIENT PATIENTS

Marcel Levi[1], C. Erik Hack[2], Jan Paul de Boer[2], Dees P.M. Brandjes[1], Harry R. Büller[1] and Jan Wouter ten Cate[1]

1. Center for Hemostasis, Thrombosis, Atherosclerosis and Inflammation Research, Academic Medical Center, University of Amsterdam, the Netherlands and 2. Department of Autoimmune Diseases, Central Laboratory of the Netherlands Red Cross Blood Transfusion Service and Laboratory for Clinical and Experimental Immunology, Amsterdam, the Netherlands

SUMMARY: The contribution of activation of the contact system to activation of the fibrinolytic system in vivo was investigated in healthy volunteers and in factor XII deficient patients.

The plasminogen activating activity in normal plasma was only partially blocked (for 77%) with specific antibodies to tissue-type plasminogen activator (t-PA) and urokinase-type plasminogen activator (u-PA). The residual activity could be quenched by a monoclonal antibody that inhibits factor XII activity and was not present in patients with a factor XII deficiency. The formation of plasmin upon the DDAVP stimulus as reflected by circulating plasmin-α2-antiplasmin (PAP) complexes was lower in factor XII deficient patients than in healthy volunteers.

These results indicate that in vivo the plasminogen activating activity is partially dependent on activation of the contact system. This fibrinolytic activity is impaired in factor XII deficient patients which may explain the occurrence of thromboembolic complications in these patients.

INTRODUCTION

The activation of plasminogen in vivo may occur by plasminogen activators such as t-PA or u-PA (1) but quenching experiments with specific antibodies have revealed that these plasminogen activators do not account for all plasminogen activating activity observed (2), indicating the existence of a third pathway of plasminogen activation.

This third pathway of plasminogen activation has been claimed to be dependent on activation of the contact system of blood coagulation (3). To determine the role of contact activation in fibrinolysis we investigated the contribution of factor XII to the plasminogen activator activity induced in plasma of healthy subjects and individuals with mild or severe factor XII deficiency.

METHODS

Study subjects and DDAVP test

Six healthy volunteers (age 21 to 33 years) and in addition six subjects with a known deficiency of coagulation factor XII were studied. Of the deficient subjects, three patients (age 21-28) had factor XII activity levels below 1% (severe factor XII deficiency) while three other patients (age 18-44) had factor XII activity levels ranging from 20% to 35% (mild factor XII deficiency).

All study subjects received Desamino D-Arginine Vasopressin (DDAVP, Desmopressin, MINRIN[R], Ferring, Sweden), at a concentration of 0.4 μg/kg bodyweight in 50 ml of saline over 15 minutes intravenously.

Assays

Plasminogen activator activity was assayed by an amidolytic assay (4). The assay was performed in the absence and presence of specific antibodies against t-PA (0.25 μg/ml), u-PA (0.25 μg/ml) or factor XII (0.25 μg/ml) and mixtures of these antibodies. Results were expressed in percentage of plasminogen activator activity in the post-DDAVP plasma samples in the absence of antibodies.

T-PA antigen and u-PA antigen was measured with ELISA techniques, as described before (5,6).

Plasmin-α2-antiplasmin complex levels were determined by a radioimmunoassay (RIA) as previously described (7).

RESULTS

Fibrinolytic activity in normal subjects and in patients with factor XII deficiency

The infusion of DDAVP in healthy volunteers resulted in a significant nearly 7-fold increase in fibrinolytic activity as reflected by the increase in plasminogen activating activity. Plasma levels of t-PA antigen and u-PA antigen increased 3.7-fold and 1.7-fold respectively. Figure 1 shows the effect of the addition of anti-t-PA, anti-u-PA or mixtures of these antibodies on plasminogen activating activity in post-DDAVP plasma of healthy volunteers (left bars). Addition of anti-t-PA antibody resulted in an inhibition of plasminogen activating activity of 59% (SEM 4.4) whereas addition of anti-u-PA antibody reduced plasminogen activating activity with 24% (SEM 4.9). The combination of anti-t-PA and anti-u-PA antibodies did not completely inhibit plasminogen activating activity (mean inhibition 77%, SEM 2.7), indicating the presence of non-t-PA or u-PA dependent fibrinolytic activity in post-DDAVP plasma. This residual plasminogen activating activity could be quenched by addition of a monoclonal antibody against factor XII activity to the combination of anti-t-PA and anti-u-PA antibodies (mean inhibition 98%, SEM 2.0).

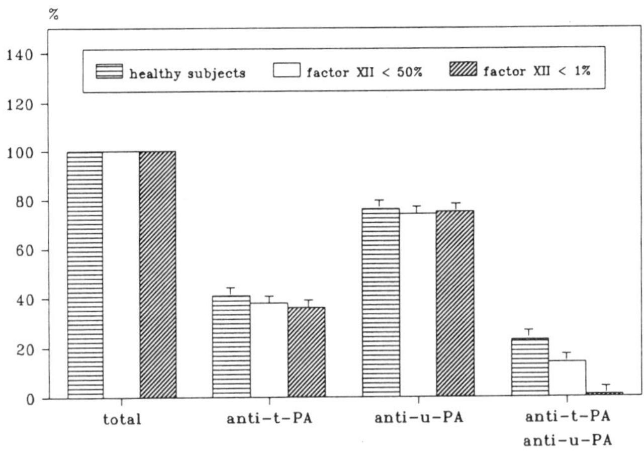

Figure 1. Plasminogen activator activity in healthy individuals and in factor XII deficient patients in the presence of antibodies (anti-t-PA, anti-u-PA and the combination of anti-t-PA and anti-u-PA).

The effect of the addition of anti-t-PA, anti-u-PA or the combination of both antibodies on the plasminogen activating activity in post-DDAVP plasma of patients with mild (middle bars) or severe (right bars) factor XII deficiency in comparison to that of healthy volunteers is shown in figure 1. There was no significant difference in the inhibition of plasminogen activating activity by either anti-t-PA or anti-u-PA antibodies between the healthy subjects and the factor XII deficient subjects. However, the residual plasminogen activating activity observed after the addition of both anti-t-PA and anti-u-PA antibodies was significantly reduced in plasma of patients with mild factor XII deficiency (14%, SEM 1.2, p<0.05 Student's t-test) compared to that in healthy volunteers (23%, SEM 2.1) and was completely absent in patients with severe factor XII deficiency (0%, SEM 0.3, p<0.05).

The increase in plasminogen activating activity resulted in the formation of plasmin as indicated by the increase in plasma levels of PAP complexes upon the infusion of DDAVP. Response of PAP complexes in plasma upon DDAVP in healthy subjects and factor XII deficient individuals is shown in figure 2. PAP complexes increased from 5.2 nM (SEM 0.7) to 28.3 nM (SEM 2.3) after DDAVP infusion in healthy volunteers. In patients with severe factor XII deficiency this increase in PAP com-

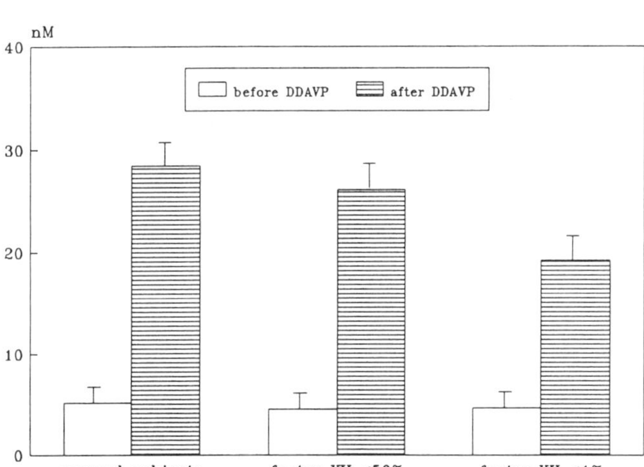

Figure 2. Plasma levels of PAP complexes induced by DDAVP in normal individuals and factor XII deficient patients.

plexes upon DDAVP was significantly reduced (preinfusion level 4.7 nM (SEM 1.0) vs. post-infusion level 19.7 nM (SEM 1.8), $p < 0.05$ compared to normal subjects, Student's t-test). The level of PAP complexes in plasma after DDAVP in patients with mild deficiency of factor XII was between that observed in patients with severe deficiency of factor XII and that seen in healthy subjects (figure 2, preinfusion level 4.9 nM (SEM 1.1) vs. post-infusion level 26.6 nM (SEM 1.7)).

DISCUSSION

Deficiency of factor XII results in a prolongation of coagulation tests in vitro, which may suggest the assocoation with a bleeding tendency in affected individuals. However, in vivo these individuals rather seem to have a higher incidence of thromboembolism (8,9). The data presented here show that activation of the contact system contributes to plasminogen activation. The relevance of this factor XII dependent plasminogen activator activity in vivo was demonstrated by the observation that activation of plasminogen in vivo as reflected by the increase in PAP complexes was significantly reduced in severely factor XII deficient patients compared to healthy controls. Therefore, we propose that the thromboembolic events that are observed in factor XII deficient individuals are due to impaired fibrinolysis.

Earlier observations revealed the absence of prothrombin activation (no generation of prothrombin fragment F_{1+2}) and fibrinogen conversion to fibrin (no generation of fibrinopeptide A) in vivo upon administration of DDAVP (7) suggesting that the activation of the contact system observed in this situation does not result in significant activation as previously described. Hence, these results support the hypothesis that the function of the contact system in vivo is a profibrinolytic rather than a procoagulant one.

Several mechanisms by which the contact system may induce plasminogen activation can be envisaged. Active factor XII, plasma kallikrein and factor XIa are all able to directly convert plasminogen into plasmin (10,11) although in vivo at a limited rate but a combined effect of factor XIIa, kallikrein and factor XIa may potentially cause contact activation dependent fibrinolytic activity. Another possibility is the involvement of a proposed but not yet completely identified plasminogen activator which is dependent on factor XII (12).

In conclusion, infusion of DDAVP induces plasminogen activator activity which is related to activation of the contact system and in particular factor XII and which occurs in addition to an increase in t-PA and u-PA activity. Therefore, we suggest that the contact system should be considered as a fibrinolytic rather than a blood coagulation system and that the association between thromboembolic disease and deficiencies of the contact system are due to an impaired fibrinolytic capacity in these patients.

REFERENCES

1. Collen D. On the regulation and control of fibrinolysis. Thromb Haemostas 1980; 43:77-89.

2. Levi M, ten Cate JW, Dooijewaard G, Sturk A, Brommer EJP, Agnelli G. DDAVP induces systemic release of urokinase-type plasminogen activator. Thromb Haemostas 1989; 62:686-689.

3. Kluft C, Dooijewaard G, EmeisJJ. Role of the contact system in fibrinolysis. Seminars Thromb Hemostas 1987; 13:50-68.

4. Verheijen JH, Mullaart E, Chang GTG, Kluft C, Wijngaards G. A simple spectrophotometric assay for extrinsic (tissue-type) plasminogen activator applicable to measurement in plasma. Thromb Haemostas 1982; 48:266-269

5. Holvoet P, Cleemput H, Collen D. Assay of human tissue-type plasminogen activator (t-PA) with an enzyme-linked immunosorbent assay (ELISA) based on three murine monoclonal antibodies to t-PA. Thromb Haemostas 1985; 54:684-687.

6. Binnema DJ, van Iersel JJL, Dooijewaard G. Quantitation of urokinase antigen in plasma and culture media by use of an ELISA. Thromb Res 1986; 43:569-577.

7. Levi M, de Boer JP, Roem D, ten Cate JW, Hack CE. Plasminogen activation in vivo upon intravenous administration of DDAVP. Quantitative assessment of plasmin-α2-antiplasmin complexes with a novel monoclonal antobody based radioimmunoassay. Thromb Haemostas 1992, in press.

8. Goodnough LT, Hidehiko S, Ratnoff OD. Thrombosis or myocardial infarction in congenital clotting factor abnormalities and chronic thrombocytopenias: A report of 21 patients and a review of 50 previously reported cases. Medicine 1983; 62:248-255.

9. Lammle B, Wuillemin WA, Huber I, Krauskopf M, Zurcher C, Pflugshaupt R, Furlan M. Thromboembolism and bleeding tendency in congenital factor XII deficiency- A study on 74 subjects from 14 Swiss families. Thromb Haemostas 1991; 65:117-121.

10. Colman RW. Surface-mediated defense reactions. The plasma contact activation system. J Clin Invest 1984; 73:1249-1253.

11. Mandle Jr RJ, Kaplan AP. Hageman factor dependent fibrinolysis. Generation of fibrinolytic activity by the interaction of human activated factor XI and plasminogen. Blood 1979; 54:850-861.

12. Binnema DJ, Dooijewaard G, van Iersel JJL, Turion PNC, Kluft C. The contact-system dependent plasminogen activator from human plasma: identification and characterization. Thromb Haemostas 1990; 64:390-397.

VARIABLE DEPLETION OF ENDOGENOUS FACTOR XII-DEPENDENT FIBRINOLYTIC ACTIVITY FOLLOWING THROMBOLYTIC THERAPY OF MYOCARDIAL INFARCTION AND ITS RELATION TO REINFARCTION

C. Kluft (1,2), S. Munkvad (1), J. Gram (1), J. Jespersen (1)

(1) South Jutland University Centre and Department of Clinical Chemistry,
Ribe County Hospital in Esbjerg, Denmark;
(2) Gaubius Laboratory, IVVO-TNO, Leiden, The Netherlands

INTRODUCTION

Three, partially interlinked pathways have been found to be involved in the activation of plasminogen in plasma. Of these three pathways, the factor XII-dependent one is not yet fully characterized (1), and possible pathophysiological consequences of significant deviations of this pathway are not elucidated.

As indicated in figure 1, the factor XII-dependent plasminogen activator activity can be assessed using excesses of neutralizing antibodies directed towards the well-known plasminogen activators t-PA and u-PA. Using this methodology we have evaluated the behaviour of the factor XII-dependent component of the fibrinolytic system in patients who undergo thrombolytic treatment, because this treatment induces excessive systemic effects of the haemostatic system possibly including effects on factor XII-dependent fibrinolysis.

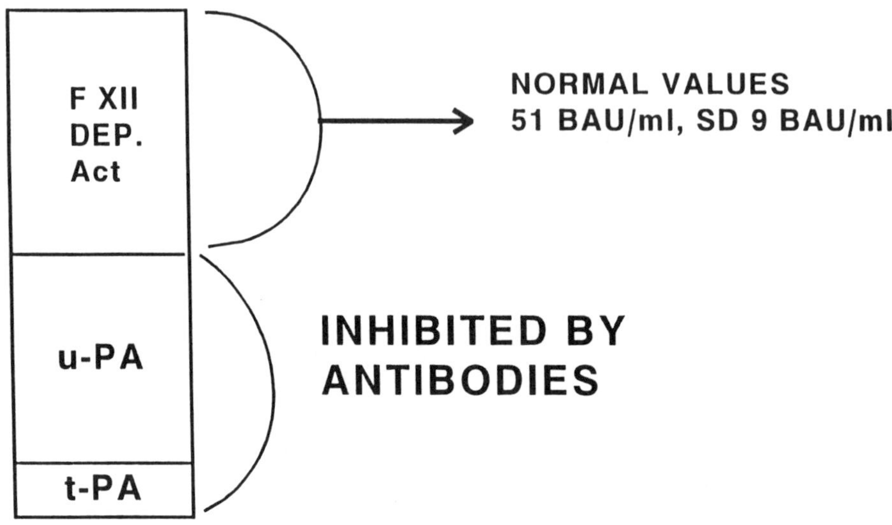

Figure 1. The factor XII-dependent plasminogen activator activity is assayed in euglobulin fractions of plasma; activation is achieved by dextran sulphate; activity is measured on plasminogen-rich fibrin plates and expressed in arbitrary blood activator units (BAU) (2).

CHANGES INDUCED BY THROMBOLYTIC TREATMENT

In a placebo-controlled study it was observed that during the natural course of myocardial infarction the factor XII-dependent activity did not change significantly. In contrast, coronary thrombolysis with t-PA or streptokinase induces a pronounced decrease of factor XII-dependent fibrinolytic activity (figure 2c) within the first 4 hours after initiation of treatment, followed by a long lasting depression (2).

RELATION TO REINFARCTION

In a small group of 20 patients with uncomplicated myocardial infarction treated with rt-PA and 24 hour heparin we studied the possible relation of the above-mentioned depletion of activity to the evolution of reinfarction within the first eight weeks (3). We observed a recurrence of in eight of the 20 patients diagnosed either by ECG and enzyme studies (n=5) or by sudden death preceded by severe chest pain according to the death certificates (n=3).

The factor XII-dependent plasminogen activator activity was assessed in the post-treatment period with sampling moments at 12 hours after the treatment and at the first, third and fourth post-treatment days. The activity remained reduced over this entire period and the patients with reinfarction (33 ± 14 (SD) BAU/ml) showed a significantly ($p < 0.05$) lower mean activity than patients with no evidence of a recurrence (46 ± 15 BAU/ml)

This observation would agree with the assumption that endogenous fibrinolytic potential is of importance in counteracting thromboembolic events. It provides the first experimental evidence that an intact factor XII-dependent plasminogen activator fibrinolytic system protects against myocardial infarction and thrombosis.

MECHANISMS OF DEPLETION

In an investigation on the mechanism of depletion of the factor XII-dependent plasminogen activator activity by rt-PA treatment, we observed a relationship between systemic plasmin formation and the depletion (4).

The above-mentioned group of eight patients with a reinfarction showed a larger systemic generation of plasmin and consumption of α-2-antiplasmin. In addition, the decrease in factor XII-dependent plasminogen activator activity correlated significantly ($r = 0.77$, $p < 0.001$) with the decrease in α-2-antiplasmin during rt-PA treatment in the whole group of 20 patients.

It was hypothesised that plasmin might be responsible for both the activation and subsequent depletion of the factor XII-dependent activity. However, in a group of seven patients treated with rt-PA we observed, as shown in figure 2A and B, that the plasma levels of factor XII and prekallikrein do not change significantly, while α-2-antiplasmin activity decreases strongly (figure 2D). Although some variability in factor XII and prekallikrein levels were present in the patients (see figure 2A,B) the depletion in factor XII-dependent plasminogen activator activity was not related to these levels.

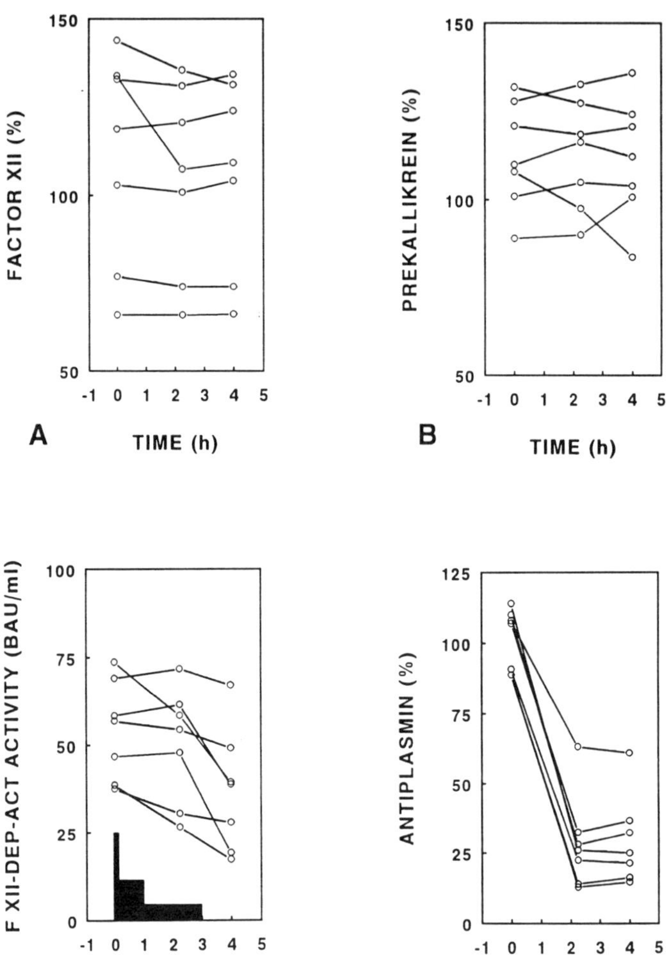

Figure 2.   Plasma levels of factor XII (immunological assay,(2)) and prekallikrein (functional assay,(2)) in relation to treatment and changes in α-2-antiplasmin activity (functional assay,(2)) and factor XII-dependent plasminogen activator activity (functional assay,2). Values are corrected for haematocrite variations (2). Seven patients treated with rt-PA (10 mg bolus, 50 mg in first hour and 20 mg/hour in the second and third hour; see black box in C) were sampled before treatment, during treatment (t = 2 1/4 h) and 1 h after termination of treatment.

The depletion of factor XII-dependent plasminogen activator activity seems to be delayed compared with the main action of the infused thrombolytic agent. At the 2 1/4 hour sampling moment during the treatment the activity is not yet greatly reduced (Fig 2C). At this sampling moment, the treatment has already resulted in administration of 85 mg rt-PA and only 15 mg is administered subsequently at a low infusion rate (20 mg/h).

The main depletion apparently occurs between this moment and 1 hour post-treatment.

Obviously, the mechanism of depletion requires further elucidation. One possibility concerns a direct effect of plasmin on the postulated plasminogen proactivator of the factor XII-dependent pathway (1), resulting in a depletion.

In this respect it should be assumed that, in view of the relatively late effects in the factor XII pathway, insufficiently controlled plasmin action in the late phase of therapy is responsible. This is consistent with a further observation that, in particular the strong depletion of α-2-antiplasmin, likely to be more prominent in the late phase of treatment, is associated with the depletion (4).

Another possibility is that plasmin acts via activation of factor XII and prekallikrein (mainly when plasmin action is relatively unrestrained in the late phase of treatment). Since plasmin does not result in a significant consumption of circulating factor XII and prekallikrein (figure 2A,B), it should be assumed that the process occurs locally. This is consistent with known mechanisms of factor XII activation which involve surface-bound processes.

To further advance the study of the mechanisms involved it is important to study activation products such as inhibitor complexes from active factor XII and kallikrein.

CONCLUDING REMARKS

The recent data on factor XII-dependent plasminogen activator activity in relation to thrombolytic treatment of patients with myocardial infarction indicate a therapy-induced effect. The actual mechanism behind the effect requires further elucidation, but the degree of systemic plasmin generation appears of importance.

The depletion of factor XII-dependent plasminogen activator activity is variable and is associated with the risk of reinfarction. This is the first association between deviations of the factor XII-dependent fibrinolytic pathway and clinical events. We suggest that the factor XII-dependent pathway might be of biologic importance in endogenous fibrinolysis. Further studies are warranted.

REFERENCES

1. Kluft C, Dooijewaard G, Emeis JJ. Role of the contact system in fibrinolysis. Semin Thromb Hemostas 1987; 13: 50-68.

2. Munkvad S, Jespersen J, Gram J, Kluft C. Long-lasting depression of the Factor XII-dependent fibrinolytic system in patients with myocardial infarction undergoing thrombolytic therapy with recombinant tissue-type plasminogen activator: a randomized placebo-controlled study. J Am Coll Cardiol 1991; 17: 957-62.

3. Munkvad S, Jespersen J, Gram J, Kluft C. Depression of Factor XII-dependent fibrinolytic activity characterizes patients with early myocardial reinfarction after recombinant tissue-type plasminogen activator therapy. J Am Coll Cardiol 1991; 18: 454-8.

4. Munkvad S, Jespersen J, Gram J, Kluft C. Association between systemic generation of plasmin and activation of the factor XII-dependent fibrinolytic proactivator system in coronary thrombolysis. Fibrinolysis, 1992, in press.

AAS 38/II
Recent Progress on Kinins

FIBRINOLYSIS AND EXTRACORPOREAL CIRCULATION

C. Kluft

Gaubius Laboratory, IVVO-TNO, Leiden, The Netherlands

INTRODUCTION

Changes in fibrinolysis can contribute to a haemorrhagic diathesis due either to an increase in fibrinolytic activation or a reduction in inhibitory capacity (or a combination of both). The purpose of this paper is to discuss which aspects of fibrinolysis can be affected by extracorporeal circulation and potentially contribute to bleeding problems.

For this purpose, the contact activation component of the fibrinolytic cascade is placed in the centre (see Fig. 1) and the consequences of its activation are discussed.

As discussed previously (1), the activation of the contact system by the foreign surface of the extracorporeal tubing is distant from the sites in the body with active haemostatic processes from the surgery. It is, therefore, important to identify which active factors, generated at the site of the contact activation, enter the circulation and can contribute at a distance to haemostatic mechanisms.

CONTACT ACTIVATION OF FIBRINOLYSIS

Early activation steps

The result of contact activation of the three early contact factors, factor XII (or Hageman factor), prekallikrein (or Fletcher factor) and high-molecular-weight (HMW) kininogen is

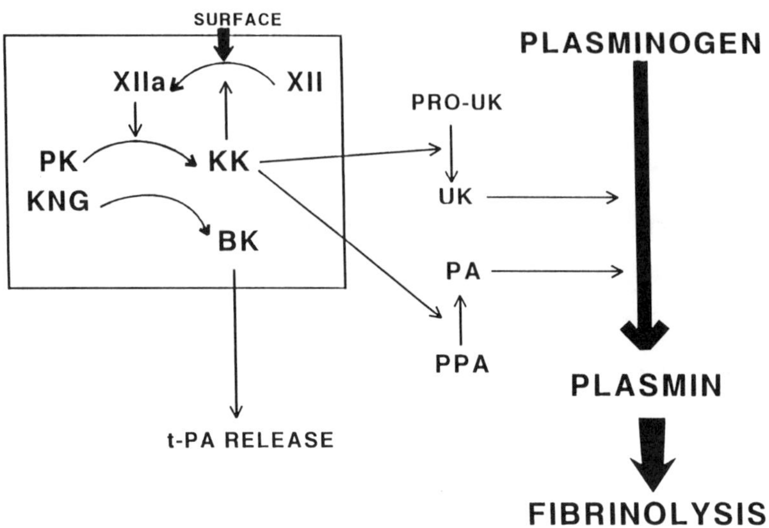

Figure 1. Contact activation and its consequences for fibrinolysis. Contact on a surface of three components: factor XII, prekallikrein (PK) and HMW kininogen (KNG) results in three activation products: factor XIIa, kallikrein (KK) and bradykinin (BK). These activation products induce t-PA release and the activation of pro-urokinase (pro-UK) to urokinase (UK) and of a factor XII-dependent plasminogen proactivator (PPA).

the generation of active enzymes and of the nonapeptide bradykinin. From these activation products, kallikrein (in part ?) and bradykinin can enter the circulation. Depending upon the extent of proteolysis of factor XII by kallikrein, either the part which contains the active site of factor XIIa remains attached to the heavy chain that contains the surface binding domain (α-factor XIIa), or is separated from the heavy chain and called β-factor XIIa. Activation is usually limited, as evidenced by low levels of conversion of prekallikrein in simulated and actual extracorporeal circulation (2,3). Thus only small amounts of these early activation products can be expected to enter the circulation and possibly exert an effect. However, because effects of such early products are amplified in further cascade processes final effects may not be negligible.

Further activation steps

Subsequent effects of kallikrein relate to the activation of circulating factors, and both kallikrein and factor XIIa may contribute to clot lysis. Bradykinin contributes to an increased level of t-PA by means of its capacity to acutely release t-PA from endothelial stores.

The effects of circulating kallikrein, as well as surface-bound kallikrein, on circulating factors concern the activation of pro-urokinase and the factor XII-dependent plasminogen proactivator (see Fig. 1). Neither effect has yet been documented, although the methodology exists for evaluating such activation of pro-urokinase (4).

The main effect of circulating kallikrein (or factor XIIa via kallikrein) on clot lysis is the activation of a thusfar incompletely-characterized process involving a postulated plasminogen proactivator (5). It is expected that in clot lysis the activation of pro-urokinase to urokinase by kallikrein (or indirectly by factor XIIa) is likely to be inferior to the effect of plasmin formed by the lysis process (6). It is, however, possible that small, initial effects of kallikrein (factor XIIa) accelerate the process in the early phase.

INHIBITION OF FIBRINOLYSIS DURING EXTRACORPOREAL CIRCULATION

The survival of activated components is usually reduced by inactivation. During extracorporeal circulation this aspect is of particular relevance for the activation products generated in the artificial loop, and these should reach a site of active haemostatic processes.

Of the early activation products, bradykinin normally shows a short lifetime due to being largely inactivated on its first passage through the lung and because of circulating inactivating enzymes. During ECC this inactivation is obviously impaired by excluding the lung circulation, while circulating inactivating enzymes are also reduced in concentration (hemodilution and impaired lung synthesis).

Factor XIIa and kallikrein are mainly inactivated by C1-inactivator (half life between two and five minutes). This inactivation is compromised due to both hemodilution and the lowering of temperature, which strongly affects the inactivation rate of C1-inactivator.

Regarding the later activation products, it is notable that when pro-urokinase becomes activated the active enzyme in circulation is not effectively inactivated by its main inhibitor

PAI-1 (plasminogen activator inhibitor-1). The increased t-PA during ECC will readily neutralize the circulating PAI-1 and the urokinase generated will have an increased survival. Another important aspect of fibrinolysis inhibition concerns the α_2-antiplasmin and factor XIII situation and the supply of PAI-1 from platelets.

In the case of fibrin clot formation the fibrin becomes temporarily stabilized due to the incorporation of inhibitors. In this inhibition α_2-antiplasmin plays an important role, in particular the binding of this inhibitor to the fibrin by factor XIII retards lysis. During ECC both the factors mentioned are reduced in concentration due to hemodilution, these concentrations appear to be of importance for the functioning of both factors, as suggested by data on congenital deficiencies with symptoms in the case of 50% levels (7,8).

The main contribution to the inhibition of plasminogen activators is from PAI-1 released locally from platelets. It should be noted that platelets are strongly affected during ECC and that this possibly involves a reduced PAI-1 supply to fibrin clots by the platelets (9). Specific assessment of platelet PAI-1 during ECC, however, is not yet available.

CONCLUDING REMARKS

From the above summary it appears that the main change in fibrinolysis during ECC concerns the status of fibrinolysis inhibition. Major reductions in fibrinolysis inhibition appear to occur. This, in itself, can cause premature lysis of fibrin clots formed during ECC. In addition, the balance is shifted further in favour of active fibrinolysis by low grade activation of the contact system, which may exert a more powerful effect since inhibition is reduced.

REFERENCES

1.   Kluft C. Pathomechanisms of defective hemostasis during and after extracorporeal circulation: Contact phase activation. In: Blood use in cardiac surgery (Friedel N, Hetzer R, Royston D, eds). Steinkopff Verlag, Darmstadt, 1991, pp 10-15.

2. Wachtfogel Y T, Harpel P C, Edmunds L H Jr, Colman R W. Formation of Cls-Clr-inhibitor, kallikrein-C1-inhibitor, and plasmin-α_2-plasmin-inhibitor complexes during cardiopulmonary bypass. Blood 1989; 73: 468-71.

3. Fuhrer G, Heller W, Hoffmeister H-E. Das Verhalten von Plasma-Präkallikrein/-kallikrein bei Patienten mit aorta-koronarer Bypass-Operation unter Anwendung zweier verschiedener Aprotinin-Dosierungsschemata. In: Proteolyse und Proteinaseninhibition in der Herz- und Gefasschircurgie (Dudziak R, Kirchhoff P G, Reuter H D, Schumann F, eds). Schattauer, Stuttgart, New York, 1985, pp 255-61.

4. Binnema D J, Dooijewaard G, Van Iersel J J L, Turion P N C. Sensitive biological immunoassay for the detection of single-chain-(scu-PA) and two-chain urokinase-type plasminogen activator (Tcu-PA) in plasma. In: The intrinsic system of fibrinolysis: Components and mechanisms (Thesis, Leiden University, Binnema D J), 1991, pp 21-35.

5. Binnema D J, Dooijewaard G, Van Iersel J J L, Turion P N C, Kluft C. The contact-system dependent plasminogen activator from human plasma: Identification and characterization. Thromb Haemostas 1990; 64: 390-7.

6. Binnema D J, Dooijewaard G, Turion P N C. An analysis of the activators of single-chain urokinase-type plasminogen activator (scu-PA) in the dextran sulphate euglobulin fraction of normal plasma and of plasmas deficient in factor XII and prekallikrein. Thromb Haemostas 1991; 65: 144-8.

7. Kluft C, Vellenga E, Brommer E J P, Wijngaards G. A familial hemorrhagic diathesis in a Dutch family: an inherited deficiency of α_2-antiplasmin. Blood 1982; 59: 1169-80.

8. Egbring R, Seitz R, Guerten G V, Koether M, Barthels M, Fuchs G, Lerch L, Kroeninger A. Bleeding complications in heterozygotes with congenital factor XIII deficiency. In: Fibrinogen 3. Biochemistry, biological functions, gene regulation and expression (Mosesson M W, Amram D L, Siebenlist K R, DiOrio J P, eds). Elsevier Science Publishers B.V., Amsterdam, 1988, pp 341-6.

9. Gomez M J, Carroll R C, Hansard M R, Kidd M, Goldman M H. Regulation of fibrinolysis in aortic surgery. J Vasc Surg 1988; 8: 384-8.

PROCOAGULANT CHANGES INDUCED BY ORAL CONTRACEPTIVES ARE BALANCED BY AN INCREASED FIBRINOLYTIC TENDENCY

I.J. Mackie, S. Campbell, M. Gallimore, *G. Robinson, S.J. Machin

Haematology Department, University College and Middlesex School of Medicine, 98 Chenies Mews, London WC1E 6HX and *The Margaret Pyke Centre, London, U.K.

SUMMARY: Oral contraceptives caused increased fibrinogen, FVII, FX, and fibrinolysis. The latter was associated with elevated FXII and PKK, while C1-INH was decreased, ATIII and α_2M were unchanged; it could not be accounted for by changes in t-PA, u-PA, PAI, plasminogen, α_2-AP, proteins C or S. HCII and α_1-PI were increased and may regulate the availability of thrombin and FXIa. The increased FXII/PKK dependent fibrinolytic potential and HCII may offset any increase in thrombin generation, while α_1-PI limits intrinsic coagulation.

INTRODUCTION

The use of combined oral contraceptives (COCs) is associated with an increased incidence of venous thromboembolism (1-3), which has been decreased, but not abolished (2,4), by reduction of the oestrogen content to 30ug. Certain haemostatic parameters have been implicated in the mechanism of this increased thrombotic risk; elevated levels of factors II, VII, IX, X, and fibrinogen during COC medication are well documented and many reports show decreased antithrombin III (ATIII) (5-11), although this may depend on age, oestrogen content and progestogen type.

Fibrinolysis is increased during COC use (2,12,13), and has been attributed to increased levels of tissue-plasminogen activator (t-PA) (14), or FXII (8,15) and decreased levels of plasminogen activator inhibitor (PAI) (14). Prekallikrein (PKK) may be increased (16) or unchanged (8,15). We have recently reported increased fibrinolysis in association with elevated factor XII (FXII) and PKK (17), and have extended these studies to investigate other components of haemostasis in a serial study of 26 women before and while receiving COC's.

MATERIALS AND METHODS

26 healthy, non-smoking women, less than 30 years old, who had not received COC's for the previous six months were studied. Samples were collected before treatment, in the luteal phase, and after three cycles (days 18-21) and six cycles (days 18-21) of treatment with monophasic COC's containing 30ug oestrogen. Blood was collected by venepuncture and anticoagulated with a one-tenth volume of 0.106M tri-sodium citrate. After centrifugation at 2000g for 15 minutes at room temperature, plasma was separated and stored in aliquots at -70°C.

Fibrin plate lysis was performed on euglobulin precipitates with and without activation by dextran sulphate (17). Results were calculated as a percentage of lysis by a large pool normal plasma (Reference Plasma 100%, Immuno Ltd, Dunton Green, Kent), which was arbitrarily said to have 100% fibrin plate lysis activity.

Amidolytic substrate assays were performed by microtitre techniques, or using the ACL 300R analyser (Instrumentation Laboratory Ltd, Warrington, Cheshire). Amidolytic assay reagents were obtained from Channel Diagnostics (Walmer, Kent) and substrates from Pentapharm (Basle, Switz.), except where specified. FXII was assayed (18) with the substrate 2AcOH.H-D-CHT-Gly-Arg-pNA, FXII activator and Kallikrein inhibitor. PKK was measured (19,20) using the substrate MBz-Pro-Phe-Arg-pNA and PKK activator, without acidification of the plasma. α_2-Macroglobulin (α_2-M) and α_1-proteinase inhibitor (α_1-PI) were assayed by a modified method (21) with Bz-Val-Lys-Arg-pNA and porcine trypsin. In the α_2-M assay, soybean trypsin inhibitor, was used to block excess porcine trypsin, so that only α_2-M /trypsin complex could cleave the substrate. In the α_1-PI assay, methylamine (Sigma Chemical Co, Poole, Dorset) was used to prevent complex formation between α_2-M and trypsin, so that the residual free trypsin was inversely proportional to α_1-PI. ATIII was measured (19) using bovine thrombin (Diagnostic Reagents Ltd, Thame, Oxon) and the substrate, S2238 (Kabi Diagnostica, Stockholm, Sweden). C1-INH activity and PAI activity were assayed using commercial kits (Immuno Ltd and Kabi Diagnostica, respectively). Heparin cofactor II (HCII) was measured using human thrombin, dermatan sulphate, and 2AcOH.H-D-CHG-Gly-Arg-pNA (22). Plasminogen was measured as a complex with streptokinase (Kabi Diagnostica) using 2AcOH.HD-Ala-CHT-Lys-pNA, and α_2-antiplasmin (α_2-AP) was measured in terms of residual plasmin activity (19) on 2AcOH.HD-Ala_CHT-Arg-pNA. Protein C (PC) (19) was measured using activator from Southern Copperhead snake venom and 2AcOh.H-D-Lys(Cbo)-Pro-Arg-pNA. PAI-3 and heparin independent protein C inhibitors were measured using activated human protein C (APC) and 2AcOh.H-D-Lys(Cbo)-Pro-Arg-pNA, in the presence and absence of heparin.

Urokinase-plasminogen activator (u-PA) was measured with an ELISA kit (Technoclone, Vienna, Austria) which measures both single and two chain forms. t-PA antigen was also measured by ELISA (Biopool, Umea, Sweden). C1-INH antigen (C1-INH Ag) was measured by ELISA (17) using polyclonal antibodies (Dako Ltd, High Wycombe, Bucks). Protein S was measured by ELISA (23) using polyclonal antisera (Dako Ltd), before (total PS) and after (free PS) PEG precipitation. Fibrinogen was assayed as clottable protein (24), and factors VII and X were measured by 1-stage coagulation assay (19).

All the above assays were standardised against a Reference Plasma 100% (Immuno Ltd). A potency of 100 U/dl or 100% was assumed for factors where no reference values were given. All other reagents were Analar grade (BDH Ltd, Poole, England). Data was analysed by Wilcoxon signed Rank test and Spearman's Correlation.

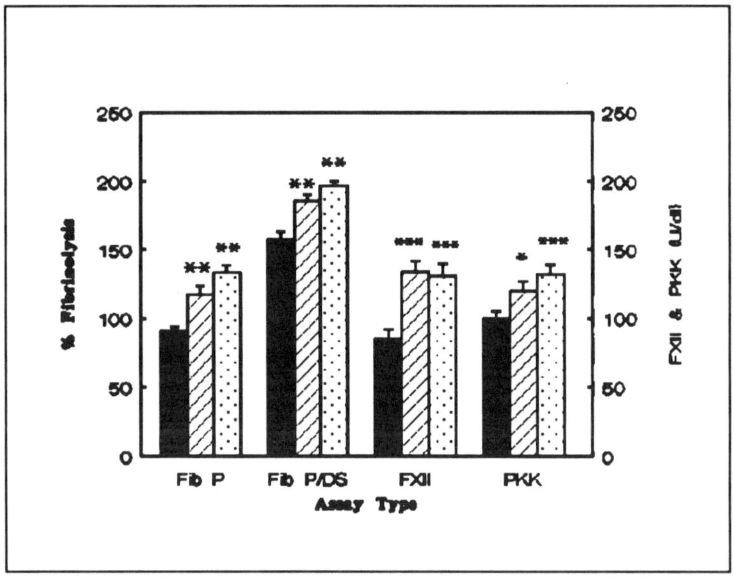

Figure 1. Fibrinolysis and Contact Factors. Mean and standard errors; Fib P = Fibrin Plate lysis, Fib P/DS = Lysis by dextran sulphate activated samples; solid bar = pre COC, hatched bar = cycle 3, dotted bar = cycle 6; * p<0.05 ** p<0.01 *** p<0.001.

RESULTS AND DISCUSSION

The use of combined oral contraceptives has been associated with an increased risk of venous thromboembolism (1-4) and this prompted us to pay particular attention to parameters which when abnormal, may cause a predisposition to thrombotic episodes, ie. fibrinogen, FVII, ATIII, HCII, PC, PS, and fibrinolysis.

COC's caused elevated plasma levels of fibrinogen, FVII, FX, FXII and PKK (Table 1, Fig 1), which agrees with previous findings (5-9,11,15), except that others have reported PKK as unchanged using a different amidolytic assay for PKK (15), or clotting and antigen assays (8). The studies of COC's and haemostasis differ in age, oestrogen content, progestogen type, and whether the women acted as their own controls, or were separate groups, each of which can influence the results. Our results support and extend those previously published (17), showing that the increase in FXII and PKK occurs in parallel and is significant. Fibrinolysis was also increased and was potentiated by dextran sulphate (Fig 1). Plasminogen levels were increased and α_2-AP was unchanged (Table 1); and these proteins would not have influenced overall fibrinolysis as α_2-AP is lost during euglobulin preparation, and plasminogen is already present in the fibrin plate, which acts predominantly as a measure of plasminogen activators. The increased fibrinolysis with and without dextran sulphate activation, showed a significant correlation with FXII (r=0.25, p<0.01; r=0.55, p<0.001) and PKK levels (r=0.3, p<0.01; r=0.29, p<0.01).

Table 1.   Mean values and standard errors in all 26 patients.

		PRE PILL	CYCLE 3	CYCLE 6
Fg	Mean	1.91	2.29***	2.39***
(g/l)	sem	0.07	0.09	0.11
FVII	Mean	83.0	89.0	97.0*
(IU/dl)	sem	2.6	3.7	3.9
FX	Mean	98.0	113.0**	116.0**
(IU/dl)	sem	3.6	3.8	5.1
Pg	Mean	102.0	110.0	122.0*
(U/dl)	sem	5.1	4.0	4.4
α_2-AP	Mean	106.0	104.0	105.0
(U/dl)	sem	2.8	3.0	3.0

*p<0.05, **p<0.01, ***p<0.005

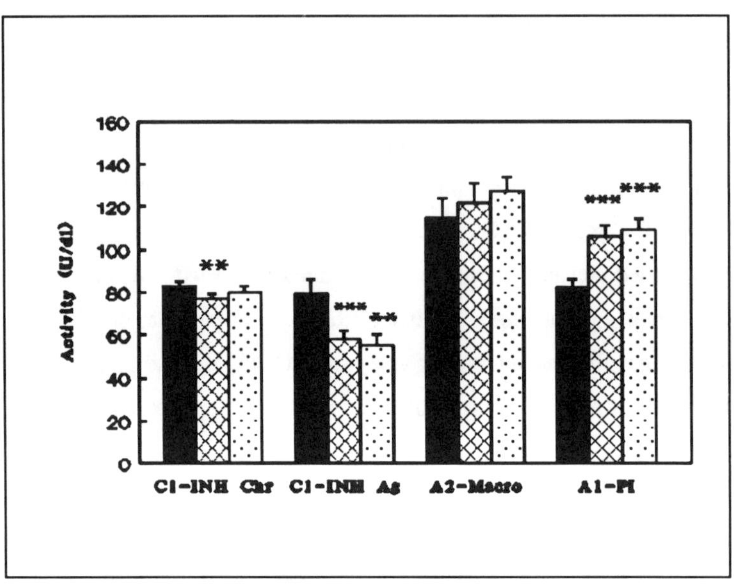

Figure 2 - Contact Factor Inhibitors. Legend as for Fig 1.

C1-INH Ag was markedly decreased by the pill, but C1-INH activity (fig 2) only showed a small decrease. This may be due to interference in the C1-INH amidolytic assay by another protease inhibitor. α_2M showed a small but non-significant rise and ATIII was unchanged (Table 2 and Fig 2). C1-INH, α_2M, and ATIII are the main inhibitors of FXIIa and kallikrein (KK) in normal plasma (25). PAI-3 has recently been recognised as another KK inhibitor (26-29). When PAI-3 was measured by its property of heparin dependent APC inhibition (30), a small but non-significant decrease was seen (Table 2).

The increased fibrinolysis was not associated with an increase in t-PA Ag, u-PA Ag, or with a decrease in PAI activity (Table 3), in fact t-PA antigen was significantly decreased. Jespersen and colleagues (14) found a similar decrease in t-PA Ag, but reported increased t-PA activity. This may be an due to interference in the assay system by FXII and PKK, particularly if inhibitors were removed by acidification, and the samples were chilled.

The enhanced fibrinolysis was not due to an increase in PC, total (not shown) or free PS, which remained unchanged (Table 3). Increased levels of PC antigen have been reported (31,32), but unchanged PC antigen (33) and activity (11) have also been observed in women receiving

COC's. A significant fall in total PS has been found, accompanied by unchanged or decreased C4b-BP, and non-significant changes in free PS (33,34).

	PRE PILL	CYCLE 3	CYCLE 6
ATIII Mean	108.0	113.0	110.0
(IU/dl) sem	3.5	3.7	3.8
HCII Mean	88.0	112.0***	101.0**
(U/dl) sem	3.2	3.1	7.9
PAI-3 Mean	91.0	83.0	80.0
(U/dl) sem	5.8	6.9	4.2
PCHIDi Mean	89.0	58.0**	64.0*
(U/dl) sem	8.0	7.8	2.7

Table 2 - Mean values and standard errors for ATIII (n=26), HCII (n=10), Heparin dependent (PAI-3) and independent (HI-PCi) PC inhibitors, (n=10). * = p<0.05, ** = p<0.01, *** = p<0.005.

Measurement of PC inhibition yielded variable results (Table 2 & Fig 2), PAI-3 (heparin dependent PC inhibitor or PCI-1) and heparin independent PC inhibition were decreased during cycles 3 and 6, while α_1-PI (PCI-2) was significantly increased. This was a surprising result, since α_1-PI is said to account for most of the heparin independent inhibition of APC (35,36). Clearly the mechanisms of APC inhibition are more complex than originally appreciated, and other PC inhibitors have been implicated (36).

In contrast to ATIII, which blocks the contact system as well as thrombin and FXa, HCII is a specific inhibitor of thrombin. HCII was significantly increased (Table 2) as previously reported in other groups of women receiving COC's (37,38), whereas ATIII was unchanged.

In conclusion, COC's cause an increase in fibrinogen and factors VII and X. This increase in the potential to generate thrombin and cause fibrin clot formation is offset by increased levels of the thrombin specific inhibitor HCII and increased fibrinolytic potential. The increased fibrin plate lysis could not be accounted for by any change in t-PA, u-PA, PAI, or PC, and was associated with increased levels of FXII and PKK. It appears to represent fibrinolysis throough the intrinsic pathway dependent on an uncharacterised pro-activator (39,40). α_1-PI is a potent inhibitor of FXIa (41,42) and may limit the generation of FXa through the intrinsic system.

Table 3. Mean values and standard errors for fibrinolytic parameters

	PRE PILL	**CYCLE 3**	**CYCLE 6**
t-PA No. (ng/ml) Mean sem	9 3.73 0.6	9 1.54* 0.18	9 2.11* 0.46
u-PA No. (ng/ml) Mean sem	8 1.43 0.3	8 1.35 0.24	8 1.01 0.25
PAI No. (AU/ml) Mean sem	10 12.7 1.6	10 12.3 1.1	10 14.0 1.1
PC No. (IU/dl) Mean sem	26 89.0 3.0	26 90.0 4.3	26 96.0 4.7
Free PS No. (U/dl) Mean sem	10 69.0 1.9	10 65.0 4.8	10 67.0 5.7

*$p<0.05$

REFERENCES

1. Bottiger LE, Boman G, Ekland G, Westerholm B. Oral contraceptives and thromboembolic disease: effects of lowering oestrogen content. Lancet 1980; i: 1097-1101.

2. Daly L & Bonnar J. Comparative studies of 30ug ethinyl estradiol combined with gestodene and desogestrel on blood coagulation, fibrinolysis, and platelets. Am J Obstet Gynecol 1990; 163: 430-437.

3. Meade TW, Greenberg G, Thompson SG. Progestogens and cardiovascular reactions associated with oral contraceptives and a comparison of the safety of 50 and 30ug preparations. BMJ 1980; 280: 1157-1161.

4. Kelleher CC. Clinical aspects of the relationship between oral contraceptives and abnormalities of the hemostatic system: Relation to the development of cardiovascular disease. Am J Obstet Gynecol 1990; 163: 392-395.

5. Meade TW, Brozovic M, Chakrabarti R, Howarth DJ, North WRS, Stirling Y. An epidemiological study of the haemostatic and effects of oral contraceptives. Brit J Haematol 1976; 34: 354-364.

6. Mammen EF. Oral contraceptives and blood coagulation: a critical review. Am J Obstet Gynecol 1982; 142: 781-790.

7. Poller L. Oral contraceptives, blood clotting and thrombosis. Brit Med Bull 1978; 34: 151.

8. Gorden EM, Ratnoff OD, Saito H, Donaldson VH, Pensky J, Jones PK. Rapid fibrinolysis, augmented Hageman factor (factor XII) titres, decreased C1 esterase inhibition titres in women taking oral contraceptives. J Lab Clin Med 1980; 96: 781-790.

9. Sabra A & Bonnar J. Haemostatic system changes induced by 50ug and 30ug oestrogen/progesteron oral contraceptives. J Reproductive Med 1983; 28: 85-91.

10. Robinson GE, Bounds W, Mackie IJ, Stocks J, Burren T, Machin S, Guillebaud J. Changes in metabolism induced by oral contraceptives containing desogestrel and gestodene in older women. Contraception 1990; 42: 263-273.

11. Cohen H, Mackie IJ, Walshe K, Gillmer MDG, Machin SJ. A comparison of the effects of two triphasic oral contraceptives on haemostasis. Brit J Haematol 1988; 69: 259-263.

12. Abbate R, Pinto S, Rostagno C, Bruni V, Rosati D, Mariani G. Effects of long-term gestodene-containing oral contraceptive administration on hemostasis. Am J Obstet Gynecol 1990; 163: 424-429.

13. Wessler S & Gital SN. Thrombotic complications of oral contraceptives. In: Hemostasis and Thrombosis. Colman RW, Hirsh J, Marder VJ, Salzman EW, editors. Philadelphia: Lippincott, 1987: 1158-1164.

14. Jespersen J, Petersen KR, Skouby SO. Effects of newer oral contraceptives on the inhibition of coagulation and fibrinolysis in relation to dosage and type of steroid. Am J Obstet Gynecol 1990; 163: 396-403.

15. Jespersen J & Kluft C. Increased Euglobulin Fibrinolytic Potential in women on oral contraceptives low in oestrogen-levels of extrinsic and intrinsic plasminogen activators, PKK, FXII and C1 inhibitor. Thrombos Haemostas 1985; 54: 454-459.

16. Adam A, Albert A, Boulanger J, Genot D, Demoulin A, Damas J. Influence of oral contraceptives and pregnancy on constituents of the kallikrein-kinin system in plasma. Clin Chem 1985; 31:1533-1536.

17. Campbell SJ, Mackie IJ, Robinson GE, Machin SJ. Contact factor mediated fibrinolysis is increased by the combined oral contraceptive pill. Br J Obs Gynecol 1992; in press.

18. Walshe KJ, Mackie IJ, Gallimore M, Machin SJ. A microtitre chromogenic substrate assay for factor XII. Thromb Res 1987; 47: 365-371.

19. Machin SJ & Mackie IJ. Haemostasis. In: Laboratory Haematology: an account of laboratory techniques, Chanarin I (Ed), Edinburgh, Churchill Livingstone, 1989: 263-399.

20. Gallimore MJ & Friberger P. Simple chromogenic peptide substrate assays for determining prekallikrein, kallikrein inhibition and kallikrein "like" activity in human plasma. Thromb Res 1982; 25: 293-298.

21. Gallimore MJ, Aurell L, Friberger P, Gustavsson S. Chromogenic peptide substrate assays for determining funtional activities of a alpha-2-macroglobulin and alpha-1-antitrypsin using a new trypsin substrate. Thrombos Haemostas 1983; 50: 230.

22. Abildgaard U & Larsen ML. Assay of dermatan sulphate cofactor (heparin cofactor II) activity in human plasma. Thrombosis research 1984; 35: 257-266.

23. Woodhams BJ. The simultaneous measurement of total and free protein S by ELISA. Thromb Res 1988; 50: 213-220.

24. von Clauss A. Gerinnungsphysiologische schnellmethode zur bestimmung des fibrinogens. Acta Haematol (Basel) 1957; 17: 237-246.

25. Mackie IJ & Bull H. Normal haemostasis and its regulation. Blood Reviews 1989; 3: 237-250.

26. Meijers JCM, Kanters DHA, Vlooswijk RAA, van Erp HE, Hessing M, Bouma BN. Inactivation of human plasma kallikrein and factor XIa by protein C inhibitor. Biochemistry 1988; 27: 4231-4237.

27. España F, Berrettini M, Griffin JH. Purification and characterization of plasma protein C inhibitor. Thromb Res 1989; 55: 369-384.

28. España F, stelles A, Griffin JH, Aznar J. Interaction of plasma kallikrein with protein C inhibitor in purified mixtures and in plasma. Thrombos Haemostas 1991; 65: 46-51.

29. Laurell M & Stenflo J. Protein C inhibitor from normal plasma: characterization of native and cleaved inhibitor and demonstration of inhibitor complexes with plasma kallikrein. Thrombos Haemostas 1989; 62: 885-891.

30. Heeb MJ, España F, Geiger M, Collen D, Stump DC, Griffin JH. Immunological identity of heparin-dependent plasma and urinary protein C inhibitor and plasminogen activator inhibitor-3. J Biol Chem 1987; 262: 15813-15816.

31. Meade TW, Stirling Y, Wilkes H, Mannucci PM. Effects of oral contraceptives and obesity on protein C antigen. Thrombos Haemostas 1985; 53: 198-199.

32. Gonzalez R, Alberca I, Vicente V. Protein C levels in late pregnancy, postpartum and in women on oral contraceptives. Thromb Res 1985; 39: 637-640.

33. Huisveld IA, Hospers JEH, Meijers JCM, Starkenburg AE, Erich WBM, Bouma BN. Oral contraceptives reduce total protein S, but not free protein S. Thrombos Res 1987; 45: 109-114.

34. Boerger LM, Morris PC, Thurnau GR, Esmon CT, Comp PC. Oral contraceptives and gender affect protein S status. Blood 1987; 69: 692-694.

35. Heeb MJ & Griffin JH. Physiologic inhibition of human activated protein C by α_1-antitrypsin. J Biol Chem 1988; 263: 11613-11616.

36. van der Meer FJM, van Tilburg NH, van Wijngaarden A, van der Linden IK, Briet E, Bertina RM. A second plasma inhibitor of activated protein C: α_1-antitrypsin. Thrombos Haemostas 1989; 62: 756-762.

37. Mackie IJ, Segal H, Burren T, Gallimore M, Walshe K, Robinson G, Machin S. Heparin cofactor II levels are increased by the use of oral contraceptives. Blood Coagulation & Fibrinolysis 1990; 1: 647-651.

38. Toulon P, Bardin J, Blumenfeld N. Increased Heparin Cofactor II levels in women taking oral contraceptives. Thrombos Haemostas 1990; 64: 365-368.

39. Kluft C, Trumpi-Kalshoven MM, Jie AFH and Veldhuyzen-Stolk EC. Factor XII-dependent fibrinolysis: A Double function of plasma kallikrein and the occurence of a previously undescribed factor XII- and kallikrein-dependent plasminogen proactivator. Thrombos Haemostas 1979; 41: 756-773.

40. Binnema DJ, Dooijewaard G, Van Lersel JJL and Kluft C. The contact-system dependant plasminogen activator from human plasma: Identification and characterisation. Thrombos Haemostas 1990; 64: 390-397.

41. Heck LW & Kaplan AP. Substrates of Hageman factor: I. Isolation and characterization of human factor XI (PTA) and inhibition of the activated enzyme by alpha-1-antitrypsin. J Exp Med 1974; 140: 1615-1974.

42. Scott CF, Schapira M, James HL, Cohen AB, Colman RW. Inactivation of FXIa by plasma protease inhibitors: predominant role of alpha-1-protease inhibitor and protective effect of high molecular weight kininogen. J Clin Invest 1982; 69: 844-852.

AAS 38/II
Recent Progress on Kinins
© 1992 Birkhäuser Verlag Basel

STUDIES ON BLOOD COAGULATION-FIBRINOLYSIS SYSTEM REGARDING KALLIKREIN-KININ SYSTEM IN THE UTERO-PLACENTAL CIRCULATION DURING NORMAL PREGNANCY, LABOR AND PUERPERIUM

S. Mutoh[1], M. Kobayashi[1], J. Hirata[2], N. Itoh[3], M. Maki[4], Y. Komatsu[1], A. Yoshida[1], H. Sasa[1], K. Kuroda[1], Y. Kikuchi[2], I. Nagata[2], Y. Ohno[5]

[1]Devision of Perinatal and Maternal Medicine and Department of Ob-Gynaecology, [2]National Defense Medical College Saitama, [3]Teijin Inc., Tokyo; [4]Department of Ob-Gynaecology, Akita University School of Medicine Akita, and [5]Sekisui Chemical Inc., Tokyo/Japan

SUMMARY:

In our previous study (Adv. Exp. Med & Biol., 247B. 569. 1989, 198B. 41. 1986, blood & vessel, 17: 51. 1986), we reported on the mechanism of coagulation-fibrinolysis system and kallikrein-kinin system in the utero-placental circulation during normal pregnancy, labor and puerperium. The samples were collected from the uterine artery (UA), uterine vein (UV) and peripheral vein (PV). In this study, we tried to elucidate the mechanism of coagulation-fibrinolysis with relation to kks by measuring of Thrombin/ Antithrombin III complx (TAT), tissue plasminogen activator (tPA)·plasminogen activator inhibitor 1 (PAI) complex (tPA·PAI·C), active plasminogen activator inhibitor 1 (active PAI), α 2-plasmin inhibitor/plasmin complex (PIC).

In 20 normal pregnant women, the levels of TAT, tPA·PAI·C and active PAI significantly increased the first trimester (TAT 4.31± 2.05 ng/ml, tPA·PAI·C 39.52± 17.34 ng/ml, active PAI 39.58± 15.29 ng/ml, n=20 M± SD P<0.001) to the third trimester (TAT 6.39± 1.93 ng/ml, tPA·PAI·C 57.94± 30.80 ng/ml, active PAI 304.24± 148.64 ng/ml, n=20 M± SD P<0.001) as compared with those of non-pregnant women (TAT 1.60 ± 0.89 ng/mg, tPA·PAI·C 11.72± 4.59 ng/ml, active PAI 11.53± 7.48 ng/ml, n=16 M± SD).

In utero-placental circulation, the levels of TAT significantly increased (TAT 22.12 ± 20.03 ng/ml n=20 M$\pm$ SD P<0.001) in UV, and tPA $\cdot$ PAI $\cdot$ C and PIC $\cdot$ markedly increased (tPA $\cdot$ PAI $\cdot$ C 93.38 ± 56.05 ng/ml, PIC 1.03 ± 0.94 μ g/ml n=20 M$\pm$ SD P<0.02) in UV, but active PAI markedly decreased (active PAI 244.18 ± 87.55 ng/ml n=20 M$\pm$ SD P<0.02) as compared with those in PV (TAT 6.1 ± 2.09 ng/ml, tPA $\cdot$ PAI $\cdot$ C 59.34 ± 18.99 ng/ml, PIC 0.49 ± 0.24 μ g/ml, active PAI 349.14 ± 157.34 ng/ml, n=20 M$\pm$ SD).

These findings suggest that the significant increase in those complexes in UA has produced a deposition of fibrin clots in the area in contact with utero-placental blood vessel, although the marked increase in tPA $\cdot$ PAI $\cdot$ C and PIC incompletly inhibited the fibrinolytic activity of tPA by the active PAI. The kks shows a consumption of prekallikrein, LMW-kininogen and HMW-kininogen, and an overproduction of kinin in UV.

INTRODUCTION

In our previous study, we reported on the blood coagulation-fibrinolysis, kks and kininase based on analysis in the utero-placental circulation, during normal pregnancy and labor, and in puerperium (Adv. Exp. Med & Biol., Vol. 247B. 569-578. 1989, Vol. 198B. 41-44.1986, blood & Vessel. Vol. 17. 51-58. 1986).

The purpose of this study is to further investigate clinical significance of blood coagulation-fibrinolysis regarding kks, especially that of the mechanism of inhibition of tPA and the formation of complexes of tPA with the active inhibitor.

MATERIAL AND METHODS

Sixteen non-pregnant women were chosen as normal controls. measurements were made of blood parameters in the PV of 20 normal gravidas from early pregnancy to term along with 20 additional measurements in the utero-placental circulation.

Blood samples were taken in siliconized vacutainer tubes containing 1/10 volume of 0.15 M sodium citrate (PH 7.0-8.5) and immediately cooled on melting ice. Plasma was obtained by

centrifugation at -4℃ for 10 minutes at 3.000 r.p.m as soon as
possible, and plasma aliquots were divided and were stored frozen at-
80℃ until analysis. Specific assays were perfomed for plasma
Thrombin/Antithrombin Ⅲ complex (TAT), tissue-plasminogen activator
(tPA)/plasminogen activator inhibitor 1 (PAI-1) complex (tPA・PAI・
C), active plasminogen activator inhibitor (active PAI) and α 2-
plasmin inhibitor/plasmin complex (PIC) regarding kks.

Table 1. Method for measurement

TAT (ng/ml)	ELISA assay	Teijin Co., Ltd., Japan
t-PA・PAI-I・C (TDC-88)(ng/ml)	ELISA assay	Teijin Co., Ltd., Japan
active PAI-I (TDC-88)(ng/ml)	ELISA assay	Teijin Co., Ltd., Japan
PIC (TD-80C)(μg/ml)	ELISA assay	Teijin Co., Ltd., Japan

Student's test was used in statistical analysis with one
standard deviation indicated in all data

RESULTS

<u>Changes of plasma and urinary coagulation-fibrinolysis system</u>
<u>during normal pregnancy</u>
    1. These factors and complexes during in the plasma normal
pregnancy, as compared with non-pregnant values, markedly increased
in the first trimester (FAP 10%, TAT 169%, tPA 16%, Bβ 15-42 24%,
PIC 62%, D-dimer 71%, tPA・PAI・C 237%, active PAI 243%) and
significantly increased from the second to the third trimester (FPA
170%, TAT 298%, tPA 46%, Bβ 194%, D-dimer 529%, tPA・PAI・C 394%,
active PAI 2.540%), although the plasma of blood PIC gradually

decreased from the second trimester and α 2PI remained unchanged
during normal pregnancy (Fig.1).

2. These factors and complexes in the urine during normal
pregnancy, as compared with non-pregnant values, gradually increased
from the first trimester (u-FPA 15%, UK 14%, Bβ 15-42 120%, PIC 242%)
and significantly increased in the third trimester (u-FPA 100%,
Bβ 15-42 144%, PIC 680%), but the levels of urinary α 2PI remained
unchanged during normal pregnancy (Fig.2).

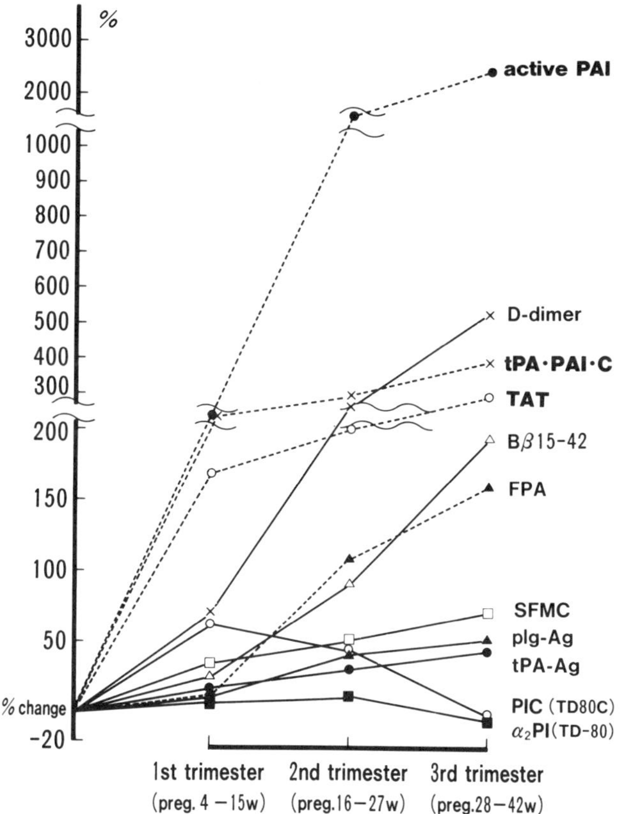

Fig. 1. Physiological changes of blood induced by pregnancy (non-pregnant (NP)
to 42 weeks of pregnancy). Increment and decrement in various parameters are
shown in percentage term compared with non-pregnant baseline

3. The levels of tPA · PAI · C and active PAI during normal
pregnancy markedly increased from the first trimester (tPA · PAI · C
39.52± 17.34 ng/ml, active PAI 39.58± 15.29 ng/ml) and significantly
increased in the third trimester (tPA · PAI · C 57.94± 30.80 ng/ml,
active PAI 304.25± 148.63 ng/ml) as compared with non-pregnant
values (tPA · PAI · C 11.72± 4.59 ng/ml, active PAI 11.53± 7.49 ng/ml)
(Fig.3, Table 2).

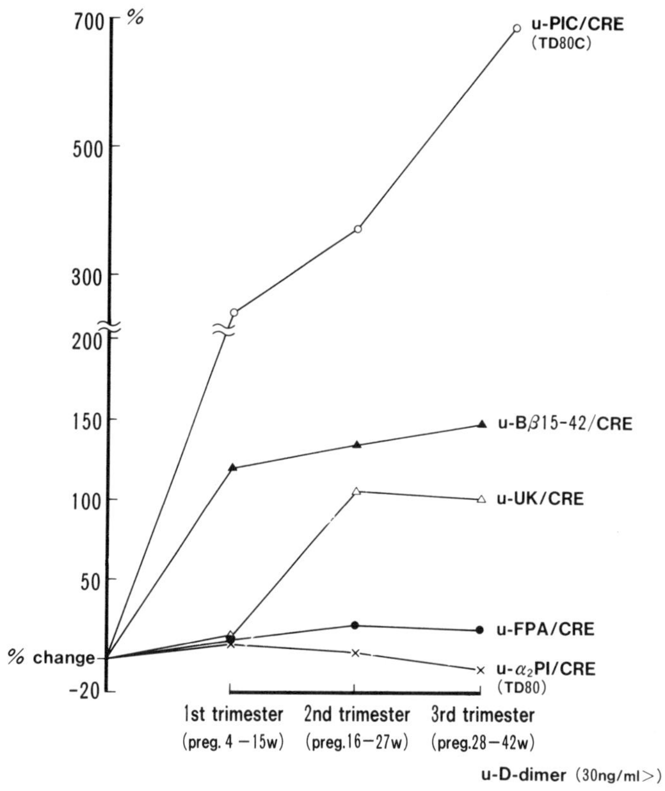

Fig. 2. Physiological changes of urine induced by pregnancy (non-pregnant (NP) to 42 weeks of pregnancy). Increment and decrement in various parameters are shown in percentage term compared with non-pregnant baseline

The changes of plasma coagulation-fibrinolysis system in the utero-placental circulation

1. The levels of TAT and FPA in UV (TAT 22.1 ± 20.0 ng/ml 262% n-20 p<0.001, FPA 10.0 ± 5.8 ng/ml 317% n=20 P<0.001) significantly

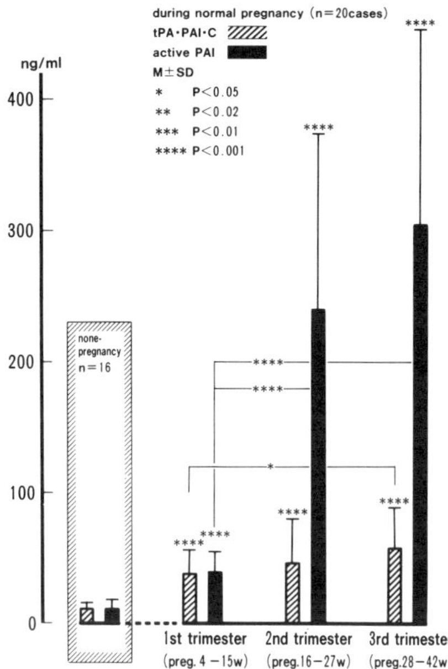

Fig. 3. Fluctuation of tPA-PAI-I complex and active PAI-I levels in plasma during normal pregnancy

Table 2. Fluctuation of plasma tPA-PAI-I and active PAI-I levels in plasma during normal pregnancy

	none-pneg. (control) n=16	during normal pregnancy (n=20cases)		
		1st trimester (preg. 4 —15w)	2nd trimester (preg.16—27w)	3rd trimester (preg.28~42w)
tPA·PAI·C ng/ml	11.72±4.59	**** 39.52±17.34	**** 47.08±23.46	**** 57.94±30.80
active PAI ng/ml	11.53±7.49	**** 39.58±15.29	**** 239.71±133.89	**** 304.24±148.62

Companison of these factors in control and during normal pregnancy   M±SD

* P<0.05
** P<0.02
*** P<0.01
**** P<0.001

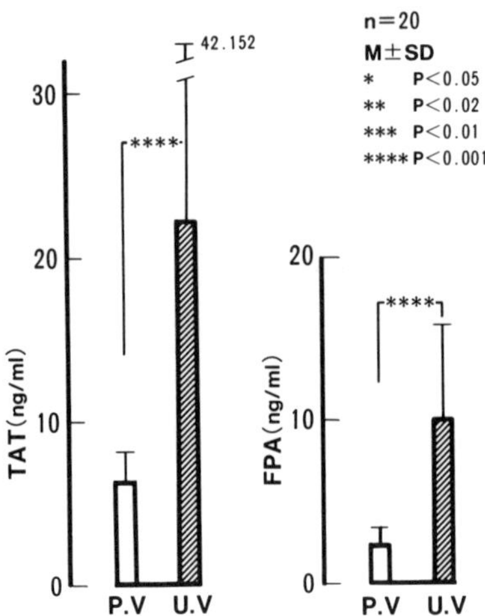

Fig. 4. Comparison of plasma TAT and FPA between peripheral vein (P.V) and uterine vein (U.V) in full term pregnancy

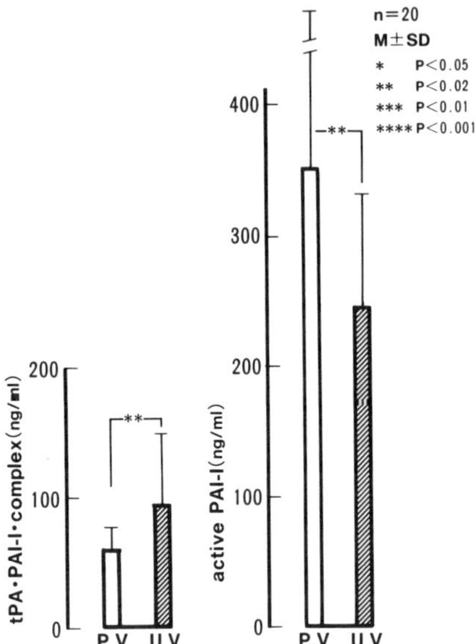

Fig. 5. Comparison of plasma tPA-PAI-I complex and active PAI-I between peripheral vein (P.V) and uterine vein (U.V) in full term pregnancy

increased as compared with those of PV (TAT 6.1 ± 2.09 ng/ml n=20 M$\pm$ SD, FPA 2.4 ± 1.1 ng/ml M$\pm$ SD) at term (Fig.4).

2. The levels of tPA $\cdot$ PAT $\cdot$ C in UV (93.4 ± 56.1 ng/ml 57% n=20 M$\pm$ SD P<0.02) markedly increased as compared with PV (tPA $\cdot$ PAI $\cdot$ C 59.3 ± 19.0 ng/ml n=20 M$\pm$ SD). The levels of active PAI in UV (244.2 ± 87.6 ng/ml -30% n=20 M$\pm$ SD P<0.02) markedly decreased as compared with PV (349.1 ± 157.3 ng/ml n=20 M$\pm$ SD) (Fig.5).

3. The levels of Bβ 15-42 and PIC in UV (Bβ 12.8 ± 5.7 ng/ml 68% n=20 P<0.01, PIC 1.03 ± 0.94 μ g/ml 110% n=20 M$\pm$ SD P<0.02) markedly increased as compared with those in PV (Bβ 7.6 ± 3.9 ng/ml n=20 M$\pm$ SD, PIC 0.49 ± 2.24 μ g/ml n=20 M$\pm$ SD) at term (Fig.6).

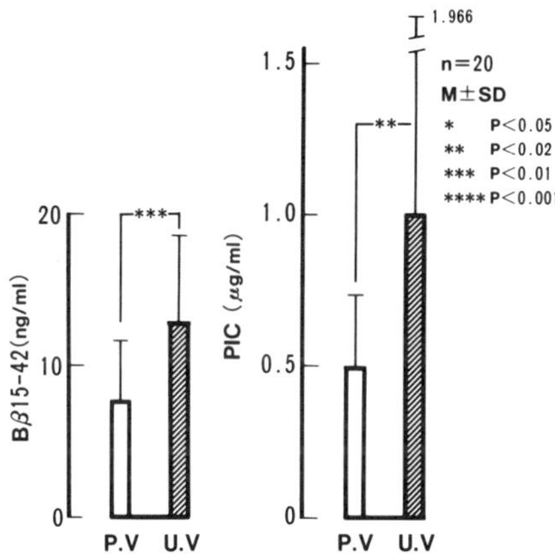

Fig. 6. Comparison of plasma Bβ15-42 and PIC between peripheral vein (P.V) and uterine vein (U.V) in full term pregnancy

DISCUSSION

<u>The relationship between the blood coagulation and fibrinolysis system during normal pregnancy</u>

The changes of plasma coagulation system showed that TAT and FPA gradually increased from the first trimester and significantly increased in third trimester. The changes of plasma fibrinolysis system showed that tPA, tPA $\cdot$ PAI $\cdot$ C, Bβ 15-42, SFMC and PIC gradually increased from the first trimester and significantly

increased in the third trimester but plasma PIC gradually decreased
from the second trimester, and urinary PIC markedly increased from
the first trimester and significantly increased in the third
trimester. The changes of plasma fibrinolytic inhibitor showed that
active PAI significantly increased from the first trimester and
α 2PI remained unchanged. These patterns suggested that the
regulation of the fibrinolysis system was preserved during the
functional state of hemostatic balance for the hypercoagulable state.

Overview of physiological plasmin-dependent fibrinolysis in the utero-placental blood circulation

Plasma levels of lipoprotein, hormones (estrogen-progesterone),
and immuno-reactive and other substrates progressively rise during
normal pregnancy. These substances are reported to be associated
with diminished plasma fibrinolysis and increased risk of venous
thromboembolic complications. The deposition of fibrin clots in the
area in contact with vessels in the utero-placental blood circulation
occurs. In the relationship between the placenta and uterus, the
placenta produces a placental activator inhibitor and the uterus
contains massive amounts of tPA.

The endogenous plasmin-dependent fibrinolytic pathway has two key
functions: (1) to generate plasmin activity within the fibrin clots
in the area of contact between the uterus and placenta at a rate
commensurate with normal wound healing: i.e., neither so rapidly that
fibrin clots dissolve before vascular repair is complete, nor so
slowly that abnormal intravascular accumulations of fibrin develop;
(2) to prevent plasmin activity from extending to non-fibrin
substrates such as fibrinogen and clotting factors V and VIII
(fibrinogenolysis), with undesirable consequences for normal
hemostasis. These demanding requirements are met through two
mechanisms. Fist, the major physiologic activator of plasminogen
(plg), tPA, preferentially activates fibrin-bound rather than free
plg, so that plasmin is generated primarily within fibrin clots and
not in the systemic circulation. Second, tPA and plasmin are
regulated by rapid, specific inhibitors: active PAI-1 and α 2PI,
respectively. Fibrinolysis is initiated when plg (synthesized by
liver) and tPA (released by vascular endothelial cells) bind to

fibrin. Since most of the tPA in normal plasma is complexed with active PAI-1 and therefore inactive, it is likely that local events occuring at the site of fibrin formation are responsible for generating the free, active tPA necessary to initiate fibrinolysis. These events are not well understood, but probably include stimulation of both tPA and active PAI-1 release from intact endothelium adjacent to the clot by thrombin, and simultaneous inactivation of PAI-1 by protein C activated by thrombin bound to the endothelial cell-surface cofactor thrombomodulin. This sequence of events provides one possible mechanism for the generation of free tPA acivity from intact vascular endothelium in response to clot formation. The active PAI-1 has been shown to be present in the subendothelial matrix, where it presumably functions to inhibit the initiation of fibrinolysis at sites of vascular injury. α 2PI is secreted by the liver into the circulating blood, where it rapidly inactives any free plasmin which escapes from the fibrin clot, thus preventing fibrinogenolysis. α 2PI further inhibits fibrinolysis by binding to some circulating plg, thereby preventing it from binding to fibrin.

These findings suggested that the significant increase in TAT and FPA in UV as compared with PV produced a deposition of fibrin clots in the area in contact with the utero-placental vessels, although the marked increase in B β 15-42, tPA・PAI・C and PIC incompletely inhibited the tPA activity by active PAI. The kks showed a consumption of prekallikrein, LMW-kininogen, HMW-kininogen, and a significantly increase of kinin in UV when compared with those in PV in full term pregnancy.

REFERENCES

1. S. Mutoh, M. Maki, Y. Ohno, Adv. Exp. Med. Bio. 41-44, 1986.
2. S. Mutoh, M. Maki, S. Takahashi: Acta. Obst. Gynaec Jap. 369-377, 1982.
3. S. Mutoh, A. Teh, Y. Ohno: Blood & Vessel. 51-58, 1986.
4. S. Mutoh: Acta Obst. Gynaec Jap. 2203-2212, 1979.
5. Robert B, Francies Jr: Blut. 1-14, 1989.
6. M. J rgensen, M. Philips, S. Thorsen: Thrombosis and Haemostasis. 872-878, 1987.
7. B. Wiman, D. Collen: Nature. 549-550, 1978.
   E.K.O. Kruithof, C.T. Thang, A. Gudinchet: Blood. 460-466, 1987.

AAS 38/II
Recent Progress on Kinins
© 1992 Birkhäuser Verlag Basel

URINARY COAGULATION-FIBRINOLYSIS, KALLIREIN-KININ SYSTEMS AND KININASE IN CASES OF PRECLAMPSIA

S. Mutoh[1], M. Kobayashi[1], J. Hirata[2], N. Itoh[3], M. Maki[4], Y. Komatsu[1], A. Yoshida[1], H. Sasa[1], K. Kuroda[1], Y. Kikuchi[2], I. Nagata[2], Y. Ohno[5]

[1]Devision of Perinatal and Maternal Medicine and Department of Ob-Gynaecology, [2]National Defense Medical College Saitama, [3]Teijin Inc., Tokyo; [4]Department of Ob-Gynaecology, Akita University School of Medicine Akita, and [5]Sekisui Chemical Inc., Tokyo/Japan

SUMMARY:

Urinary kallikrein and kallikrein activity significantly decreased in cases of preeclampsia (u-kall./CRE · index 42.39 ± 9.66 ng/mg, u-kall. act./CRE · index 0.26 ± 0.06 ng/min/mg), and urinary kininase II and kininase activity significantly increased (u-kininase /CRE · index 10.91 ± 1.26 x10^{-3} IU/min/mg, u-kininase act./CRE · index 506.37 ± 178.45 pg/min/mg) when compared with those of normal gravidas from 28 weeks to 42 weeks of gestation (u-kall./CRE · index 189.31 ± 14.17 ng/mg, u-kall. act./CRE index 1.08 ± 0.10 ng/min/mg, u-kininase /CRE · index 6.24 ± 0.31 x10^{-3} IU/min/mg, u-kininase act./CRE · index 15.64 ± 0.10 pg/min/mg). Urinary FPA, Bβ 5-42, α 2-PI, and α 2PI-plasmin-complex (PIC) significantly increased in preeclampsia (u-FPA/CRE · index 23.59 ± 8.47 ng/mg, u-Bβ /CRE · index 105.26 ± 29.30 ng/mg, u-α 2PI/CRE · index 121.53 ± 43.57 ng/mg, u-PIC/CRE index 278.39 ± 60.50 ng/mg) when compared with those of normal control group (u-FPA/CRE · index 0.92 ± 0.04 ng/mg, u-Bβ /CRE · index 12.15 ± 0.44 ng/mg, u-α 2PI/CRE · index 4.18 ± 0.33 ng/mg, u-PIC/CRE · index 5.98 ± 1.15 ng/mg). Urinary urokinase markedly increased and urinary D-dimer was detected in severe cases of preeclampsia (u-UK/CRE · index 58.20 ± 43.69 ng/mg, u-D-dimer 54.76 ± 9.89 ng/ml) when compared with those of normal control group.

These findings suggest that deficiency in urinary kinin excretion may induce hypertension in addition to the changes of urinary coagulation-fibrinolysis system that represents the occurrence of either the endothelial cell injury in the glomerulus or the renal tulbular damage in mild cases of preeclampsia, eventually resulting in the intra-renal vascular coagulation.

INTRODUCTION

The hypertensive disorders in pregnancy are common complicaitons of gestation and form one of the major factors that continue to result in the majority of maternal deaths. Furthermore, hypertensive disorders are major causes of perinatal mortality and severe morbidity. Diagnotic criteria of preeclampsia denote pregnancy-induced hypertension with proteinuria and/or edema.

In our previous study 2),3),4), we reported the changes of blood coagulation-fibrinolysis system, kallikrein-kinin system (kks) and pathophysiological findings of the kidney in preeclampsia. These chages suggested that blood coagulation-fibrnolysis system demonstrated the presence of chronic disseminated intravascular coagulation (DIC) and marked increase in urinary FDP. Furthermore, blood kks showed overproduction of kinin in severe cases of preeclampsia.

In this study, we tried to investigate the pathophysiological mechanism for the occurrence of hypertension, edema and the intraglomerulo-endothelial injury, eventually resulting in the intra-renal coagulation as judged by the assessment of urinary coagulation-fibrinolysis, urinary kks and urinary kininase in preeclampsia.

MATERIAL AND METHODS

The study patients consisted of 78 normal gravidas from 28 weeks to 42 weeks of gestation and 60 preeclamptic patients (36 mild and 24 severe toxemias). The fresh urinary samples were collected at 9 to 10 a.m and kept in ice and centrifuged at -4° C for 10 minutes at 3,000 r.p.m as soon as possible, and then stored at -70° to -80° C until use.

Specific assays were performed for urinary fibrinopeptide A (FPA), fibrin derived peptide Bβ 15-42 (Bβ 15-42), urokinase (UK), α 2-plasmin inhibitor (α 2PI), α 2PI-plasmin-complex (PIC), fragment D-dimer, urinary kallikrein activity and kallikrein (anti-human urinary kallikrein antibody), kinin, kininase activity, kininase Ⅱ and creatininine.

Table 1.　Method for measurement

u-FPA/CRE. index (ng/mg)	RIA (PEG separation)	IMCO Co., Ltd., Sweden
u-Bβ15-42/CRE. index (ng/mg)	RIA (PEG separation)	IMCO Co., Ltd., Sweden
u-urokinase/CRE. index (ng/mg)	RIA (secondary-antibody separation)	
u-$\alpha$$_2$PI(TD-80)/CRE. index (ng/mg)	TD-80	Teijin Co., Ltd., Japan
PIC(TD-80C)/CRE. index (ng/mg)	TD-80C	Teijin Co., Ltd., Japan
u-D-dimer (ng/ml)	ELISA assay	AGEN Co., Ltd., Australia
u-kallikrein activity/CRE. index (ng/min/mg)	RIA (PEG separation)	
u-kallikrein /CRE. index (ng/mg)	RIA (PEG separation)	
u-kinin/CRE. index (ng/mg)	RIA (PEG separation)	
u-kininase activity/CRE. index (pg/min/mg)	RIA (PEG separation)	
u-kininase II /CRE. index ($\times 10^{-3}$IU/min/mg)	Kasahara's method	

The ratios of these factors to creatinine (CRE) were shown in Table 1 as the indices. Student's test was used for statistical analysis with the standard error indicated in all data.

RESULTS

<u>I. The urinary coagulation-fibrinolysis system</u>

1) Fig.1 shows that the levels of u-FPA/CRE · index significantly increased (23.59± 8.47 ng/mg, n=24, M± SM, P<0.001) in severe preeclampsia, and markedly increased (2.14± 0.34 ng/mg, n=36, M± SE,

P<0.001) in mild preeclampsia as compared with those of normal gravidas from 28 weeks to 42 weeks of gestation (0.92 ± 0.04 ng/mg, n=78, M$\pm$ SE). Levels of u-FPA/CRE · index in severe preeclampsia markedly increased as compred with those of mild preeclampsia (P<0.02) (Tables 2 and 3).

 2) The levels of u-Bβ 15-42/CRE · index also significantly increased (105.26 ± 29.30 ng/mg, n=24, M$\pm$ SE, P<0.001) in severe preeclampsia and (28.13 ± 3.16 ng/mg, n=36, P<0.001) in mild preeclampsia as compared with control levels (12.15 ± 0.44 ng/mg, n=78). Levels of u-Bβ 15-42/CRE · index in severe preeclampsia markedly increased as compared with those of mild preeclampsia (P<0.02) (Fig.1, Tables 2 and 3).

 3) Fig.2 showed that the levels of u-UK/CRE · index markedly increased (58.20 ± 43.69 ng/mg, n=18, M$\pm$ SE, P<0.05) in severe preeclampsia, but remained unchanged (7.33 ± 1.04 ng/mg, n=23) in mild preeclampsia as compared with control levels (7.20 ± 1.00 ng/mg, n=78) (Tables 2 and 3).

 4) Fig.3 showed that the levels of u-α 2PI/CRE · index significantly increased (121.53 ± 43.57 ng/mg, n=18, P<0.001) in severe preeclampsia and significantly increased (8.50 ± 2.23 ng/mg, n=23, P<0.01) in mild preeclampsia as compared with normal control levels (4.18 ± 0.33 ng/mg, n=78). Levels of u-α 2PI/CRE · index in severe cases markedly increased as compared with those of mild preeclampsia (P<0.02) (Tables 2 and 3).

 5) The levels of u-PIC/CRE · index also significantly increased (278.39 ± 60.50 ng/mg, n=18, P<0.001) in severe preeclampsia and (71.58 ± 28.09 ng/mg, n=23, P<0.01) in mild preeclampsia as compared with control levels (5.98 ± 1.15 ng/mg, n-78). Levels of u-PIC/CRE · index in severe preeclampsia markedly increased as compared with those of mild preeclampsia (Fig.3, Tables 2 and 3).

 6) Fig.3 showed that the levels of urinary D-dimer markedly increased (54.76 ± 9.89 ng/ml, n=21, P<0.01) in severe preeclampsia but remained unchanged in mild preeclampsia as compared with control levels (D-deimer 30> , n=78) (Fig.4, Tables 2 and 3).

II . urinary kallikrein-kinin system and kininase

 1) Fig.5 showed that urinary kallikerein activity/CRE · index in severe preeclampsia (0.26 ± 0.06 ng/min/mg, n=18, M$\pm$ SE, P<0.001)

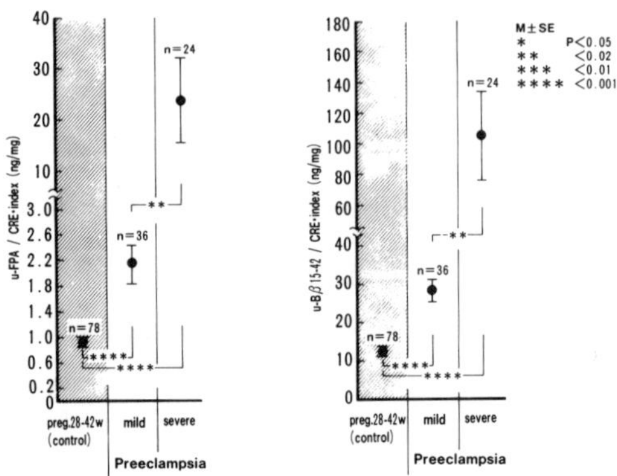

Fig. 1. Comparison of urinary fibrinopeptid A (FPA)/CRE-index (ng/mg) and urinary fibrin-derived peptide Bβ15-42 (Bβ15-42)/CRE-index (ng/mg) between preeclampsia and normal control (28 - 42 weeks)

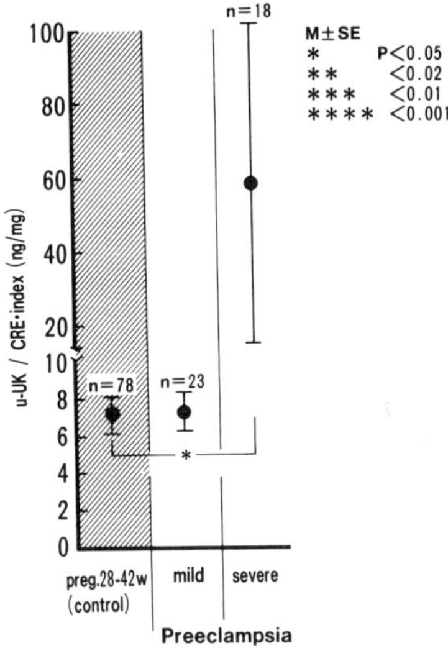

Fig. 2. Comparison of urinary urokinase/CRE-index (ng/mg) between preeclampsia and normal control (28 - 42 weeks)

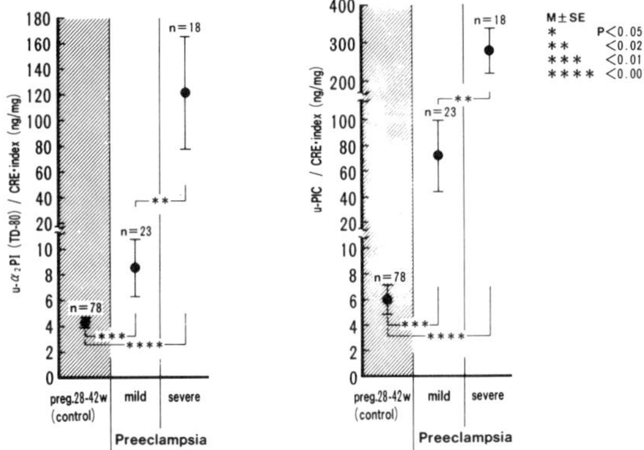

Fig. 3. Comparison of urinary α_2-plasmin inhibitor (TD-80)/CRE-index (ng/mg) and urinary PIC (TD-80C)/CRE-index (ng/mg) between preeclampsia and normal control (28 - 42 weeks)

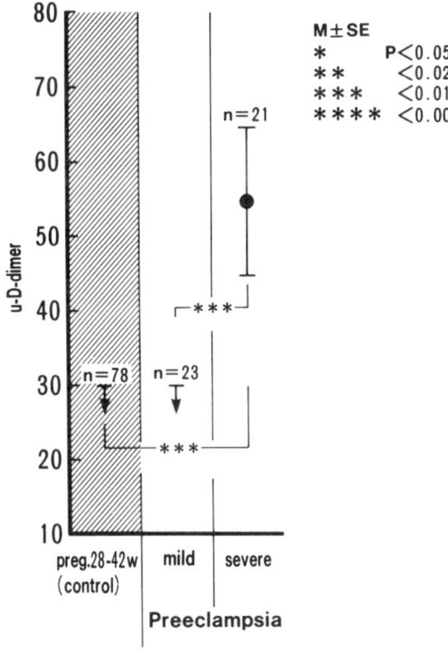

Fig. 4. Comparison of urinary D-dimer (ng/ml) between preeclampsia and normal control (28 - 42 weeks)

and in mild preeclampsia (0.23 ± 0.03 ng/min/mg, n=23, M$\pm$SE, P<
0.001) significantly decreased when compared with the those of
normal control group (1.08 ± 0.10 ng/min/mg, n=78, M$\pm$SE) (Fig,5,
Tables 2 and 3).

2) The levels of u-kall./CRE · index significantly decreased ($42.39
\pm 9.66$ ng/mg, n=26, P<0.001) in severe preeclampsia and ($58.53 \pm
12.7$ ng/mg, n=33, P<0.001) in mild preeclampsia as compared with
control levels (189.31 ± 14.17 ng/mg, n=78). The levels of u-kall./CRE ·
index in severe preeclampsia showed in a slight tendency to decrease
than in mild preeclampsia (Fig.5, Tables 2 and 3).

3) Fig.6 showed that the levels of urinary kinin/CRE · index
significantly decreased (4.58 ± 0.63 ng/mg, n=26, M$\pm$SE, P<0.001)
in severe preeclampsia and (6.21 ± 0.75 ng/mg, n=33, P<0.001) in mild
preeclampsia as compared with normal levels (11.25 ± 0.68 ng/mg, n=33,
M$\pm$SE). The levels of u-kinin/CRE · index in severe preeclampsia
slightly decreased as compared with those of mild preeclampsia, but
not significantly (Fig.6, Tables 2 and 3).

4) Fig.7 Showed that the levels of u-kininase act./CRE · index
significantly increased (506.37 ± 178.45 pg/min/mg, n=18, P<0.001)
in severe preeclampsia and (150.82 ± 101.30 pg/min/mg, n=23, P<0.001)
in mild preeclampsia when compared with those of normal control group
(15.65 ± 0.10 pg/min/mg, n=78). The u-kininase act./CRE · index in
severe preeclampsia markedly increased as compared with that of mild
preeclampsia (P<0.02) (Tables 2 and 3).

5) The levels of u-kininase II /CRE · index significantly increased
(10.91 ± 1.26 x10^{-3} IU/min/mg, n=26, M$\pm$SE, P<0.001) in severe
preeclampsia and markedly increased (10.24 ± 0.88 x10^{-3} IU/min/mg,
n=33, P<0.01) in mild preeclampsia as compared with normal levels
(6.24 ± 0.31 x10^{-3} IU/min/mg, n=78) (Fig.7, Tables 2 and 3).

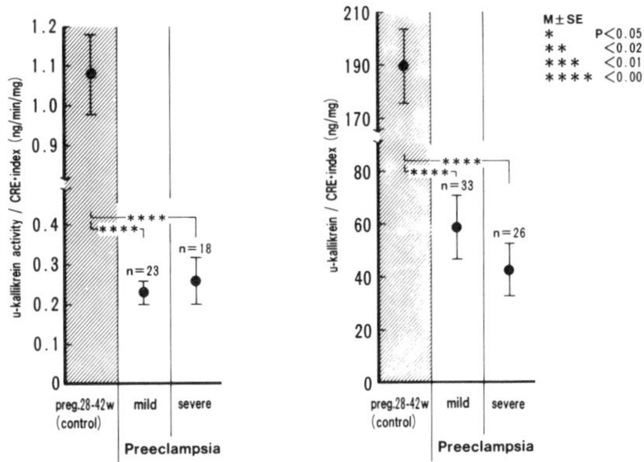

Fig. 5. Comparison of urinary kallikrein activity/CRE-index (ng/min/mg) and urinary kallikrein/CRE-index (ng/mg) between preeclampsia and normal control (28 - 42 weeks)

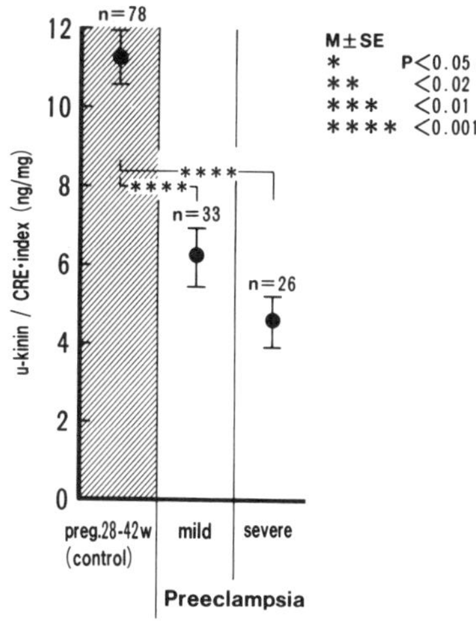

Fig. 6. Comparison of urinary kinin/CRE-index (ng/ml) between preeclampsia and normal control (28 - 42 weeks)

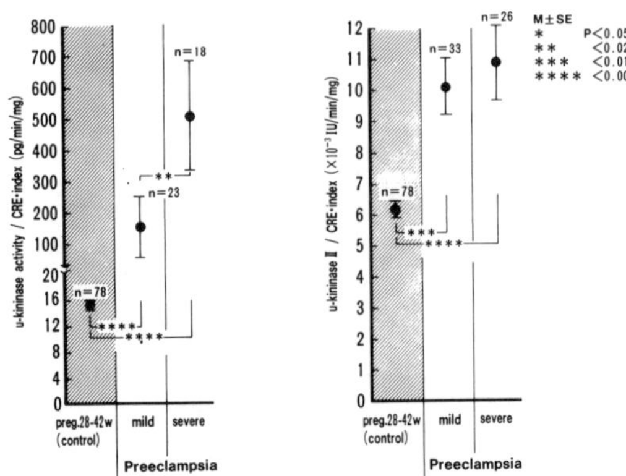

Fig. 7. Comparison of urinary kininase activity/CRE-index (pg/min/ml) and urinary kininase II/CRE-index (x10^{-3} IU/min/mg) between preeclampsia and normal control (28 - 42 weeks)

Table 2. Comparison of urinary coagulation-fibrinolysis system, kallikrein-kinin system between preeclampsia and normal control (28 - 42 weeks)

	preg. 28—42weeks (control)	Preeclampsia	
		mild	severe
u-FPA/CRE. index (ng/mg)	n=78 0.92±0.04	n=36 2.14±0.34	n=24 ** 23.59±8.47
u-Bβ15-42/CRE. index (ng/mg)	n=78 12.15±0.44	n=36 28.13±3.16	n=24 ** 105.26±29.30
u-urokinase/CRE. index (ng/mg)	n=78 7.21±1.00	n=23 7.33±1.04	n=18 58.20±43.69
u-α₂-PI(TD-80) /CRE. index (ng/mg)	n=78 4.18±0.33	n=23 8.50±2.23	n=18 ** 121.53±43.57
u-PIC(TD- 80C) /CRE. index (ng/mg)	n=78 5.98±1.15	n=23 71.58±28.09	n=18 *** 278.39±60.50
u-D-dimer (ng/ml)	n=78 30>	n=23 30>	n=21 *** 54.76±9.89
u-kall. activity/ CRE. index (ng/min/mg)	n=78 1.08±0.10	n=23 0.23±0.03	n=18 0.26±0.06
u-kall. /CRE. index (ng/mg)	n=78 189.31±14.17	n=33 58.53±12.07	n=26 42.39±9.66
u-kinin/CRE. index (ng/mg)	n=78 11.25±0.68	n=33 6.21±0.75	n=26 4.58±0.63
u-kininase activity /CRE. index (pg/min/mg)	n=78 15.64±0.10	n=23 150.82±101.30	n=18 ** 506.37±178.45
u-kininase-II /CRE. index (×10⁻³IU/min/mg)	n=78 6.24±0.31	n=33 10.24±0.88	n=26 10.91±1.26

Comparison of these factors in between preeclampsia and control;
Comparison of these factors in between mild preeclampsia and severe preeclampsia
M±SE   * P<0.05;   ** P<0.02   *** P<0.01   *** P<0.001

Table 3. Comparison of urinary coagulation-fibrinolysis system, kallikrein-kinin system between preeclampsia and normal control (28 - 42 weeks)

		Preeclampsia	
		mild	severe
urinary-coagulation-fibrinolysis system	u-FPA/CRE. index (ng/mg)	↑	↑↑
	u-Bβ15-42/CRE. index (ng/mg)	↑	↑↑
	u-urokinase/CRE. index (ng/mg)	→	↑
	u-α_2PI(TD-80)/CRE. index (ng/mg)	↑	↑↑
	u-PIC(TD-80C)/ CRE. index (ng/mg)	↑	↑↑
	u-D-dimer (ng/mg)	→	↑
urinary-kallikrein-kinin system	u-kall. activity/CRE. index (ng/min/mg)	↓	↓
	u-kall. /CRE. index (ng/mg)	↓	↓
	u-kinin/CRE. index (ng/mg)	↓	↓
	u-kininase activity/CRE. index (pg/min/mg)	↑	↑↑
	u-kininase II /CRE. index ($\times 10^{-3}$IU/min/mg)	↑	↑

DISCUSSION

In our previous study, we reported that the comparison of the
results of blood coagulation-fibrinolysis system, kks and
pathophysiological finding of the kidney in severe preeclampsia,
and in normal gravidas from 28 weeks to 42 weeks of gestation and
suggested the presence of chronic DIC status with secondary
hyperfibrinolytic state, markedly increased urinary FDP and the
consumption of prekallikrein, HMW-kininogen and LMW-kininogen and
overproduction of kinin. In the pathological changes of renal
glomerular lesions of toxemia, Mackay, Morrill, Vassalli and other
workers 8),9) suggested that toxemia predisposes to a state of
continued slow but intravascular coagulation which produced
deposition of fibrin or fibrin-like material in the glomerulus.
In eclampsia, the process is massive and sudden, leading to
intracapillary thrombosis which is visible by light microscopy. The

clotting process is slow and incomplete, but progessive, and doses
not lead to the capillary occlusion but deposition of macromolecular
aggregates of fibrin on the capillary basement membrane, which can
only be visualized by electron microscopy and immunohistochemical
techninques.

I . Analysis of the urinary coagulation-fibrinolysis system of
    preeclampsia

1. Mild preeclampsia

Urinrary levels of FPA/CRE, Bβ/CRE and α2PI/CRE indices markedly
increased, urinary urokinase/CRE · index remained unchanged and
urinary D-dimer was not detected when compared with normal control
levels.

The marked and rapid increase in the urinary excretion of Bβ and
PIC by glomrular filtration and overactive metabolism in the proximal
tubule of the kidney because plasma Bβ and PIC maredly increased,
although plasma FPA reamined unchanged and plasma α2PI markedly
decreased when compared with those of the normal control group. For
this reason, the marked and rapid increase in urinary excretion of
FPA and α2PI results from the leakage from plasma FPA and α PI.

2. Severe of preeclampsia

Urinary FPA/CRE, Bβ/CRE, PIC/CRE and α2PI/CRE indices
significantly inceased, urinary UK/CRE · index markedly increased
and urinary D-dimer was detected when compared with that of normal
levels. During pregnancy 1), urinary urokinase tended to increase
from first trimester to term,. The marked increase in the levels of
urinary urokinase appears to reflect closely the extent of
intraglomerular coagulation and fibrinolysis.

The appearance of urinary fragment D-dimer, and the significant
increase in urinary levels of FPA, Bβ , PIC, and α2PI results from
the digestion of cross-linked fibrin and/or fibrin-like material
deposited in the intraglomerular endothelial cell, providing
additional information on the balance between fibrin formation and
its removal. These findings suggested the occurrence of either
intraglomerular endothelial injury or the renal tubular damage in
mild preeclampsia, eventually resulting in the intra-renal vascular
coagulation.

<u>Ⅱ . Analysis of urinary kks. and kininase of preeclampsia</u>

Kinins are potent vasodilatory peptides. It is well known that kinins are produced in the kidney, and may also be formed in the distal part of the nephron. There is evidence that urinary kinin excretion is directly related to intrarenl kinin formation. It has been reported that the excretion of kinins is decreased in patients with essential hypertension and end-stage renal disease. It has recently been suggested that the renal kks, together with the renin-angiotensin and prostaglandin systems, is an integral part of the intrarenal hormonal system that controls water and electrolyte excretion, thus participating in the regulation of blood pressure. Our study showed that in preeclampsia, defective urinary kinin excretion is related to significantly decreased urinary kallikrein and significantly increased urinary kininase.

REFERENCES

1. S. Mutoh, Y. Ohno, N. Itoh: Adv. Exp. Med. Biol. 569, 1989.
2. S. Mutoh, A. Teh, M. Saitoh: Perinatal Care and Gestosis. 381, 1985.
3. S. Mutoh, Y. Ohno, M. Maki: Adv. Exp. Med. Biol. 44, 1986.
4. S. Mutoh, M. Maki: Acta Obst. Gynaec Jpn. 1519, 1982.
5. S. Mutoh, Y. Ohno: Thromb Haemostas. 451, 1989.
6. A. Greco, G. Porcelli: Adv. Exp. Med. Biol. 645, 1979.
7. Marc S. Weinberg, Peter Azar: Kidney International. 975, 1985.
8. Mckay, D.G., Mlerrill, S.J.: Am J Obstet Gymecol. 507, 1953.
9. Morris, R.H., Vassalli, P.: Obstet Gymecol. 32, 1964.

AAS 38/II
Recent Progress on Kinins
© 1992 Birkhäuser Verlag Basel

STUDIES OF BLOOD COAGULATION-FIBRINOLYSIS REGARDING KALLIKREIN-KININ SYSTEM IN SEVERE PREECLAMPSIA

S. Mutoh[1], M. Kobayashi[1], J. Hirata[2], N. Itoh[3], M. Maki[4], Y. Komatsu[1], A. Yoshida[1], H. Sasa[1], K. Kuroda[1], Y. Kikuchi[2], I. Nagata[2], Y. Ohno[5]

[1]Devision of Perinatal and Maternal Medicine and Department of Ob-Gynaecology, [2]National Defense Medical College Saitama, [3]Teijin Inc., Tokyo; [4]Department of Ob-Gynaecology, Akita University School of Medicine Akita, and [5]Sekisui Chemical Inc., Tokyo/Japan

SUMMARY: In our previous study 1), 2), 3) we reported the changes of coagulation-fibrinolysis, kallikrein-kinin system and kininase in preclampsis. In this study, we tried to obtain systemic information of chronic DIC status with regard to kallikrein-kinin system in severe preeclampsia. This systemic information was evaluated in 20 cases of normal gravidas from 28 to 42 weeks of gestation as a control by measuring plasma Thrombin/Antithrombin III complex (TAT), tissue plasminogen activator (tPA) plasminogen activator inhbitor (PAI) complex, active plasminogen inhibitor-1 (active PAI), 2PI plasmin complex (PIC). Results: The levels of plasma TAT and tPA significantly increased (TAT=10.9±8.3ng/ml n=24 M±SD P<0.02, tPA=6.1±3.2ng/ml n=10 M±SD P<0.01), tPA PAI C and active PAI markedly increased (tPA PAI C=85.07±50.01ng/ml n=24 P<0.05, active PAI=407.4±166.0ng/ml n=24 P<0.205), and PIC and D-dimer=435.1±145.2ng/ml n=8 M±SD P<0.001) in severe preeclampsia as compared with those of normal values (TAT=6.1 2.0ng/ml, tPA=3.6±1.5ng/ml, tPA PAI C=57.9±30.8ng/ml, active PAI=304.2±148.6ng/ml, PIC=0.49±0.24 mg/ml, D-dimer=282.9±75.3ng/ml). These findings suggest that patients with severe preeclampsia are in chronic DIC status and in profound alteration of the fibrinolytic system as characterized by strong increase in the levels of active PAI, tPA PAI C, PIC, B and D-dimer, although these alterations do not affect the overall fibrinolytic activity.

INTRODUCTION

In our previous study, we reported the changes of blood coagulation-
fibrinolysis and kallikrein-kinin systems in preeclampsia. The
results suggested that preeclamptic patients appeared to be in
chronic DIC status with regard to the consumption of prekallikrein,
LMW-kininogen, HMW-kininogen and overproduction of kinin in cases of
preeclampsia (Acta Obst Gynec Jap. 34:1519. 1982, Perinatal Care
and Gestosis. 381. 1985). The purpose of this study is to further
investigate clinical significance of plasma coagulation-fibrinolysis
regarding kks in severe cases of preeclampsia, especially on its
plasma concentration and kinetics and mechanism of tPA, inhibition
of tPA and the formation of complexes of tPA with the active
inhibitor, complexes of antiplasmin with rapidly inactivating free
plasmin which escapes from the fibrin clots, thus preventing
fibrinolysis in the circulating blood and D-dimer, a specific
fragment resulting from the degradation of cross-linked fibrin.

MATERIAL AND METHODS

The systemic information was comparatively assessed in 20 severe
preeclamptic patients with 30 normal gravidas from 28 to 42 weeks
gestation as a control group. Blood samples were taken in
siliconized vacutainer tubes containing 1/10 volume of 0.15 M sodium
citrate (PH 7.0-8.5) and immediately cooled on melting ice. Plasma
was obtained by centrifugation at -4℃ for 10 minutes with 3,000
r.p.m as soon as possible, and plasma aliquotes were divided and
stored frozen at -80℃ until analysis. Specific assays were
performed on plasma Thrombin/Antithrombin Ⅲ complex (TAT), tissue
plasminogen antigen (tPA), tissue plasminogen activator (tPA)/

plasminogen activator inhibitor-1 (PAI-1) complex (tPA PAI C),
active plasminogen inhibitor-1 (active PAI-1), α 2-plasmin inhibitor
/plasmin complex (PIC) and fragment D-dimer regarding kks.

Table 1. Method for measurement

TAT	(ng/ml)	ELISA assay	Teijin Co., Ltd., Japan
t-PA antigen	(ng/ml)	ELISA assay	Biopool Co., Ltd., Sweden
t-PA·PAI-I·C	(ng/ml)	ELISA assay	Teijin Co., Ltd., Japan
active PAI-I	(ng/ml)	ELISA assay	Teijin Co., Ltd., Japan
PIC	(μg/ml)	ELISA assay	Teijin Co., Ltd., Japan
D-dimer	(ng/ml)	ELISA assay	AGEN Co., Ltd., Australia

Student's test was used in statistical analysis with one
standard deviation indicated in all data

RESULTS

   1. The levels of TAT and FPA significantly increased (TAT=10.9$\pm$
1.7 ng/m1. 79%. P<0.02, FPA=4.7$\pm$0.6 ng/m1. 81%. P<0.01) in severe
preeclampsia as ampared with those of normal gravidas from 28 to 42
weeks of gestation (TAT=6.1$\pm$0.4 ng/m1, FPA=2.6$\pm$0.3 ng.m1) (Fig.1,
Table 2).
   2. The levels of tPA and Bβ 15-42 significantly increased (tPA=
6.1$\pm$1.0 ng/m1. 68%. P<0.01, Bβ =23.0$\pm$1.8 ng/m1. 147%. P<0.001)
in severe preeclampsia as compared with control leveles (tPA=3.6$\pm$
0.3 ng/m1, Bβ =9.3$\pm$0.8 ng/m1) (Fig.2, Table 2).

3. The levels of tPA PAI C and active PAI markedly increased (tPA PAI C=85.1± 10.2 ng/m1. 47%. P<0.05, active PAI=407.4± 33.9 ng/m1. 34%. p<0.05) as compared with control levels (tPA PAI C=57.9± 6.9 ng/m1, active PAI=304.2± 33.23 ng/m1) (Fig.3, Table 2).

4. The levels of PIC and D-dimer significantly increased (PIC= 0.8± 0.1 μ g/m1. 71%. P<0.001, D-dimer=435.1± 51.3 ng/m1. 54%. P<0.001) in severe preeclampsia as compared with those of normal levels (PIC=0.49± 0.1 μ g/m1, D-dimer=282.9± 16.8 ng/m1) (Fig.4, Table 2).

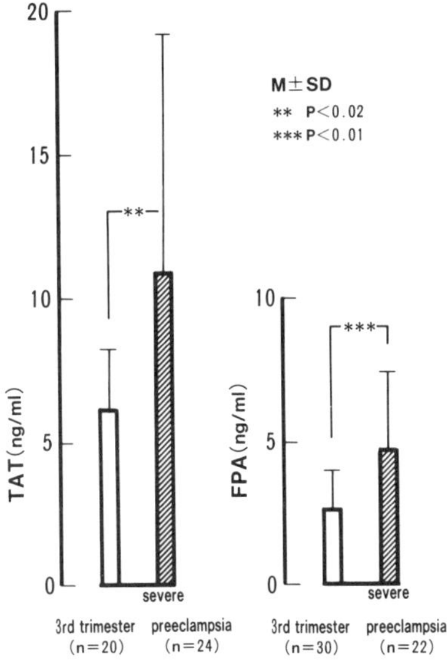

Fig. 1. Comparison of plasma TAT and FPA between preeclampsia and normal control (28 - 42 weeks)

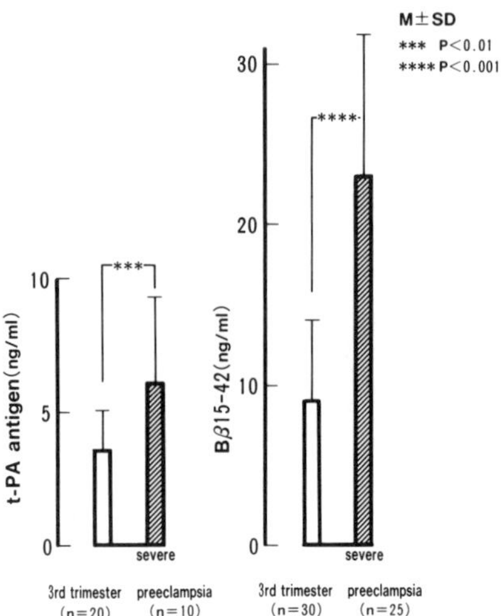

Fig. 2. Comparison of plasma t-PA antigen and Bβ15-42 between severe preeclampsia and normal control (28 - 42 weeks)

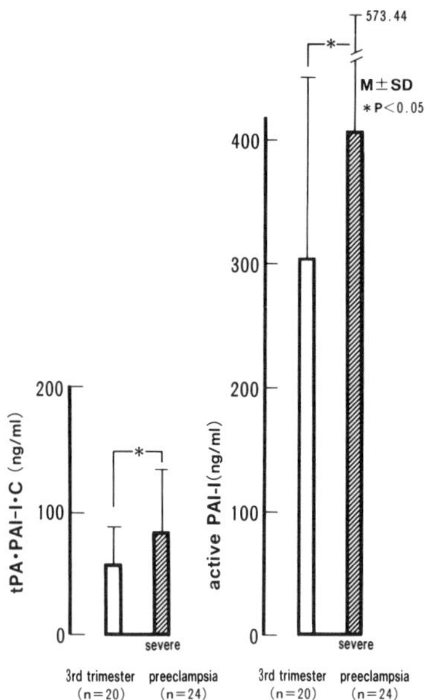

Fig. 3. Comparison of plasma tPA-PAI-I-complex and active PAI-I between severe preeclampsia and normal control (28 - 42 weeks)

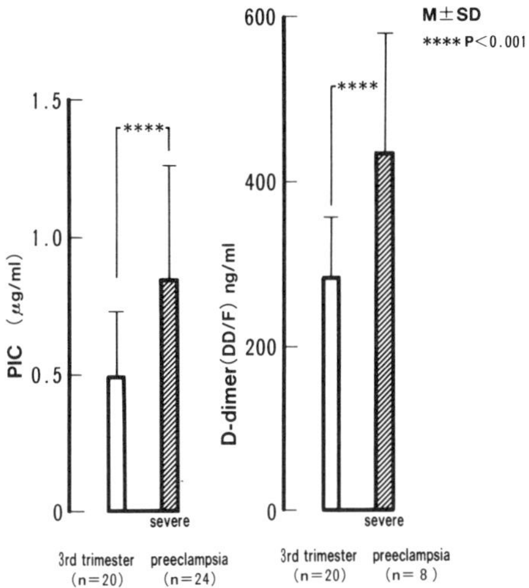

Fig. 4. Comparison of plasma PIC and D-dimer (DD/F) between severe preeclampsia and normal control (28 - 42 weeks)

Table 2. Comparison of plasma coagulation-fibrinolysis system between severe preeclampsia and normal control (28 - 42 weeks)

		preg. 28-42weeks of normal gestation (control)		severe preeclampsia	
		n	M±SD	n	M±SD
TAT	ng/ml	20	6.10±1.98	24	10.9±8.3[**]
FPA	ng/ml	30	2.6±1.3	22	4.7±2.7[***]
tPA-Ag	ng/ml	20	3.6±1.5	10	6.1±3.2[***]
Bβ15-42	ng/ml	30	9.3±4.6	25	23.0±8.9[****]
tPA·PAI·C	ng/ml	20	57.9±30.8	24	85.1±50.0[*]
active PAI	ng/ml	20	304.2±148.6	24	407.4±166.0[*]
PIC	μg/ml	20	0.49±0.24	24	0.84±0.42[****]
D-dimer	ng/ml	20	282.9±75.3	8	435.1±145.2[****]

Comparison of these factors in
between severe preeclampsia and control

M±SD
*   P<0.05
**   P<0.02
***   P<0.01
****P<0.001

DISCUSSION

In our previous stuey 1),2),3), we reported that the changes in
coagulation-fibrinolysis regarding kks in patients with severe
preeclampsia included the discrepancy between the intrinisic and the
extrinisic coagulating factors, significant increase in the
intrinisic coagulating factor, exhaustion of the extrinisic factors,
a depletion of ELT, a rise in SFMC, significant increase in FPA, Bβ
15-42 and FDP, significant decrease in plg, AT-III and α 2PI,
significant decrease in prekallikrein, marked decrease in HWM-
kininogen, consumption of LWM-kininogen and significant increase of
kinin, indicating the presence of chronic DIC status with an
overproduction of kinin.

The present study confirms previous reports indicating that
patients with severe preeclampsia show the significant changes in
coagulation-fibrinolysis factors when compared with normal pregnant
women of similar gastational ages. In this study, the levels of
TAT, tPA, PIC, and D-dimer significantly increased, and tPA PAI C
and active PAI markedly increased in severe preeclampsia when
compared with those of normal gravidas from 28 to 42 weeks of
gestation.

The physiologic plasmin-dependent fibrinolysis is initiated when
plasminogen (synethesized by liver) and tPA (released by vascular
endothelial cells) bind to fibrin. Since most of the tPA in normal
plasma forms complexes with active PAI and therefore inactive, it is
likely that local events occuring at the site of fibrin formation
are responsible for generating free, active tPA necessary to
initiate fibrinolysis. Active PAI-1 is also produced by platelets.
Recently, active PAI-1 has been shown to be present in
subendothelial matrix, where it presumably functions to inhibit the
initiation of fibrinolysis at siotes of vascular injury. The high
PAI-1 levels are associated with poor prognosis. PIC formed in the
circulation dissociated in the presence of fibrin, because plasmin
has a greater affinity for fibrin than for its inhibitors.
In contrast, plasmin which is released from digested fibrin is
rapidly and irreversibly neutralized by α 2PI in the circulation.
Bβ 15-42 appeares to result from degradation of fibrin by plasmin.

D-dimer, a specific fragment results from the degradation of cross-linked fibrin by plasmin. Our results show that patients with severe preeclampsia are in the state of chronic DIC and profound alteration of the fibrinolysic system characterized by strong increase in the levels of the active PAI, tPA PAI C, PIC, Bβ an D-dimer, although these changes do not affect the overall fibrinolytic activity.

REFERENCES

1. S. Mutoh, A. Teh, M. Saito : Perinatal care and gestosis, 381-384, 1985.
2. S.Mutoh, M. Maki, S. Takahashi : Acta Obst Gynaec Jpn. 1519-1527, 1982.
3. S.Mutoh, M. Maki, Y. Ohno : Aav. Exp. Med. Biol, 41-44, 1986.
4. S. Mutoh, A. Teh, Y. Ohno : Blood & Vessel, 51-58, 1986.
5. A. Estllés, J. Gilabert, J. Aznar : Blood, 1332-1338, 1986.
6. E.K.O. Kruithof, C.T. Thang, A. Gudinchet : Blood 460-466, 1987.
7. Robert B, Francis Jr. : Blut, 1-14, 1989.
    E.K.O. Kruithof : Fibrinolysis, 59-70, 1988.

AAS 38/II
Recent Progress on Kinins
© 1992 Birkhäuser Verlag Basel

DETERMINATION OF CATHEPSINS B, H, L AND KININOGEN IN BREAST CANCER PATIENTS

D. Gabrijelčič, B. Svetic, D. Spaić, J. Škrk*, J. Budihna*, V. Turk

Dept. of Biochemistry, Jozef Stefan Institute, Jamova 39, 61000 Ljubljana, *Institute of Oncology, 61000 Ljubljana, Slovenia

SUMMARY: In 20 matched pairs, an increase of all cathepsins was measured in carcinoma tissue compared with normal tissue of the same breast. On contrary, the mean value for kininogen was almost 2 fold lower than mean value determined in normal cytosols. From all proteins tested, the amount of cathepsin B correlated mostly with the degree of malignancy inside the group of invasive ductal carcinoma ($n=90$, $p<0.01$).

INTRODUCTION

Numerous studies have been prepared dealing with a possible role of different proteinases in pathology of malignant growth, invasivenes and metastasis (1,2). The metastatic cascade consists of sequence of steps, which probably include the secretion of several proteinases, like serine proteinase plasminogen activator (3), metallo enzymes, such as collagenases (4), and lysosomal proteinases: cathepsin D (5) and cathepsins B (6) and L (7). All these enzymes are able to cleave and degrade basement membranes.

If lysosomal enzymes are involved in spread of breast cancer, measurements of their levels in primary tumors might indicate metastatic potential. Most of the studies have been done on cathepsin as prognostic marker (8,9), and lately also on cysteine proteinases, as potentially important clinical parameters in breast carcinoma (10,11,12).

On cysteine proteinase inhibitors in human tumors there are very limited data (13,14). Lah et al. (15) found a significant decrease in CPI activities in paralel with an increase in the activities of cathepsins B and L in human breast carcinoma. It has been also shown (15) that the patients bearing tumors with decreased CPI levels, had a poorer prognosis.

High molecular weight CPI activity has been found in tumor and normal tissue extracts. The kininogens may come from serum in the tissues or be of intracellular origin (16).

In our study, we determined the total amount of cathepsins B, H and L in different breast tumor cytosols. We correlated the quantities of proteinases with total CPI activities. We also investegated the LMW kininogen in normal and malignant breast tissue in order to find out any possible correlation of proteinases and inhibitor content with known histopathologic characteristics of breast carcinoma.

MATERIALS AND METHODS

<u>Patients data and preparation of tissue homogenates</u>: 90 patients with primary breast cancer (all invasive or infiltrative ductal carcinoma), surgically treated at the Institute of Oncology, Ljubljana, Slovenia, were included in the study. Data available for each case were: age, histologic type, histologic grading from I to III (well, moderately and poorly differentiated, respectively), involvement of the regional lymph nodes and steroid hormonal receptors.

Samples of tumorous and non-tumorous (free of tumor cells) tissues from the same breast, representing a matched pair, were obtained immediately after surgical removal and immersed in liquid nitrogen.

Tissue homogenates (also called cytosolic fractions) were prepared from those tissue samples by homogenation and centrifugation (40000g) as reported by Mc Guire et al. (17). One part of the homogenate was used for steroid hormonal receptor determination, the rest of the volume was used for biochemical studies.

<u>Protein determination</u>: Protein content in tumor tissue homogenates was determined using the method described by Bradford (18). Bovine serum albumine was used as standard.

<u>Enzymes and Inhibitors</u>: Cathepsin B was isolated from human liver as described by Zvonar (19). Cathepsins H and L were purified from human kidney according to Popovic (20) and Mason (21), respectively. HMW and LMW kininogens and their rabbit antisera were kindly provided from MEDOR GmbH (Herrsching, Germany). Kininogen domains were isolated according to Salvesen method (22), slightly modified (23). Recombinant cystatin C was performed as described by Cimerman et al. (24).

<u>Cathepsin B activity assay</u>: Cathepsin B activity was measured specifically, using Z-Arg-Arg-AMC (Serva, Heidelberg, Germany), according to Barrett (25).

<u>Immunoreactivity</u>: Immunoreactivity studies were performed using immunoselective polyclonal antibodies against cathepsins B, H and L, and LMW kininogen raised in rabbits and sheep. Immunization procedure and preparation of sera were performed as reported (26). Immunoselective antibodies were purified from rabbit and sheep antisera using as immunoadsorbent column containing human liver cathepsin B, human kidney cathepsins H or L and human plasma LMW kininogen bound to CNBr activated Sepharose 4B (Pharmacia, Uppsala, Sweden). Cathepsins were quantitatively determined in breast tumor and non-tumor cytosols by enzyme immunoassays, according to procedures reported previously (27).

LMW kininogen was determined by newly developed sandwich ELISA, using immunoselective rabbit anti-LMW kininogen IgGs for coating in concentration 2.5g/l. An optimal dilution of 1/2500 of peroxidase-labeled anti-LMW kininogen IgG conjugate (28) was used for detection.

<u>Statistical methods</u>: Summary data are expressed as the mean values +/- standard error (SE) unless otherwise noted. For comparison of the data on matched pairs of carcinoma and normal breast tissue, the Student-t test was used. The difference between mean values was used to establish statistical significance. Values of 0.05 or less were considered significant.

RESULTS AND DISCUSSION

Cathepsins B, H, L and kininogen concentrations have been determined immunologically in matched pairs of tumor and non-tumorous tissue samples of the same breast. ELISA tests for cathepsins B, H and L have been performed as described in l.c. (27). LMW kininogen sandwich ELISA has been developed and optimized as demonstrated in Fig.1. The test has a sensitivity range from 5 ug/l to 800 ug/l and a detection limit of 8 ug/l of LMW kininogen. Recovery of antigen was found to be between 92% and 105%.

The specificity and cross reactivity of isolated immunospecific anti-kininogen immunoglobulins were controlled by enzyme immunoassay test, using different antigens. Beside LMW kininogen, kininogen domains D_1, D_2 and D_3, and recombinant cystatin C were used. As can be seen from Fig.2, anti-LMW kininogen IgGs are not specific; they cross react with HMW kininogen and with domains (30%-60%), but not with recombinant cystatin C. As proved by Western blot analysis (not shown), the kininogen domains were not in the free form present in the breast cancer homogenates.

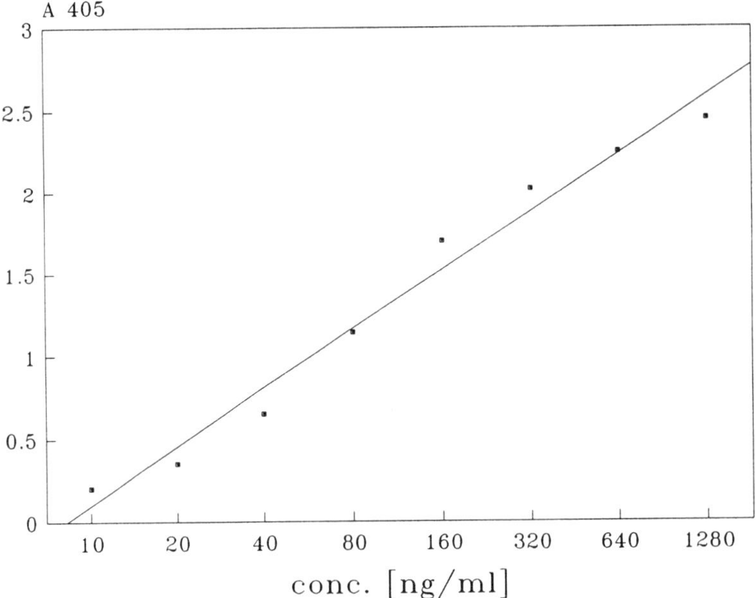

Figure 1. Binding curves of LMW kininogen in the enzyme immunoassay for LMW kininogen

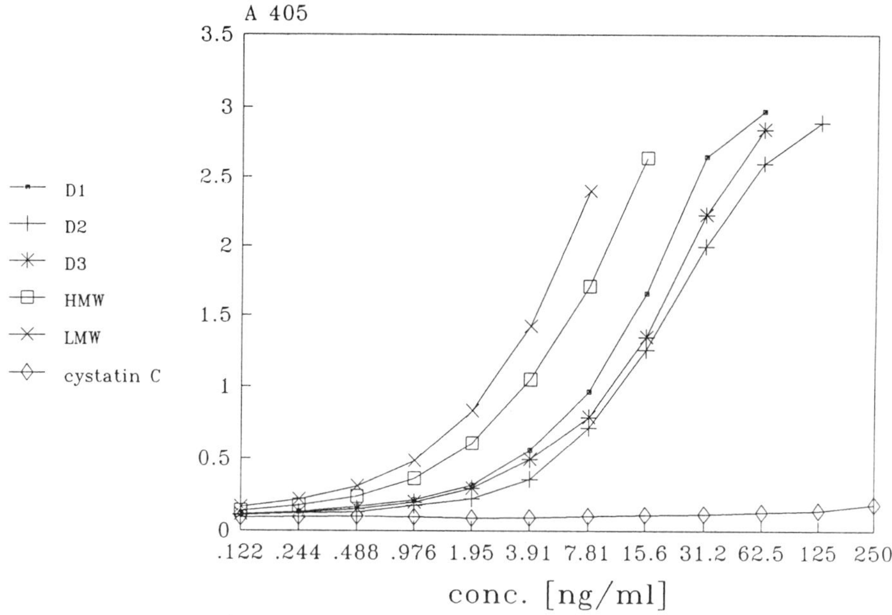

Figure 2. Binding curves of LMW kininogen(1), HMW kininogen(2), kininogen domains D_1(3), D_2(4) and D_3(5) and recombinant cystatin C(6) in the enzyme immunoassay with anti-LMW kininogen IgGs

With sandwich ELISA for LMW kininogen, the inhibitor was measured in 20 matched pairs of tumor and non-tumorous tissue cytosols (Table 1). Results shown in Table 1 demonstrate an approximately 2 fold average decrease on quantity of kininogen, measured in tumor cytosols, when compared with normal tissue samples. Till now, no data in literature on kininogen concentration in breast cancer homogenates are available.

Table 1. Kininogen content determined immunologically in breast cancer cytosols compared with non-malignant samples from the same patients (n=20).

	concentrations	
	normal (mg/g)[*]	tumor (mg/g)[*]
kininogen	4.98 ± 1.2	2.45 ± 0.9

[*] values are given as mean +/- standard error

In the same samples cathepsin B was immunologically determined (Table 2). Cathepsin B amounts were found to be on the average about 9 fold higher in tumor tissue cytosols, compared with normal tissue of the same breast (p<0.01). The activity levels were found to be 23 fold elevated when measured with Z-Arg-Arg-AMC (p<0.01). Similar results for cathepsin B activity in breast tumor cytosols were reported by Vashista et al. (11) and Lah et al. (15).

Table 2. Cathepsin B content determined quantitatively and enzymatically in breast cancer cytosols compared with non-malignant samples from the same patients (n=20).

	enzyme immuno assay (µg/g)[*]	specific enzyme activity (mU/g)
normal	14.15 ± 2.56	98 ± 37
tumor	125.2 ± 27.39	2225 ± 461
	T=8.8 p<0.01	T=22.7 p<0.01

[*] values are given as the mean +/- standard error

Cathepsin L values in tumor cytosols ranged from 21 µg/g to 80 µg/g. The mean of 37.85 µg/g was determined, which is almost 3 fold higher than cathepsin L values obtained in tumor sera (11.5 µg/g 1.7) (27). To give statistically relevant values we need a higher sample population, but up to now we did not find correlations of cathepsin L values with any of known clinical parameters (morphological grading, lymph node involvement, etc.), although the cathepsin L activity in breast tumor cytosols is elevated on average 52.5 fold (15), when compared with normal breast tissue.

Table 3 summarizes cathepsin H values obtained on 75 samples of breast carcinoma. It can be clearly seen that cathepsin H values are higher in malignant then in non-malignant samples. Inside the group of invasive ductal carcinoma, the values for cathepsin H increase with the pathological grading (x III/x I = 6.5 fold, Table 3). It is the first time that cathepsin H has been demonstrated and determined in breast carcinoma.

Table 3. Values of cathepsin H in different cytosols of breast cancer patients

tumor grade	No	concentrations x (µg/g)[*]
I	12	369 ± 14
II	35	1023 ± 243
III	26	2385 ± 1020

[*] values are given as the mean +/- standard error

Table 4A shows the relation of cathepsin B values with pathological grading inside the group of invasive ductal carcinoma and with regional lymph node involvement. From the results obtained, a strong positive correlation of the average amount of cathepsin B measured immunologically with the stage of tumor dedifferentiation (T I/III = 2.31, p<0.05) could be seen. Negative correlation of cathepsin B values with the involvement of regional lymph nodes was also observed inside the same group (T = 1.99, p<0.05, Table 4B). Up to now, there are no quantitative data available, showing direct correlation of cathepsin B (or other cysteine proteinase) with the degree of malignancy in breast carcinoma patients. There are a few reports showing that the release of cysteine proteinases from breast tumor tissue could play an important role in tumor growth, invasivenes and metastasis, based on activity measurements (11).

Table 4A. Concentration of cathepsin B in different cytosols of breast cancer patients, devided according to histologic grading.

breast tumor cytosols tumor grade	No	concentrations cathepsin B x $(\mu g/g)^*$
I	17	75.92 ± 6.3
II	42	117.74 ± 27.4
III	31	161.98 ± 69

[*] values are given as the mean +/- standard error

T I/III=2.31, p<0.05;   T I/II=0.87, N.S.

Table 4B. Concentration of cathepsin B in different cytosols of breast cancer patients devided according to the involvement of regional lymph nodes.

No	involvement of lymph nodes	concentration $(\mu g/g)^*$
38	+	87.35 ± 11.3
37	-	162.91 ± 25.5

[*] values are given as the mean +/- standard error

In this report we showed that in breast carcinoma patients all three cysteine proteinases, cathepsins B, H and L, are elevated in tumor tissue, when compared with normal tissue. On the contrary, the kininogen values are reduced. We showed also that cathepsin B is directly connected with the stage of tumor

  D. Gabrijelčič et al.

dedifferentiation. Our results prove that cathepsin B participates in the processes of tumor growth and metastasis in breast carcinoma.

REFERENCES

1. Tryggvasom K, Hoyhtya M, Salo T. Proteolytic degradation of extracellular matrix in tumor invasion. Biochim. Biophys. Acta 1987; 907:191-217.
2. Mullins DE, Rohrlich ST. The role of proteinases in cellular invasiveness. Biochim. Biophys. Acta 1982; 695:177-214.
3. Reich R, Thompson E.W, Iwamoto Y, Martin GR, Deason JR, Fuller GC, Miskin R. Effects of plasminogen activator serine proteinases, and collagenase IV on the invasion of basement membranes by metastatic cells. Cancer Res. 1988; 48:3307-3312.
4. Liotta LA, Stetler-Stevenson WG. Metallo-proteinases and cancer invasion. Semin. Cancer Biol. 1990; 1:99-106.
5. Briozzo P, Morisset M, Capony F, Rougeot C, Rochefort H. In vitro degradation of extracellular matrix with 52000 cathepsin D secreted by breast cancer cells. Cancer Res. 1988; 48:3688-3692.
6. Sloane BF, Rozhin J, Hatfield JS, Crissman JD, Honn KV. Plasma membrane-associated cysteine proteinases in human and animal tumors. Expl. Cell Biol. 1987; 55:209-224.
7. Rozhin J, Wade RL, Honn KV, Sloane BF. Membrane-associated cathepsin L: a role in metastasis of melanomas. Biochem. Bioph. Res. Commun. 1989; 164: 556-561.
8. Spyratos F, Maudelonde T, Brouillet JP, Brunet M, Defrenne A, Andrieu C, Hacene K, Desplaces A, Rouesse J, Rochefort H. Cathepsin D: an independent prognostic factor for metastasis of breast cancer. The Lancet 1989; 11: 1115-1118.
9. Thorpe SM, Rochefort H, Garcia M, Freiss G, Christensen IJ, Khalaf S, Paolucci F, Pau B, Rasmussen BB, Rose C. Association between high concentrations of Mr 52000 cathepsin D and poor prognosis in primary human breast cancer. Cancer Res. 1989; 49:6008-6014.
10. Krepela E, Vicar J, Cernoch M. Cathepsin B in human breast tumor tissue and cancer cells. Neoplasma 1989; 35:41-52.
11. Vasishta A, Baker PR, Preece PE, Wood RAB, Cuschieri A. Inhibition of proteinase-like peptidase activities in serum and tissue from breast cancer patients. Anticancer Res. 1988; 8:785-790.
12. Gabrijelčič D, Annan-Prah A, Škrk J, Kramberger M, Šebek S, Turk V. Determination of cathepsins B and H in sera and tissues of breast cancer patients. In: Proteinases and their inhibitors: Recent developments Auerswald E, Fritz H, Turk V, editors. WEKA-Druck GmbH, Linnich: KFA Juelich. 1989: pp.9-12.
13. Okumichi T, Nishiki M, Takasugi S, Yamane M, Ezaki H. Purification of thiol proteinase inhibitor from human lung cancer tissue. Hiroshima J. Med. Sci. 1984; 33:801-808.
14. Sheashan K, Shuja K, Murnane MJ. Cysteine proteinase activities and tumor development in human colorectal carcinoma. Cancer Res. 1989; 49:3809-3814.
15. Lah TT, Kokalj-Kunovar M, Štrukelj B, Pungerčar J, Barlič-Maganja D,   Drobnič-Košorok M, Kastelic L, Babnik J, Golouh R, Turk V. Stefins and lysosomal cathepsins B, L and D in human breast carcinoma. Int. J. Cancer 1991;in press.
16. Tsushima H, Hopsu-Havu VK. Cysteine proteinase inhibitors in human squamous cell carcinoma. Acta Histochem. 1989; 85:23-28.
17. Mc Guire WL. Estrogen receptors in human breast cancer. J.Clin. Invest. 1973; 52:73-77.
18. Bradford N. A rapid sensitive method for the quantitation of g quantities of protein utilizing the principle of protein-dye binding. Anal. Biochem. 1976; 72:248-254.
19. Zvonar T, Kregar I, Turk V. Isolation of cathepsin B and N-benzoyl-arginine- -naphtylamide hydrolase from bovine lymph nodes. Croat. Chem. Acta 1980; 53:509-517.
20. Popovič T, Brzin J, Kos J, Lenarčič B, Machleidt W, Ritonja A, Hanada K, Turk V. A new purification procedure of human kidney cathepsin H, its properties and kinetic data. Biol. Chem. Hoppe-Seyler 1988; 369:Suppl., 175-183.
21. Mason RW, Green GDJ, Barrett AJ. Human liver cathepsin L. Biochem. J. 1985; 226:233-241.

22.   Salvesen G, Parkes C, Abrahamson M, Grubb A, Barrett AJ. Human low-Mr kininogen contains
       three copies of a cystatin sequence that are divergent in structure and in inhibitory activity for
       cysteine proteinases. Biochem. J. 1986; 234:429-434.
23.   Rešek S. Diplome work. 1990.
24.   Cimerman N, Trstenjak-Prebanda M, Ritonja A, Turk V. Studies on the interaction of the
       recombinant cystatin C and their two modified forms with papain. 35. Congresso Nazionale, Joint
       Symposia, Abstracts, Bari, 1990: pp. 124.
25.   Barrett AJ. Fluorimetric assays for cathepsin B and cathepsin H with methylcoumarylamide
       substrates. Biochem. J. 1980; 187:909-912.
26.   Morton B, Siegel Y, Sinha N, Vanderlaan WP. Production of antibodies by inoculation into lymph
       nodes. Methods Enzymol. 1983; 93:3-12.
27.   Gabrijelčič D, Svetic B, Spaić D, Škrk J, Budihna M, Dolenc I, Popović T, Cotič V, Turk V.
       Determination of cathepsins B, H and L in breast cancer patients. Eur. J. Clin. Chem. Clin.
       Biochem. 1991; in press.
28.   Avrameas A, Ternynck T, Guesdon JL. Coupling of enzymes to antibodies and antigens. Scand. J.
       Immunol. 1978; 8, Suppl. 7:7-23.

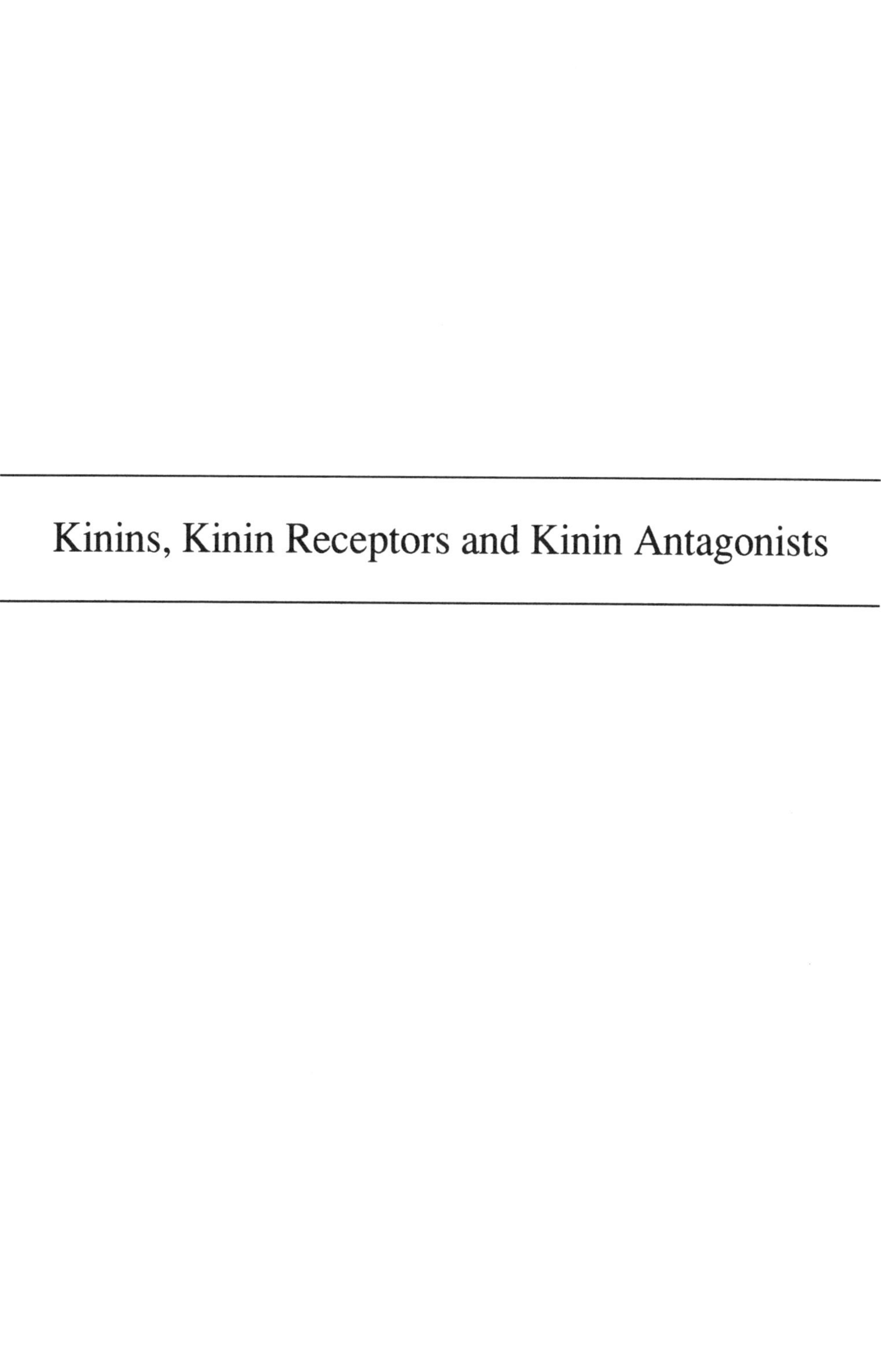

Kinins, Kinin Receptors and Kinin Antagonists

AAS 38/II
Recent Progress on Kinins
© 1992 Birkhäuser Verlag Basel

ELECTROPHYSIOLOGICAL APPROACHES TO THE STUDY OF BRADYKININ AND NITRIC OXIDE IN INFLAMMATORY PAIN

Anthony Dickenson, Jane Haley, Mel Schachter and Vicky Chapman

Dept. of Pharmacology, University College London, Gower St., London WC1E 6BT

SUMMARY: These electrophysiological studies, using desensitization and selective antagonists, demonstrate a peripheral role of bradykinin in the generation of pain in the rat. In addition, nitric oxide is shown to play a complex role in peripheral and spinal events in nociception.

BRADYKININ AS A PERIPHERAL MEDIATOR OF PAIN

Bradykinin has actions on numerous biological systems. It has been shown that peripheral bradykinin production is increased in a variety of inflammatory states (1). Although bradykinin is rapidly inactivated by proteolytic enzymes the kallikreins are inactivated much more slowly and therefore there is the capacity for maintained bradykinin production, allowing it to play a role not only in the initial phase of the inflammatory response but also the later stages of inflammation. The direct application of exogenous bradykinin stimulates nociceptors in muscle, viscera and skin. Bradykinin injected into the paw produces nociceptive behaviour in the mouse (2) and intra-arterial injection elicits vocalization in both the dog and cat (3). In addition, application of bradykinin onto a blister base in the human elicits a pain response which can be blocked by selective antagonists (4,5).The actions of bradykinin are mediated by two receptors B1 and B2. During inflammatory states bradykinin is generated in the damaged tissue and activates peripheral C-fibres which transmit pain to the spinal cord.

We report here using electrophysiological recordings of dorsal horn sensory neurones in the anaesthetized rat, (6) that bradykinin plays an important role in the transmission of painful messages from the site of inflammatory pain to the spinal cord. The model consists of the recording of nociceptive neurones in the dorsal horn, neurones that give rise to ascending pain messages and also drive the withdrawal reflex. There is considerable evidence that these neurones are important in the transmission of acute and inflammatory pain and their responses are sensitive to analgesics ranging from NSAIDS to morphine (6). Non tissue damaging electrical stimulation of tactile A-fibres and nociceptive C-fibres has been used as a comparison to the responses elicited by peripheral administration of the algogen formalin. Formalin produces an initial first peak of activity which lasts for 10 minutes followed at 20 minutes by a prolonged second phase of activity lasting for at least one hour. The first phase of the formalin response is thought to be primarily due to the direct activation of the small afferent sensory neurones by the formalin. The second phase is thought to be due to the activation of the C-fibres by inflammatory mediators such as bradykinin and prostaglandins so functional studies can be made with antagonists (7,8,9,10) applied at peripheral local, systemic or spinal sites.

RESULTS AND DISCUSSION

Injection of bradykinin (10μg in 10μl) into the peripheral receptive field resulted in an excitation of the dorsal horn neurones which did not exceed 5 minutes. Repetitive administration of the same dose of bradykinin at 10 minute intervals resulted in a loss of response of the central neurones until there was little or no response at all by the 4th and 5th injections. Subsequent formalin administration into this area resulted in a response with a slightly reduced first peak and a markedly reduced second peak to a value of 31% of control.

The B1 receptor antagonist DesArg9[Leu8]bradykinin administered directly into the receptive field 10 minutes prior to formalin did not inhibit but rather caused a dose related increase in both peaks of the response with the top dose of 200μg causing a significant increase of 136% in the second peak.

Injection of the bradykinin B2 receptor antagonist [Hyp3Thi5,8DePhe7]bradykinin (B4162) into the receptive field 10 minutes prior to formalin resulted in an inhibition of the second but not the first peak. The highest dose (50μg) inhibited the second peak by 61% whilst producing only a 4% alteration in the first peak. B4162 is a peptide analogue of bradykinin and may therefore be degraded within the tissue and in favour of this, administration 10 minutes after formalin resulted in a small increase in effectiveness. Administration of the top dose (50μg) of the B2 receptor antagonist B4162 directly into the receptive field (and site of electrical stimulation) did not inhibit the electrically evoked A and C fibre responses of the dorsal horn neurones.

The effects of the B2 receptor antagonist B4162 on the formalin response were from antagonism at the bradykinin receptor. Subcutaneous administration of saline into the receptive field 10 minutes following the first administration of bradykinin increased the next two responses to bradykinin. This sensitization was only transient with the fourth and fifth injections of bradykinin showing profound desensitization. 50μg B4162 which reduced the formalin response blocked this sensitization. Further experiments showed that the effects of B4162 on the formalin response were not due to agonist actions of the antagonist which could cause desensitization.

The recently available BK2 antagonist HOE140 was used to verify the role of bradykinin in the periphery during pain states. This compound has been shown to be a potent and long acting antagonist at the BK2 receptor in both in vivo and in vitro experiments (7,8) and so can be compared to the previous results with the less potent and less stable BK2 antagonist B4162. HOE140 was injected (50μl) into the peripheral receptive field 10 minutes pre formalin.

Table 1. The effects of HOE140 on the formalin response

DOSE	FIRST PEAK	SECOND PEAK
$0.5\mu g$	2864±843	21508±7924 n=5
$1\mu g$	4064±1165	12227±3789 n=10
$10\mu g$	999±256	1231±991 n=6
Control	7685±1926	27008±6416 n=16

Only the highest dose ($10\mu g$) of antagonist inhibited the first peak of the formalin response. The second peak is markedly inhibited by 1 and $10\mu g$ of HOE 140 with the latter causing a 95% reduction in the second phase and an 87% reduction in the first. These results can be compared to the effect of peripheral B4162 on the formalin response which significantly inhibited the second peak of the formalin response and not the first and the inhibition of the second phase was only about 60%. Although both of these compounds are selective B2 antagonists, HOE140 was approximately fifty times more potent in our experiments and longer lasting (at least three hours) as compared to the first generation antagonist B4162. These findings agree with those seen in smooth muscle assays (7). The marked inhibition of the second peak by peripheral HOE140 and B4162 strongly implicates a role of bradykinin at the B2 receptor during the second phase of the formalin response but also a role in the first phase as revealed by HOE140 (12).

Injection of formalin into the receptive field following desensitization with bradykinin resulted in a 69% reduction in the size of the second peak of the neuronal response to formalin and a 40% reduction in the first peak of the response. Thus the ability of the receptive field to respond to bradykinin is critical in the peripheral nociceptive events occurring during the formalin response, especially during the second peak.

The selective B1 receptor antagonist DesArg9[Leu8]bradykinin (1) was unable to inhibit either phase of the formalin response and resulted instead in a significant increase in the size of the second peak. Enhanced responses to bradykinin have been observed with this B1 antagonist in visceral afferent fibre recordings in the dog but even lower doses of the B1 antagonist were still unable to inhibit the activity induced by bradykinin (13). In addition the ventral root depolarizations induced by peripheral administration of bradykinin in an in vitro rat tail-cord preparation were unaltered by either the B1 agonist or antagonist (14). A human study has shown that B2 antagonists block the pain response elicited by bradykinin administered onto a blister base whilst a B1 antagonist was ineffective and a B1 agonist was unable to elicit pain (15).

The mechanism by which the bradykinin B2 receptor antagonists inhibit the formalin response is as yet undetermined. They may be blocking a direct depolarizing action of bradykinin on the afferent fibres. Alternatively they may be blocking the local vascular actions of the peptide since the same dose range of B4162 blocks bradykinin induced plasma extravasation in the rabbit (16) and reduces hyperalgesia in the rat (17). However bradykinin induced plasma extravasation in the rat was not blocked by B2 antagonists (15) although the oedema produced by carrageenan was reduced by a B2 antagonist in the dose range that inhibited the hyperalgesia (18). It is therefore possible that the antagonists may both block direct afferent stimulation by bradykinin and reduce the plasma extravasation induced by the peptide preventing inflammatory and nociceptive mediators from arriving at the site of insult via the plasma.

SOME SPINAL AND PERIPHERAL ASPECTS OF THE ROLE OF NITRIC OXIDE IN PAIN

Endothelium derived relaxing factor (EDRF) (19) is now believed to be the simple molecule nitric oxide (NO) (20,21). The inflammatory mediators bradykinin, substance P and histamine can produce vascular relaxation indirectly by stimulating the production of NO in endothelium cells and this subsequently stimulates guanylate cyclase within the smooth muscle. However, these events have now been shown to occur in several, seemingly diverse cells and tissues including the brain. The synthesis of NO from an amino acid precursor L-arginine appears to involve a enzymatic hydroxylation/oxidation reaction (22). This enzymatic synthesis of NO has now been shown in many cells including endothelium cells, macrophages and neutrophils.

Bradykinin is known to activate C fibres and to be a peripheral mediator of chemical nociception. The ability of bradykinin to generate NO and thus produce local vascular effects presents a potential role for NO in both inflammatory and nociceptive events.

An exciting development has been the discovery of NO production within the central nervous system (23), and it has been proposed that NO may be released from neurones following receptor activation. Stimulation of guanylate cyclase has been shown to occur via the generation of NO following activation of the N-methyl-D-aspartate (NMDA) excitatory amino acid receptor (24). The activation of dorsal horn neurones within the spinal cord following noxious peripheral stimulation in vivo such as the second phase of the formalin response has been shown to involve excitatory amino acid receptors, including the NMDA receptor (25). This raises the intriguing possibility that activation of the NMDA receptor within the spinal cord following peripheral noxious stimulation may result in the generation or release of NO. The recent development of inhibitors of NO synthesis (26) allows us to determine whether NO has a role in the peripheral generation or spinal processing of nociceptive information.

RESULTS AND DISCUSSION

The nitric oxide inhibitor N-nitro-L-arginine methyl ester (L-NAME) administered intravenously (10-100 mg/kg) was unable to inhibit the acute electrically evoked C fibre responses of the neurones. By contrast, when injected 40 minutes prior to the injection of formalin the second peak was inhibited with little change in the first peak. The highest dose used (100 mg/kg) produced a 74% inhibition in the the second peak but only a 45% inhibition of the first peak.

Administration of L-NAME (500 and 1500 μg) directly into the site of formalin injection as a 10 minute pretreatment inhibited the first phase of the formalin response (57% inhibition with 1500 μg). The second peak was significantly inhibited with the 1500 μg dose producing a 63% inhibition. Injection of the top dose of L-NAME into the contralateral paw 10 minutes prior to formalin injection had no significant effect on the subsequent response indicating the inhibition is unlikely to result from leakage of L-NAME into the systemic circulation. By contrast to pretreatment, administration of 1500 μg L-NAME into the receptive field 10 minutes after formalin has no effect on the second peak. Thus the ability of peripheral L-NAME to inhibit the second phase of the formalin response is dependent on its time of administration.

Injection of 1500 μg NAME directly into the site of electrical stimulation within the receptive field resulted in a rapid but transient inhibition of both the A and C fibre evoked responses of the dorsal horn neurones. The cell responses were inhibited by 35% and 12% respectively and returned to control levels by 20 minutes. Thus this reduction of the second peak of the formalin response will not result from depression of the C or A fibre activity since the inhibitory effects have worn off prior to the time of generation of the second phase although it could explain the reduced first peak.

Intrathecal L-NAME inhibited both the A and C fibre evoked responses of the neurones. The top dose of 1500 μg produced inhibitions of 24% and 30% for the A and C fibre evoked responses respectively. Intrathecal L-NAME 30 minutes prior to formalin resulted in a dose-related inhibition of both the first and second peaks of the formalin response. The top dose of 1500 μg L-NAME produced inhibitions of the first and second peak of 71% and 69% respectively.

Attempts were made to reverse the effects of L-NAME with L-arginine. Intrathecal administration of 4500 μg L-arginine reduced the electrically evoked A and C fibre responses of the neurones by 24 % and 67 % respectively. Intrathecal coadministration of 1500 μg L-NAME and 4500μg L-arginine did not significantly alter the C fibre response although the 34% reduction was very similar to that produced by 1500 μg L-NAME alone.

Intrathecal administration of 4500 μg L-arginine 30 minutes prior to formalin inhibited the first and second peaks of the response by 65% and 67% respectively. Intrathecal coadministration of 4500 μg L-arginine and 1500 μg L-NAME, 30 minutes prior to formalin, inhibited the first and second peaks of the formalin response by 58% and 61% respectively

N-nitro-L-arginine methyl ester (L-NAME) is a putative NO inhibitor (26,27) being more potent in vivo and in vitro than the widely used L-NG-monomethyl arginine. Intravenous, peripheral or intrathecal administration of L-NAME inhibited the second peak of formalin induced activity in dorsal horn neurones. However the effects of L-NAME on the first peak of the response and the electrically evoked A and C fibre responses were more varied.

Intravenous administration of L-NAME had only minor effects on the electrically evoked responses of the neurones. However, a marked inhibition of the second peak of the formalin response was observed with no significant reduction in the first peak. Using a different NO inhibitor L-NG-nitro arginine (L-NOARG) a behavioural study in mice observed preferential inhibition of the second peak of formalin induced nociception although higher doses also reduced the first peak (28). L-NOARG administered intraperitoneally is also antinociceptive in the hotplate and abdominal constriction tests in mice (28)

The inhibition of formalin evoked dorsal horn neuronal activity by L-NAME is unlikely to result from any non-specific events such as changes in blood pressure elicited by the compound since this could be expected to influence both peaks of the response.

The antinociceptive actions of intravenous L-NAME on formalin evoked dorsal horn neuronal activity may result from either peripheral or central mechanisms of action but the mechanisms by which L-NAME is inhibiting the formalin response can only be speculated upon. It is possible that NO is involved in the activation of C fibres by algogenic substances such as bradykinin but the ability of L-NAME to inhibit vasodilatation could account for the peripheral antinociception observed. The second peak of the formalin response is known to result from the development of inflammation in the periphery (9) and one of the mediators involved is now known to be bradykinin (10,11). The ability of inflammatory mediators such as bradykinin to cause local vasodilatation and presumably plasma extravasation are likely to be inhibited by L-NAME. This could prevent bradykinin and possibly other mediators gaining access to the C fibres.

Intrathecal administration of L-NAME resulted in an inhibition of both peaks of the formalin evoked dorsal horn neuronal activity and a small but significant inhibition of the electrically evoked A and C fibre responses of the neurones. Coadministration of L-NAME with a three times higher dose of L-arginine was unable to reverse the effects of the inhibitor. In addition L-arginine alone produced a significant inhibition in the A and C fibre evoked responses and both the first and second peaks of the formalin response. In agreement with this antinociceptive action of L-arginine, analgesia has been observed in humans upon systemic administration of L-arginine (29) and peripheral administration appears antinociceptive in carrageenan hyperalgesia in rats (30).

A mechanism for the inhibition produced by spinal L-NAME occurs may be proposed on the basis of recent work (23). Activation of excitatory amino acid receptors and in particular the NMDA receptor leads to NO synthesis in the cerebellum. The involvement of spinal NMDA receptors in the responses of dorsal horn neurones to formalin has been described by us (25) and so a similar mechanism may be operating in the spinal cord. The inhibition of the formalin response by intrathecal L-NAME implies the generation of NO within the spinal cord may be involved in the responses of the dorsal horn neurones to this nociceptive stimulus.

NO is known to stimulate guanylate cyclase, resulting in the generation of cGMP in the brain (23,31) However intrathecal administration of dibutyryl cyclic guanosine monophosphate (DBcGMP), a stable cGMP analogue, produces antinociception and inhibits C-fibre evoked activity of ascending axons (32). The antinociceptive actions of L-arginine may therefore result from the stimulation of cGMP production within the spinal cord.

The doses of drugs used in these experiments are extremely high but similar to those used in behavioural and in vivo studies. In addition, the selectivity of L-NAME has not yet been evaluated and whilst both L-NAME and L-NMMA have been shown to inhibit the synthesis of NO from its precursor possible actions of these compounds in other systems need investigation.

Thus whilst the responses of dorsal horn neurones to peripheral formalin administration can be modulated by a putative inhibitor of NO synthesis they can also be reduced by a precursor of NO synthesis. These apparently contradictory results are in agreement with behavioural studies in both rodents and humans (28,29,30). The antinociceptive effects of L-NAME occur both in the periphery where it may be acting on the vasculature, and spinally where it could be preventing events occurring at the synapse following NMDA receptor activation. Thus NO may be involved, in some complex way, in nociceptive events both in the periphery and within the spinal cord. It may possibly act as a mediator of the effects of bradykinin in the periphery and centrally in the NMDA receptor mediated excitation of the dorsal horn transmission neurones.

CONCLUSION

These studies show that the roles of mediators at a number of sites can be studied using these electrophysiological techniques, without many of the problems of non-specific effects of agents. The results show that the activation of C-fibres by bradykinin via the B2 receptor is vital for the dorsal horn neuronal responses to formalin and that nitric oxide is also a mediator both in the periphery and in the spinal cord where it may be involved in the NMDA receptor activation of nociceptive neurones.

ACKNOWLEDGEMENTS: These studies were supported by the MRC and SERC-CASE studentships with the Sandoz Institute for Medical Research to Dr. J. Haley and V. Chapman.

REFERENCES

1.Regoli D, Barabé J. Pharmacology of bradykinin and related kinins. Pharmacol. Rev. 1980; 32: 1-46.

2.Shibata M, Ohkubo T, Takahashi H, Inoki R. Interaction of bradykinin with substance P on vascular permeability and pain response. Japan. J. Pharmacol. 1986; 41: 427-429.

3.Guzman F, Braun C, Lim RKS. Visceral pain and the pseudaffective response to intra-arterial injection of bradykinin and other algesic agents. Arch. Int. Pharmacodyn. 1962;136: 353-384.

4.Horton EW. Action of prostaglandin E1 on tissues which respond to bradykinin. Nature (Lond.) 1963: 200: 892-893.

5.Whalley ET, Clegg S, Stewart JM, Vavrek RJ. The effect of kinin agonists and antagonists on the pain response of the human blister base. Naunyn-Schmiedeberg's Arch. Pharmacol. 1987: 336; 652-655.

6. Dickenson AH, Recent advances in the physiology and pharmacology of pain: plasticity and its implications for clinical analgesia. J. Psychopharm. 1991; 5: 342-351.

7. Wirth K, Hock FJ, Albus U et al. Hoe 140 a new potent and long lasting bradykinin-antagonist: in vivo studies. Brit. J. Pharm. 1991; 102: 774-777.

8. Lembeck F, Griesbacher T, Eckhardt M, Henke S, Briepohl G, Knolle J. New long-acting potent bradykinin antagonists. Brit. J. Pharm. 1991; 102: 297-304.

9.Hunskaar S, Hole K. The formalin test in mice: dissociation between inflammatory and non-inflammatory pain. Pain 1987; 30: 103-114.

10.Haley JE, Dickenson AH, Schachter M. (1989) Electrophysiological evidence for a role in chemical nociception in the rat. Neurosci. Lett. 1989; 97: 198-202.

11.Shibata M, Ohkubo T, Takahashi H, Inoki R. Modified formalin test :characteristic biphasic pain response. Pain 1989 38: 347-352.

12. Beresford IJM, Birch PJ. Antinociceptive activity of the bradykinin antagonist HOE140 in rat and mouse. Brit. J. Pharmacol. 1992; in press

13.Mizumura K, Minagawa M, Tsujii Y, Kumazawa T. The effects of bradykinin agonists and antagonists on visceral polymodal receptor activities. Pain 1990; 40: 221-227.

14.Dray A, Bettaney J, Forster P, Perkins MN. Activation of a bradykinin receptor in peripheral nerve and spinal cord in the neonatal rat in vitro. Br. J. Pharmacol. 1988; 95: 1008-1010.

15.Whalley ET, Nwator IA, Stewart JM, Vavrek RJ. Analysis of the receptors mediating vascular actions of bradykinin. Naunyn-Schmiedeberg's Arch. Pharmacol. 1987; 336: 430-433.

16. Griesbacher T, Lembeck F. Effect of bradykinin antagonists on bradykinin-induced plasma extravasation, venoconstriction, prostaglandin E2, nociceptor stimulation and contraction of the iris sphincter muscle in the rabbit. Brit. J. Pharm. 92: 1987; 333-340.

17.Steranka LR, Manning DC, DeHaas CJ, Ferkany JW, Borosky SA, Connor JR, Vavrek RJ, Stewart JM, Snyder SH. Bradykinin as a pain mediator: Receptors are localized to sensory neurons, and antagonists have analgesic actions. Proc. Natl. Acad. Sci., U.S.A. 1988; 85: 3245-3249.

18.Costello AH, Hargreaves KM. Suppression of carrageenan-induced hyperalgesia, hyperthermia and edema by a bradykinin antagonist. Eur. J. Pharmacol. 1989; 171: 259-263.

19.Furchgott RF.The role of endothelium in the responses of vascular smooth muscle to drugs. Ann. Rev. Pharmacol. Toxicol. 1984; 24: 175-197.

20.Ignarro LJ, Buga GM, Wood KS, Byrns RE, Chaudhuri G. Endothelium-derived relaxing factor produced and released from artery and vein is nitric oxide. Proc. Natl. Acad. Sci. U.S.A. 1987; 84: 9265-9269.

21.Palmer RMJ, Ferrige AG, Moncada S. Nitric oxide release accounts for the biological activity of endothelium-derived relaxing factor. Nature (Lond.) 1987; 327: 524-526.

22.Marletta MA. Nitric oxide: biosynthesis and biological significance. Trends. Biol. Sci. 1989;14: 488-492.

23.Garthwaite J, Charles SL, Chess-Williams R. Endothelium-derived relaxing factor release on activation of NMDA receptors suggests role as intercellular messenger in the brain. Nature (Lond.) 1988; 336: 385-388.

24.East SJ, Garthwaite J. Nanomolar NG-nitroarginine inhibits NMDA-induced cyclic GMP formation in rat cerebellum. Eur. J. Pharmacol. 1990; 184: 311-313.

25. Haley JE, Sullivan AF, Dickenson AH. Evidence for spinal N-methyl-D-aspartate receptor involvement in prolonged chemical nociception in the rat. Brain Res. 1990; 518: 218-226.

26.Rees DD, Palmer RMJ, Schulz R, Hodson HF, Moncada S.Characterization of three inhibitors of endothelial nitric oxide synthase in vitro and invivo. Br. J. Pharmacol. 1990; 101: 746-752.

27.Moore PK, al-Swayeh OA, Chong NWS, Evans RA, Gibson A. L-NG-nitro arginine (L-NOARG), a novel, L-arginine-reversible inhibitor of endothelium-dependent vasodilatation in vitro. Br. J. Pharmacol. 1990; 99: 408-412.

28.Hart SL, Oluyomi AO, Wallace P, Babbedge RC, Moore PK. L-NG-nitro arginine (L-NOARG), a selective inhibitor of nitric oxide biosynthesis exhibits antinociceptive activity in the mouse. Eur. J. Pharmacol. 1990; 183: 1440.

29. Takagi HA, Harima H, Shimizu H. A novel clinical treatment of persistent pain with L-arginine. Eur. J. Pharmacol. 1990; 183: 1443.

30.Duarte IDG, Lorenzetti BB, Ferreira SH. Peripheral analgesia and activation of the nitric oxide-cyclic GMP pathway. Eur. J.Pharmacol.1990;186: 289-293.

31.Miki N, Kawabe Y, Kuriyama K. Activation of cerebral guanylate cyclase by nitric oxide. Biochem. Biophys. Res. Commun. 1977; 75: 851-856.

32.Jurna I, Cyclic nucleotides and aminophylline produce different effects on nociceptive motor and sensory responses in the rat spinal cord. NS. Arch. Pharmacol. 1984; 327: 23-30.

AAS 38/II
Recent Progress on Kinins
© 1992 Birkhäuser Verlag Basel

EVIDENCE THAT NITRIC OXIDE OR A RELATED SUBSTANCE IS A NEUROVASODILATOR IN THE SUBMANDIBULAR GLAND OF THE CAT

M. Schachter, B. Matthews[1] and K. D. Bhoola[2]

Pharmacology Group, King's College London, Manresa Road, London SW3 6LX and Departments of Physiology[1] and Pharmacology[2], School of Medical Sciences, University of Bristol, Bristol BS8 1TD

SUMMARY: Close–arterial injection of L–N^G–nitro arginine methyl ester, a compound that inhibits the synthesis of nitric oxide (NO), caused a dose–dependent reduction in both the parasympathetic and sympathetic (rebound) nerve–induced vasodilatation within the submandibular gland of the cat. At the same time, salivary secretion produced by each nerve was relatively unaffected, and the sympathetic vasoconstriction was enhanced. These results suggest that NO or a related compound may be either a neurotransmitter or neuromodulator contributing to the autonomic nerve–induced vasodilatation in the submandibular gland of the cat.

INTRODUCTION

As far back as 1872, Heidenhain (1) observed that whereas atropine abolished the salivary secretion from the submandibular salivary gland evoked by parasympathetic (chorda typani) nerve stimulation, the accompanying vasodilatation was relatively unaffected. In an effort to explain this hitherto unaccountable event we have made use of the laevo– and dextro– guanadino substituted arginine derivatives of N^G–nitro arginine methyl ester (L– and D– NAME) (2). The prototype for this compound, L–N^G–monomethyl arginine (L–NMMA) was first introduce in 1988 (3). Since these compounds act by inhibiting the synthesis of NO from L–arginine, they seemed useful tools for assessing the role of NO or related compounds in physiological and pathological events.

METHODS

Experiments were carried out on 8 adult, male cats (4 to 6 kg in weight and 9 to 14 months old), anaesthetised with sodiun pentobarbitone (Sagital, May & Baker, Dagenham, England); the dose used for each cat was 42 mg/kg intrapritoneally, followed by 3 mg/kg intrvenously into the saphenous vein as required. Dissection, exposure of nerves, cannulation of the submandibular duct and the lingual artery, retrograde close arterial injections into the lingual artery and related procedures were performed as described by Bhoola et al. (4) and Beilenson et al. (5). Close–arterial injections of L–NAME were made retrogradely into the lingual artery, slowly over 30 sec for individual doses, whereas cummulative doses were infused over a 2.5 h period. Electrical stimuli (10 V, 1 ms pulse duration, 20 pulses/sec) were applied to each autonomic nerve from an isolated stimulator. The rate of flow of saliva and of blood were recorded using a method described by Burgen (6). Each fluid (saliva and blood) was collected in a separate reservoir on a level with the gland, and as it entered the receptacle it displaced air through a hypodermic needle. The pressure difference between the inside and outside of the bottle was recorded as a measure of the rate of flow of the fluid entering the reservoir. The outflow resistances were such that a flow of 1 ml/min produced a pressure gradient of 5 mm H_2O.

RESULTS

Close–arterial, retrograde injections of L–NAME into the lingual artery caused a dose–dependent (10, 12.5, 50 and 100 mg/kg) reduction in the vasodilatation produced by parasympathetic nerve stimulation. The responses with 12.5 and 100 mg/kg are illustrated in Fig. 1.

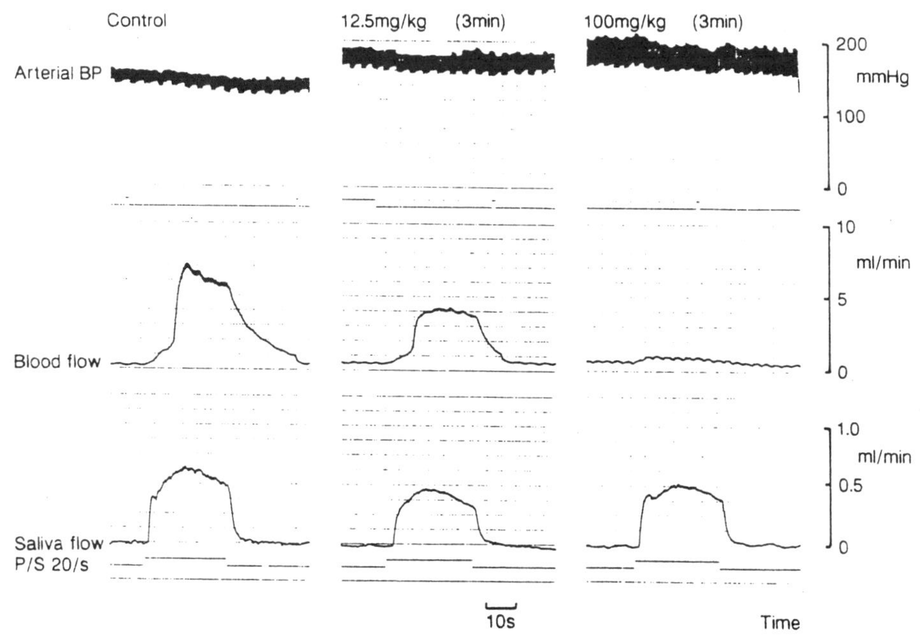

Figure 1. Dose–dependent inhibition of vasodilatation produced by parasympathetic nerve stimulation after close–arterial injection of L–NAME.

A similar, even more pronounced effect was observed with cummulative doses. The vasodilatation that followed at the end of sympathetic nerve stimulation was also reduced by L–NAME, but the sympathetic vasoconstriction was not affected. The time–course of inhibition and recovery after intra–arterial injection of L–NAME (50 mg/kg) is shown in Fig. 2. The dextro–isomer, D–NAME, when injected similarly and in equivalent doses, did not reduce the vasodilatation evoked by stimulation of either nerve. In one cat, the vasodilatation produced by parasympathetic nerve stimulation following atropinisation of the animal (0.1 mg/kg injected intravenously) was abolished by a subsequent, intra–arterial injection of L–NAME (50 mg/kg).

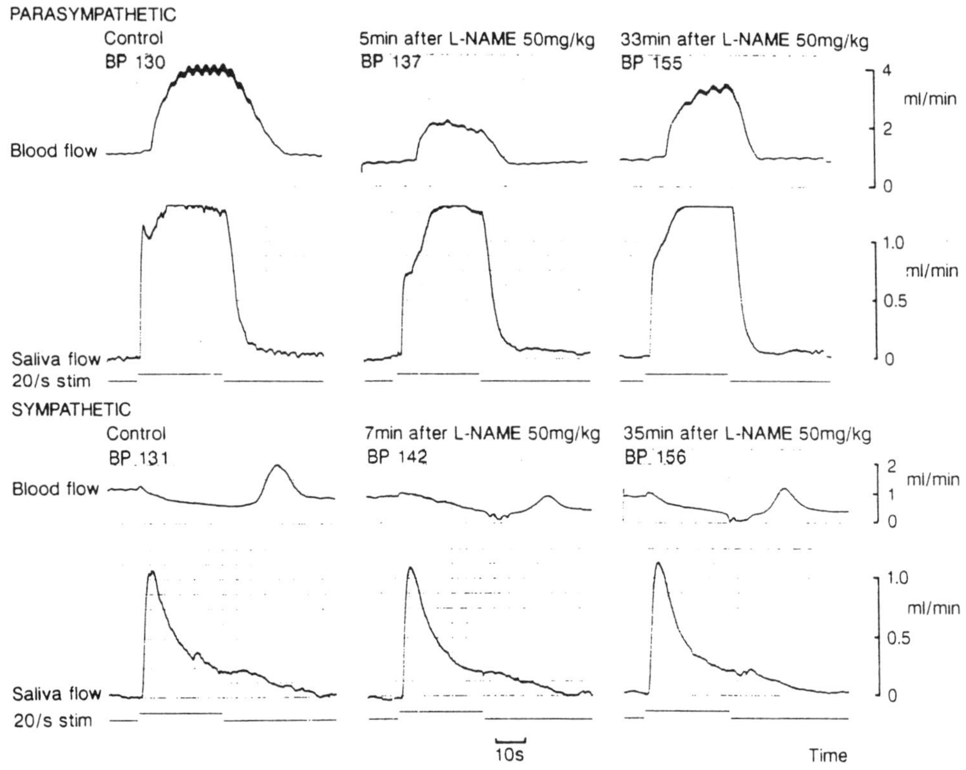

Figure 2. Inhibition and recovery of parasympathetic and sympathetic nerve induced–vasodilatation following close–arterial injection of L–NAME.

DISCUSSION

Studies with isolated, in–vitro preparations suggest that NO may be a neurotrasmitter for a number of tissues. These include the anococcygeus muscle of the rat (1), the smooth muscle of the canine ileocolonic junction (7), and the nerve endings of the mesenteric and cerebral vessels of the dog (8). Furthermore, nitric oxide synthase, the enzyme involved in the formation of NO has been shown by immunocytochemistry to occur in neurones (9). Our observations indicate that NO is involved in the parasympathetic nerve induced vasodilatation and also the vascular dilatation that follows the vasoconstriction produced by stimulation of the sympathetic nerve. However, many compounds have been proposed as the chemical mediator of the atropine–resistant parasympathetic vasodilatation in the submandibular salivary gland since 1872. These include among others, acetylcholine, bradykinin, vasoactive intestinal peptide and purinergic mediators. In every case the evidence has been circumstantial (10, 11, 12, 13). The results reported in the present study suggest a vasodilator role for NO in the atropine–resistant vasodilatation that has eluded an answer for over a hundred years. Evidence that NO may influence arterial blood pressure (14, 15) and platelet function (16, 17) suggests that it may have a wider function in health and disease.

ACKNOWLEDGEMENTS

We are very grateful to Dr. N. Vongsavan for his expert assistance during the experiments. One of us (M.S.) would like to thank Drs. Alan Gibson and Phil Moore for valuable discussions.

REFERENCES

1. Heidenhain R. Uber die Wirkung einiger Gifte auf die Nerven der Glandula submaxillaris. Arch Gesamte Physiol 1872; 5:309–318.

2. Hobbs AJ, Gibson A. L–N^G–nitro–arginine and its methyl ester are potent inhibitors of non –adrenergic, non–cholinergic transmission in the rat anococcygeus. Br J. Pharmaol 1990; 100:749–752.

3. Palmer RMJ, Rees DD, Ashton DS, Moncada S. L–arginine is the physiological precursor for the formation of nitric oxide in endothelium–dependent relaxation. Biochem Biophys Res Commun 1988; 153:1251–1256.

4. Bhoola KD, Morley J, Schachter M, Smaje LH. Vasodilatation in the submaxillary gland of the cat. J Physiol Lond 1965; 179:162–184.

5. Beilenson S, Schachter M, Smaje LH. Secretion of kallikrein and the role in vasodilatation in the submaxillary gland. J Physiol Lond 1968; 199:303–317.

6. Burgen ASV. In: Salivary Glands and their Secretions. Screebney LM, Meyer J, editors. Oxford: Pergamon Press, 1964: 303–307.

7. Bult H, Boeckstaens GE, Pelckmans PA, Jordaens FH, Van Maerke YM, Herman AG. Nitric oxide as an inhibitory non–adrenergic non–cholinergic neurotrasnmitter. Nature 1990; 345:346–347.

8. Toda N, Okamura T. Modification by L–N^G monomethyl arginine (L–NMMA) of the response to nerve stimulation in isolated dog mesenteric and cerebral arteries. Jpn J Pharmacol 1990; 52:170–173.

9. Bredt DS, Hwang PM, Snyder SH. Localisation of nitric oxide synthase indicating a neural role for nitric oxide. Nature 1990; 347:768–769.

10. Schachter M, Beilenson S. Kallikrein and vasodilatation in the submaxillary gland. Gastroenterology 1967; 52:401–405.

11. Hilton SM. The physiological role of glandular kallikreins In: Bradykinin, Kallidin and Kallikrein. Hand Exp Pharmacol, Erdös EG, editor. Berlin–New York: Springer–Verlag, 1970; 25:389–399.

12. Schachter M. Vasodilatation in the submaxillary gland of the cat, rabbit and sheep. In: Bradykinin, Kallidin and Kallikrein. Hand Exp Pharmacol, Erdös EG, editor. Berlin–New York: Springer–Verlag, 1970; 25:400–408.

13. Karpinski E, Barton S, Longridge D, Schachter M. A study of vasoactive intestinal peptide and acetylcholine as possible mediators of vasodilatation in the cat submandibular gland. Can J Physiol Pharmacol 1984; 62:650–653.

14. Vallance P, Collier J, Moncada S. Effects of endothelium–derived nitric oxide on peripheral tone in man. Lancet 1989; ii:997–1000.

15. Rees DD, Palmer RMJ, Moncada S. Role of endothelium–derived nitric oxide in the regulation of blood pressure. Proc Natl Acad Sci USA 1989; 86:3375–3378.

16. Moncada S, Radomski WW, Palmer RMJ. Endothelium–derived relaxing factor: identification as nitric oxide and a role in the control of vascular tone and platelet function. Biochem Pharmacol 1988; 37:2495–2501.

17. Bhardwaj R, May G, Page CP, Moore PK. Endothelium–derived relaxing factor inhibits platelet aggregation in human whole blood in–vitro and the rat in–vitro. Eur J Pharmacol 1988; 157:83–91.

AAS 38/II
Recent Progress on Kinins

INCREASED SENSITIVITY OF GUINEA PIG GALLBLADDER *in vitro* TO BRADYKININ

Mandy Woods and Alan W. Baird

Department of Pharmacology, University College Dublin,

Ireland

SUMMARY : Bradykinin evoked concentration dependent contractions of guinea pig gallbladder smooth muscle strips *in vitro*. Responses to kinins increase over three hours of incubation. Induction of a B_1-mediated action, waning activity of endogenous kininase(s) and involvement of eicosanoids as mediators have been investigated as potential contributing mechanisms to the four-fold, time dependent increase in response of this tissue to bradykinin.

INTRODUCTION.

Bradykinin (BK) stimulates electrogenic bicarbonate secretion in guinea pig gallbladder (1). Since alkaline fluid secretion by this organ may underlie inflammation (2), we speculated that gallbladder disease may, in part, be a consequence of kinin formation. Kinin-induced bicarbonate secretion appears to be mediated by eicosanoid synthesis since the effect was mimicked by exogenous prostaglandins and was abolished by inhibitors of cyclooxygenase. Thus measurement of gallbladder ion transport is a useful tool for pharmacological studies of kinin receptor agonists and antagonists (1).

The object of this study was to investigate effects of kinins on smooth muscle contraction in strips of guinea pig gallbladder. We have carried out experiments to compare what is already known about kinin-induced ion transport with contractile responses in the same organ. In addition, we used three pharmacological approaches to determine the mechanism(s) of increasing sensitivity of gallbladder to BK.

MATERIALS and METHODS

Gallbladders were obtained from Dunkin-Hartley guinea pigs (400-500 g.). Paired tissues from each animal were mounted in organ baths in Krebs-Henseleit solution of the following composition (mM) : Na Cl 118; KCl, 4.7; $CaCl_2$, 2.5; $MgSO_4$, 1.2; KH_2PO_4, 1.2; $NaHCO_3$, 24.8 and glucose, 11.1. Bathing solutions were maintained at 37°C and gassed with 95% O_2 / 5% CO_2. Isotonic contractions were recorded using a Washington isotonic transducer coupled to a Washington oscillograph 400 MD2. Tissues were allowed to equilibrate for thirty minutes. Contact times for agonists were five minutes within which time all responses had reached peak values.

Following equilibration, bradykinin (BK; 0.3μM) was administered at 30 min intervals for a period of 180 min with wash out after each addition. The effects of des-Arg^9-BK, a selective B_1 agonist, were also investigated in the same way.

We conducted a series of experiments in the presence of a number of endogenous peptidase inhibitors, MGTPA, captopril and phosphoramidon, which were used to inhibit kininases I and II and neutral endopeptidase, respectively. In control tissue three consecutive cumulative responses to BK (0.3μM, 1μM) were obtained at 30, 60,and 90 min intervals. In paired test tissue the second BK challenge (at 60 min)was made in the presence of one of each of the kininase inhibitors.

Inhibitors of cyclooxygenase (indomethacin and piroxicam) were employed to determine whether BK-induced contractions are mediated by eicosanoid synthesis.

To investigate the possible *de novo* synthesis of B_1 receptors, cycloheximide, an inhibitor of protein synthesis was used. In control tissue responses were obtained to BK, des-Arg^9-BK and carbachol at 30 and 180 min. In paired tissues initial control responses were obtained to kinins and carbachol at 30 min and following this the 'test' tissue was incubated with cycloheximide (70μM) for a period of two hours after which responses to kinins and carbachol were obtained. All drugs used were supplied by Sigma Chemical Co.(U.K.) unless otherwise stated. dl-2-mercaptomethyl-3-guanidinoethylthiopropionic acid (MGTPA) was purchased from Calbiochem (Nottingham, U.K.).

Results are expressed as % of maximum contraction in response to KCl (0.1M. obtained at the end of each experiment). Data is expressed as mean ± standard error of the mean. Statistical analysis was carried out using Student's paired t-test. Probability values $p < 0.05$ were considered significant.

RESULTS

Effect of bradykinin, des-Arg ^{9}-BK and prostaglandin E_2 on guinea pig gallbladder smooth muscle

Bradykinin (0.3µM, 1µM) produced a concentration dependent contraction of guinea pig gallbladder smooth muscle. Contractile responses to bradykinin increased in a time dependent manner _in vitro_ from an initial null level to an increase of 85% of maximal contractile capacity within 180 min. (Fig 1) Increased responses were not due to priming of tissue with BK as naive tissue, treated at 180 min only, produced a response of 91.9±24.8% (expressed as % of maximum contraction with KCl) which was similar to that of tissue treated periodically every 30 min for 180 min (85.3±15.7%). Guinea pig gallbladder smooth muscle did not respond to des-Arg^9-BK (3µM) after one hour equilibration _in vitro_ but significant contractile responses were recorded at 3h incubation (Fig. 1).

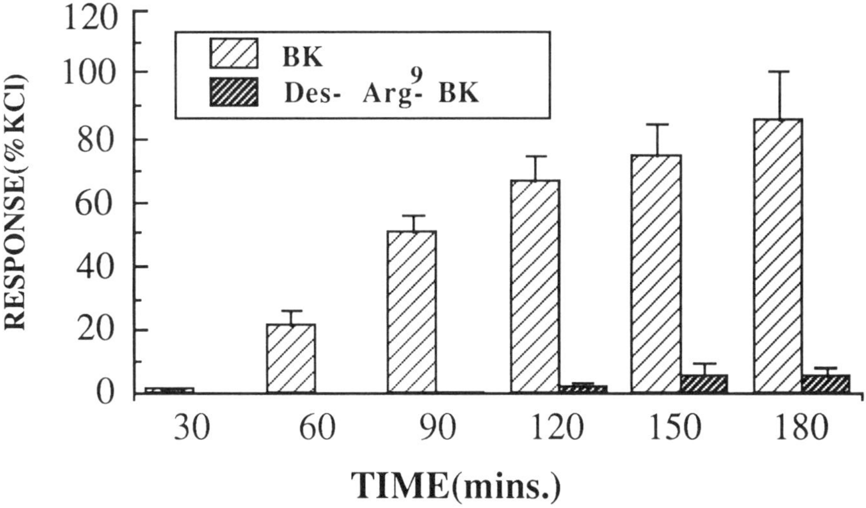

Figure 1. Kinin induced contractions increase over time

Contractions induced by BK (0.3µM; n=11) increased in a time dependent manner. Times are given relative to first establishment of fresh tissue in organ baths. In separate preparations, responses to des-Arg^9 BK (3µM; n=6) appeared gradually over the experimental period.

Prostaglandin E_2 (0.01μM, 0.03μM) produced concentration dependent contractions of guinea pig gallbladder smooth muscle which also increased over a time period of 90 min. This increased responsiveness was not a feature of all drugs which produce gallbladder contraction since KCl concentration response curves constructed at 30 & 180 min were superimposable.

Effect of peptidase inhibitors on BK induced contraction of guinea pig gallbladder smooth muscle

In this study, responses to BK were elicited at 60 minutes so that either inhibitory or potentiating actions of the drugs might be observed. Pretreatment with captopril (10μM), an inhibitor of angiotensin converting enzyme, significantly enhanced contractile effect of bradykinin by a factor of 4.1 (p <0.05). Inhibitors of neutral endopeptidase (phosphoramidon; 10μM) or of kininase I (MGTPA; 30μM) were without effect. None of the kininase inhibitors altered contractile responses of gallbladder to prostaglandin E_2 (0.1μM / 0.3μM; Fig. 2).

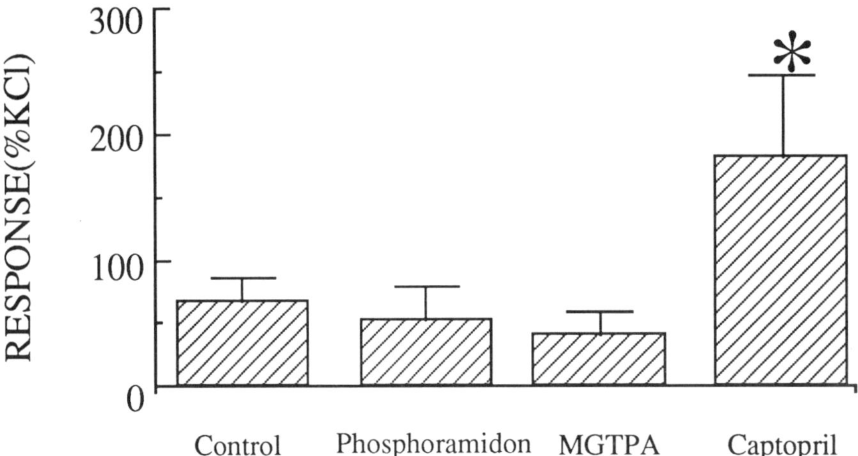

Figure 2. Kininase inhibitors

Phosphoramidon (10μM; n=5) and MGTPA (30μM; n=7) did not alter contractile responses to BK. Captopril (10μM; n=8) did significantly (p<0.05) enhance the kinin response when compared with control values. None of the kininase inhibitors altered contractile responses of gallbladder to PGE_2 (0.1μM).

Effect of inhibitors of cyclooxygenase on BK induced contractions

Pretreatment with either indomethacin (2.8μM) or piroxicam (1μM) significantly attenuated contractile responses to BK (0.3μM). Responses to BK were reduced to 28.7±13.5% in the presence of indomethacin when compared to control values of 100.7±22.3%. This effect of indomethacin was irreversible. Indomethacin had no effect on contraction induced by exogenously administered PGE_2. In the presence of piroxicam, responses to BK were reduced to 4.3±1.7% when compared to control values of 69.9±19.8%. The effect of piroxicam was reversible.

Effect of cycloheximide

Cycloheximide (70μM), an inhibitor of protein synthesis, when applied continuously throughout the experimental period did not alter the enhanced responsiveness of guinea pig gallbladder to BK (0.3μM). Responses to des-Arg^9-BK (3μM) were also unaffected by pretreatment with cycloheximide. Responses to carbachol (0.1μM) at 30 and 180 min were unaffected by cycloheximide, excluding a toxic effect of this drug on the preparation (Fig 3.)

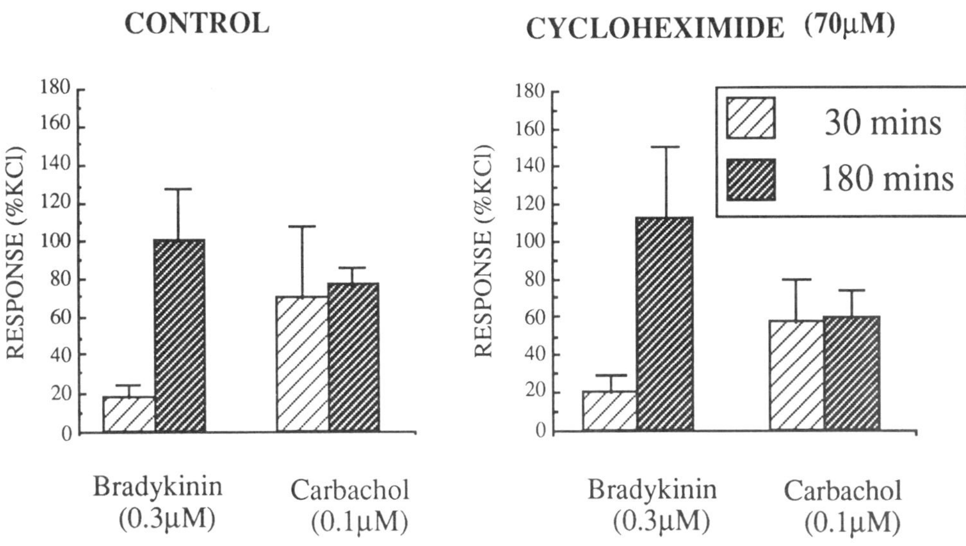

Figure 3. Effects of cycloheximide on contractile responses

Responses to BK at 180 minutes were greater than those obtained 30 minutes after setting up the preparation (p<0.05). Cycloheximide, an inhibitor of protein synthesis did not influence the enhanced responsiveness of guinea pig gallbladder to BK. Responses to carbachol (0.1 μM) applied at 30 and 180 minutes were unaffected by cycloheximide, excluding a toxic effect of this drug on the preparation

DISCUSSION

In the present study it has been demonstrated that BK evoked contraction of guinea pig gallbladder smooth muscle *in vitro*. Responses to successive applications of BK increased in a time dependent manner and this enhancement was not dependent upon repeated administrations of kinins. We have also demonstrated that this effect was not a feature of all agents which produce gallbladder contraction since responses to carbachol were not altered over time, and KCl cumulative concentration response curves at 30 and 180 min were superimposable.

We investigated whether the enhanced responsiveness to BK in this tissue was a consequence of *de novo* generation of B_1 receptors (3). Responses to the selective B_1 agonist des-Arg^9-BK appeared only during incubation *in vitro* . However the magnitude of this apparent B_1 -mediated response was not sufficient to account for the degree of enhancement of responses to BK. Cycloheximide , an inhibitor of protein synthesis, had no effect on des-Arg^9-BK or BK induced contraction of guinea pig gallbladder smooth muscle. This is in contrast with the finding that cycloheximide almost completely prevented the development of the contractile response to des-Arg^9-BK in rabbit aortic strips (4). From these results it is concluded that the proprosed *de novo* synthesis of B_1 receptors is not a major contributor to the increased responsiveness obtained with BK.

Kinin forming and inactivating activities have been reported in bile and gallbladder homogenates. (5,6). We suggest that exhaustion of endogenous kininase activity may contribute to the observed enhancement of contractile responses to BK. Captopril significantly enhanced the contractile effect of BK. Angiotensin converting enzyme (kininase II) may be a major peptidase involved in the metabolism of kinins in the gallbladder. Kininase activity present at the beginning of the experimental period may attenuate early responses to BK and gradual depletion of kininase II, or loss of enzyme activity, will unveil a relatively greater influence of exogenous kinins. Inhibitors of kininase I and of carboxypeptidase N had no influence on responses to BK suggesting that these enzymes are not involved in metabolism of kinins in guinea pig gallbladder.

Eicosanoid synthesis is a feature of kinin action in various organs (7). It has already been demonstrated that BK stimulation of ion transport across guinea pig gallbladder epithelium is dependent upon eicosanoid formation (1). In this study we demonstrated that BK-induced gallbladder smooth muscle contraction is also dependent upon PG synthesis, since inhibitors of cyclooxygenase reduced or even abolished responses to BK. Exogenous PGE_2 provoked contractions and this effect increased over time in a manner analogous to that observed with kinins.

In summary, we have described the actions of kinins on smooth muscle contraction of smooth muscle strips of guinea pig gallbladder. Features of the response (sensitivity to cyclooxygenase inhibition) are common to BK effects on epithelial cells (1) and neurons (8). In contrast to the pro-secretory action of kinins in gallbladder, which is a quantitatively reproducible effect, contractile responses increase over time. We provide evidence for a number of mechanisms each of which might contribute to the enhanced sensitivity to BK. How the distinct actions of kinins on different cell types in the same organ might be functionally coordinated will be the subject of future investigations.

ACKNOWLEDGEMENTS

We are grateful to the Health Research Board of Ireland for financial support.

REFERENCES

1. Baird A.W. & Margolius H.S. Bradykinin stimulates electrogenic ion secretion by guinea pig gallbladder. J. Pharmacol. exp. Ther. (1989) **248**; 268-272.

2. Thornell E., Jivegard L. Bukhave K. , Rask-Madsen J. & Svanvik J. Prostaglandin E$_2$ formation by the gallbladder in experimental cholecystitis. Gut (1986) **27**; 370-373.

3. Regoli D., Barabe J. & Park W.K. Receptors for bradykinin in rabbit aorta. Can. J. Physiol. Pharmacol. (1977) **55**; 855-867.

4. Bouthillier J., Deblois D. & Marceau F. Studies on the induction of pharmacological responses to des-arg^9-bradykinin in vitro and in vivo. Br. J. Pharmacol.(1987) **92**; 257-264.

5. Amundsen E. & Nustad K. Kinin forming and destroying activities of cell homogenates. J. Physiol (Lond.) (1965) **179**; 479-488.

6. Moller-Nielsen H. Kinin forming and inactivating activities in human bile and biliary tract homogenates. Scand. J. Lab. Invest. (1969) **24** (Suppl. 107); 73-74.

7. Nasjletti A. & Malik K.U. Relationships between the kallikrein-kinin and prostaglandin systems. Life Sci. (1979) **25**; 99-110.

8. Waldrop T.G. & Ordway G.A. Role of prostaglandins in initiating cardiovascular reflexes originating from the pancreas and gallbladder. Cardiovasc. Res. (1986) **20**; 312-316.

AAS 38/II
Recent Progress on Kinins
© 1992 Birkhäuser Verlag Basel

CONTRASTING PROPERTIES OF BRADYKININ RECEPTOR SUBTYPES MEDIATING CONTRACTIONS OF THE RABBIT AND PIG ISOLATED IRIS SPHINCTER PUPILLAE PREPARATION

Christopher M Everett, Judith M Hall, Debra Mitchell and Ian K M Morton

Pharmacology Group, Biomedical Sciences Division, King's College London, Manresa Road, London SW3 6LX, UK

SUMMARY: Bradykinin contracts both the pig and rabbit iris sphincter preparations. In the pig, the bradykinin antagonists Lys,Lys-[Hyp^3,Thi^{5,8},D-Phe^7]-BK and D-Arg-[Hyp^3,Thi^5,D-Tic^7,Oic^8]-BK (HOE140) inhibited responses with pK$_B$ estimates of 6.0 and 8.4, respectively. These affinities are markedly lower than in the rabbit preparation, suggesting that different receptors are present in each of the two species.

INTRODUCTION

The rabbit iris has been well studied with regards to peptide action, and it is known that bradykinin (BK) contracts the sphincter muscle indirectly via the release of neurokinins from sensory nerves (1). In contrast, in the less well studied pig preparation, BK appears to contract the sphincter by a direct action on the smooth muscle (2).

Originally, the receptors for bradykinin (BK) were divided into B$_1$ and B$_2$ subtypes (3), on the basis of activity or inactivity, respectively, of BK analogues with deleted C-terminal arginine residues. In previous studies we have found that on this basis, the BK receptors in the rabbit preparation are not of the B$_1$ subtype, so can be regarded as of the B$_2$ subtype (4). In this study, we have gone on to characterise the BK receptors in the pig preparation, and compared them with those of the rabbit.

METHODS

Paired preparations of pig sphincter pupillae muscle, either fresh or stored over night, were mounted in Krebs' solution at 37°C for isometric recording, and cumulative concentration-response curves for BK were obtained in the absence (control preparation) or presence (test preparation) of increasing antagonist concentrations (5 min pre-incubation).

Sensitivity to the B_1 agonist [des-Arg^9]-BK was determined at the beginning and end of experiments, and where it was active the B_1 antagonist [des-Arg^9,Leu^8]-BK was tested. Otherwise, BK was used in the determining affinities of the B_2 antagonists Lys,Lys-[Hyp^3,Thi^{5,8},D-Phe^7]-BK and D-Arg-[Hyp^3,Thi^5,D-Tic^7,Oic^8]-BK.

RESULTS

Only in iris preparations from certain pigs, were there reliable contractile responses to the selective B_1 agonist [des-Arg^9]-BK, when it was quite active (pD$_2$ = 7.9). Here, responses were attenuated by the B_1 antagonist [des-Arg^9,Leu^8]-BK, the Schild slope for this being flattened at higher concentration, though extrapolation from the lower part gave a pA$_2$ of 6.2 (see **Table 1**). At 10 μM, the antagonist was a partial agonist (30% carbachol max).

In the remainder of the pig iris preparations, BK was quite active in contracting preparations (pD$_2$ = 7.5; see **Table 1**) though the dose-response line showed some evidence of two phases (**Figure 1a**).

Two B_2 antagonists were compared for their activities in inhibiting bradykinin responses: the established analogue Lys,Lys-[Hyp^3,Thi^{5,8},D-Phe^7]-BK (B4310, B4311) and the novel agent D-Arg-[Hyp^3,Thi^5,D-Tic^7,Oic^8]-BK (HOE140). Schild plot analysis suggested that both had competitive kinetics of action, but their affinities were very different; giving pK$_B$ estimates of 6.0 and 8.4, respectively (see **Table 1** and **Figure 1**). The pK$_B$ for Lys,Lys-[Hyp^3,Thi^{5,8},D-Phe^7]-BK was unchanged by the peptidase inhibitors phosphoramidon, mergetpa and enalaprilat (all 1 μM; pK$_B$ = 5.96 ± 0.16; n = 6).

The activities of these various ligands in the pig preparation are summarised in **Table 1** in terms of pD$_2$ (-log EC$_{50}$) or pK$_B$ (pA$_2$), and compared with values for the rabbit.

Table 1. Activities of BK and analogues in pig and rabbit iris preparations.

Analogue		Apparent pK$_B$ or pD$_2$	
		Rabbit iris	**Pig iris**
		(± s.e.mean; n)	(± s.e.mean; n)
BK	**Agonist**	**7.8**	**7.5**
		(0.2; 15)	(0.7; 8)
[des-Arg^9]-BK	**Agonist**	**N.A**	**NA/7.9**
			(0.7; 4)
[des-Arg^9,Leu^8]-BK	**Antagonist**	**N.A**	**NA/6.2**
			(0.2; 8)
Lys,Lys-[Hyp^3,Thi^{5,8},D-Phe^7]-BK	**Antagonist**	**7.9**	**6.0**
		(0.1; 4)	(0.1; 11)
D-Arg-[Hyp^3,Thi^5,D-Tic^7,Oic^8]-BK	**Antagonist**	**10.5**	**8.4**
		(0.1; 11)	(0.1; 9)

NA - not active.

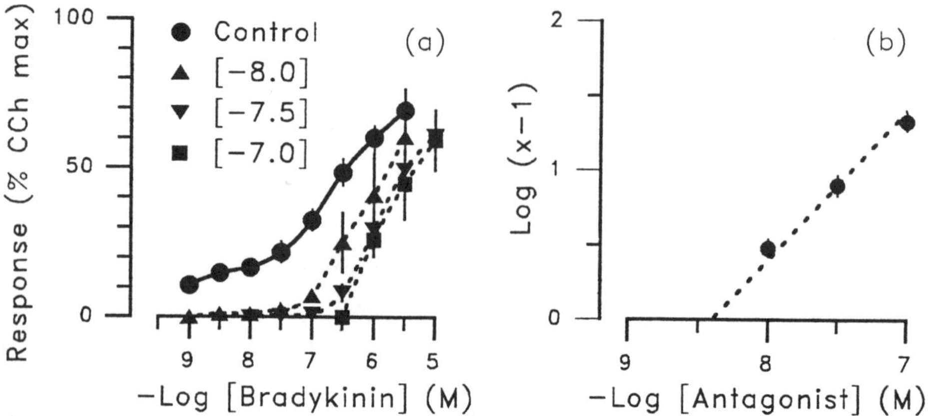

Figure 1. Antagonism by D-Arg-[Hyp^3,Thi^5,D-Tic^7,Oic^8]-BK of response to BK in the pig iris sphincter preparation. (a) Log concentration response curves for BK in the absence (Control) or presence of the indicated concentrations of antagonist. (b) Schild plot for data from individual experiments (n = 11) where there is no significant deviation of the slope from unity ($P > 0.05$) so unity is imposed; estimated pK$_B$ 8.4±0.1 (see **Table 1**).

DISCUSSION and CONCLUSION

These results highlight a number of differences between the two species. The rabbit iris provides a useful model where bradykinin acts prejunctionally as a neuroinflammatory mediator releasing neurokinins (1) to act postjunctionally at a number of subtypes of neurokinin receptor (5). In contrast, in the pig iris the action of bradykinin appears to be largely postjunctional and independent of release of neurokinins or other mediators (2).

With respect to the recognition characteristics of the bradykinin receptors in the two species, there are also clear differences. Firstly, unlike in the rabbit iris (4), in the pig preparation there was clear evidence in some animals of B$_1$ receptors with characteristics similar to B$_1$ receptors in established preparations (3). Why the B$_1$ contribution varied between pigs was not established, though it did not seem to depend on equilibration times or cold storage (data not shown). The non-B$_1$ component of the action of bradykinin was competitively antagonised by analogues having established activity at B$_2$ receptors (6,7,8,9,10). The observation that in both species there was a large difference between the affinities of the two analogues studied is not surprising, since D-Arg-[Hyp^3,Thi^5,D-Tic^7,Oic^8]-BK has proved to have a much higher affinity than members of the [D-Phe^7]-BK series in most preparations studied (7,9,10). However, what is more interesting is that our affinity estimates for both antagonists was nearly two orders of magnitude lower in the pig as compared to the rabbit. In this respect, the properties of the receptors in the pig more closely match those most commonly seen in the guinea-pig (4,7), which have been suggested to form a distinct subtype (11), rather than those of the rabbit or rat.

In view of these marked differences between the preparations from the pig and rabbit, both in the locus of action of bradykinin, and of the receptors on which its acts, it seems evident that care should be taken in projection of findings from experimental species to man.

ACKNOWLEDGEMENTS

This project is supported by the Wellcome Trust. We also thank the Sandoz Institute for Medical Research for support, and Dr Allan Hallett for supplies of peptides.

REFERENCES

(1) Wahlestedt C, Bynke G, Håkanson R. Pupillary constriction by bradykinin and capsaicin, mode of action. Eur J Pharmacol 1985; **106**:577-583.

(2) Geppetti P, Patacchini R, Ceccioni R, Tramontana M, Meini, A, Romani A, Nardi M, Maggi CA. Effects of capsaicin, tachykinins, CGRP and bradykinin in the pig iris sphincter muscle. Br J Pharmacol 1990; **341**:301-307.

(3) Regoli D, Barabé J. Pharmacology of bradykinin and related peptides. Pharmacol Rev 1980; **32**:1-46.

(4) Field JL, Fox AJ, Hall JM, Magbagbeola AO, Morton IKM. Multiple bradykinin B_2 receptors in smooth muscle preparations? Br J Pharmacol 1988; **93**:284P.

(5) Hall JM, Mitchell D, Morton IKM. Neurokinin receptors in the rabbit iris sphincter characterised by novel agonist ligands. Eur J Pharmacol 1991; **199**:9-14.

(6) Griesbacher T, Lembeck F. Actions of bradykinin antagonists on bradykinin-induced plasma extravasation, prostaglandin E_2 release, nociceptor stimulation and contraction of the rabbit iris sphincter muscle of the rabbit. Br J Pharmacol 1987; **92**:333-340.

(7) Field JL, Hall JM, Morton IKM. Bradykinin receptors in the guinea-pig taenia caeci are similar to proposed BK_3 receptors in the guinea-pig trachea, and are blocked by HOE140. Br J Pharmacol 1992; **105**:293-296.

(8) Hall JM, Morton IKM. Bradykinin B_2 receptor evoked K^+ permeability increase mediates relaxation in the rat duodenum. Eur J Pharmacol 1991; **193**:231-238.

(9) Hock FJ, Wirth K, Albus U, Linz W, Gerhards HJ, Wiemer G, Henke G, Breipohl G, König W, Knolle J, Schölkens BA. HOE 140 a new potent and long acting bradykinin-antagonist: *in vitro* studies. Br J Pharmacol 1991; **102**:769-773.

(10) Lembeck F, Griesbacher T, Eckhardt M, Henke S, Briepohl G Knolle J. New, long-acting, potent bradykinin antagonists. Br J Pharmacol 1991; **102**:297-304.

(11) Farmer SG, Burch RM, Meeker SA, Wilkins, DE. Evidence for a pulmonary B_3 bradykinin receptor. Mol Pharmacol 1989; **36**:1-8.

AAS 38/II
Recent Progress on Kinins
© 1992 Birkhäuser Verlag Basel

CHARACTERIZATION OF A KALLIDIN RECEPTOR IN THE EEL INTESTINE

N. Cougnon, C.F. Deacon, K.S. Lilley[*] and I.W.Henderson

Institute of Endocrinology, Department of Animal and Plant Sciences, Sheffield University, Western Bank, Sheffield S10 2TN, UK and * Department of Biochemistry, Leicester University, Leicester LE1 7RH, UK

SUMMARY: Edman degradation of an eel bradykinin (BK) -like peptide isolated and detected by gel filtration and HPLC and RIA gave an amino acid sequence of Arg^1-Pro-Pro-Gly-X-Ser-Pro-Leu-Arg^9. Kallidin but not BK and des-Arg^9-BK contracted eel intestine. The contractile effect of kallidin was not decreased by B_1 and B_2 receptor antagonists (up to $10^{-6}M$), nor by anticholinergics, antiadrenergics, ganglion blockers and an angiotensin II receptor antagonist but was attenuated by $10^{-5}M$ indomethacin. Kallidin appears to interact with a receptor different from the BK B_1 and B_2 receptor types and prostaglandins may participate in the response.

INTRODUCTION

The plasma kallikrein-kinin system, in mammals, has widespread physiological and pharmacological activities including vasodilation [1].

The kallikreins, a group of serine proteases, are activated, in mammalian and reptilian blood, by the Hageman factor (factor XII) and generate BK from high molecular weight kininogen. Factor XII can be activated in vitro by contact with a charged surface such as glass beads [2].

Kallikrein-kinin systems have not been fully identified in teleost fishes. Incubation of trout plasma with trypsin generates a BK-like immunoreactive peptide which does not share the pharmacological profile of BK [3].

Eel plasma incubated with glass beads to activate Hageman factor generated a immunoreactive BK-like peptide that was active upon eel intestine but not rat intestine or uterus. The BK-like immunoreactivity (BK-LI) and the biological activity were present in the same HPLC fractions [4]. Kallidin but not BK contracted eel intestine.

In this study, an attempt has been made to isolate and sequence the generated kinin-like peptide and, in addition, some pharmacological characteristics of the eel intestinal kinin receptor are described.

MATERIALS AND METHODS

Generation and purification of a kinin-like peptide

Sixty ml of plasma from anaesthetised eels, *Anguilla anguilla*, were diluted with sixty ml of 0.9% NaCl containing 2mM 1,10 phenanthroline and shaken with acid washed glass beads (30g) for 60 minutes at 37° C [5]. The reaction mixture was extracted on to Sep-Pak C_{18} cartridges. Bound material was eluted with 70% (v/v) acetonitrile and chromatographed on a column (100 x 1.6cm) of Sephadex G-25 medium equilibrated with 1 M acetic acid. The column was eluted at a flow rate of 24ml/h and fractions (2ml) were assayed for BK-LI. The fractions containing BK-LI were pooled and chromatographed on a 25 x 0.46 cm C18 reverse phase column (Jones Chromatography). The concentration of acetonitrile in the eluting solvent was raised to 70% over 30 minutes using a linear gradient. Fractions (1 min) were collected and assayed by RIA. The immunoreactive fraction was rechromatographed on a 0.46 x 25cm Supelcosil LC-3DP diphenylmethyl silylsilica column. The concentration of acetonitrile in the eluting solvent was raised to 70% over 75 minutes using a linear gradient.

The primary structure of the isolated peptide was determined by automated Edman degradation.

Bioassays on eel intestine

Segments of eel intestine were suspended in organ baths (14ml) containing oxygenated (5% CO_2, 95% O_2) Krebs solution (NaCl 117.5mM, KCl 4.7mM, KH_2PO_4 1.18mM, $MgSO_4$ $7H_2O$ 2.5mM, $CaCl_2$ $6H_2O$ 2.5mM, $NaCO_3$ 2.5mM, glucose 5.5mM), at 30°C. The eel intestine was stretched to 2g. After equilibration, the intestine was contracted with KCl and kallidin until a stable response was obtained. The drugs were dissolved in Krebs solution and applied to the bath. Contractions were recorded isometrically on a Reba par 1000 apparatus.

Analysis of data

The values were compared to the concentration elicited by 10^{-7} M kallidin (100%) using the Kruskall-Wallis test for multiple comparisons [6].

RESULTS

<u>Purification of eel kinin</u>

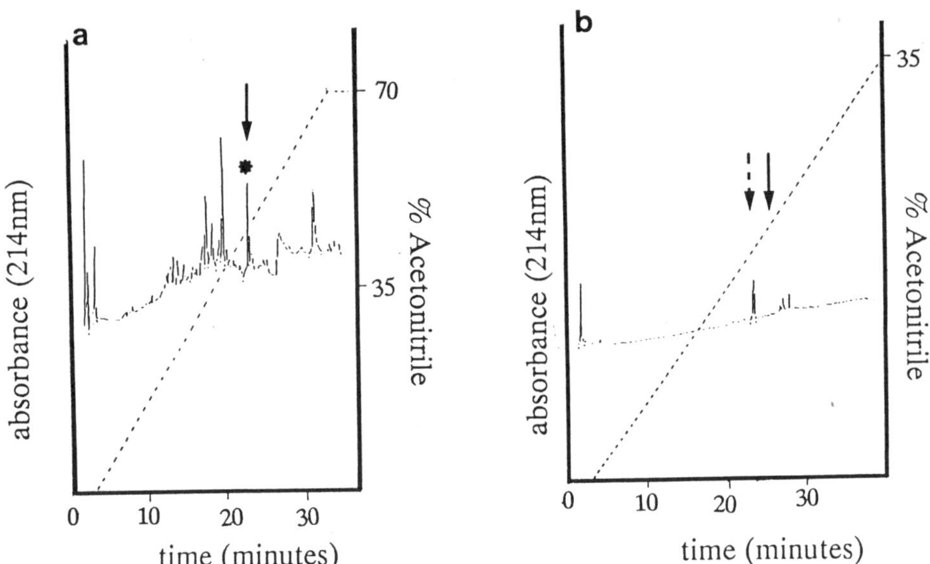

Figure 1a. Purification of eel kinin on a C18 reverse phase HPLC column. The dashed line represents the acetonitrile gradient. The arrow shows the retention time of synthetic BK. The peak denoted by the asterisk shows BK-LI.

Figure 1b. Purification of eel kinin on a Supelcosil LC-3DP reverse phase column. The dashed line represents the acetonitrile gradient. The plain arrow show the retention time of synthetic rat BK and the dashed arrow the retention time of synthetic rat kallidin.

Due to the low immunoreactivity found in the plasma only one fraction showed BK-LI after elution from a Sephadex G-25 gel permeation column. According to the elution volume of synthetic rat BK, ten fractions were pooled and chromatographed on a C18 column where they eluted as a single BK-LI peak with the same retention time as synthetic rat BK (Fig. 1a). This peak, rechromatographed on a LC-3DP column, eluted with the same retention time as kallidin (Fig. 1b).

<u>Automated Edman degradation of isolated eel kinin-like peptide</u>

Sequence analysis of the peptide showed two amino acid substitutions compared to mammalian BK, Leu for Phe in position 8 and an undetermined amino acid for Phe in position 5 (Table 1).

Table 1. Automated Edman degradation of isolated eel kinin-like peptide.

cycle	residue	amount(pmoles)
1	Arg	64.5
2	Pro	15.2
3	Pro	12.5
4	Gly	25.6
5	?	
6	Ser	3.6
7	Pro	4.6
8	Leu	3.1
9	Arg	1.3

<u>Bioassay on isolated eel intestine</u>.

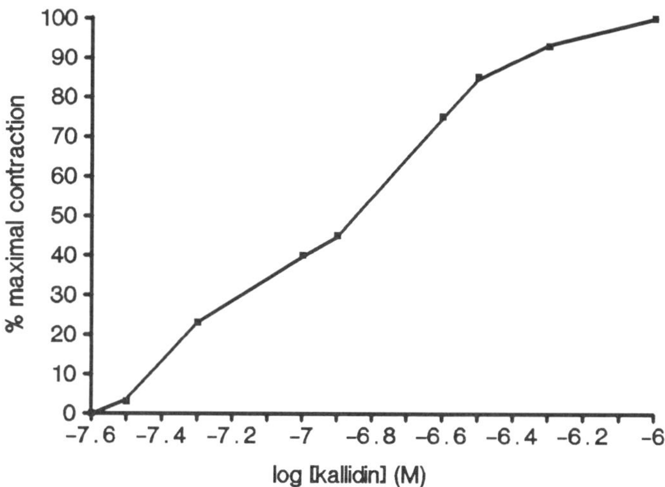

Figure 2. Dose-response curve of kallidin on isolated eel intestine.
Increasing concentrations of kallidin dissolved in Krebs were added to the bath. The tissue was washed between each dose.

The kallidin contracted eel intestine in a dose-dependent fashion with a ED_{50} of $1.2 \times 10^{-7}M$ (Fig. 2).

Des-Arg^9-BK and BK were without effect on this preparation at concentrations up to $3 \times 10^{-6}M$.

The intestinal responses were not blocked by anticholinergic, antiadrenergic and ganglion blocking drugs. In presence of $10^{-5}M$ indomethacin the kallidin response was significantly attenuated (Fig. 3).

B_1 and B_2 receptor antagonists, Des-Arg^9-Leu^8-BK and [Thi^{5,8},DPhe^7]-BK did not block the kallidin response at concentrations of up to 10^{-6} and $10^{-5}M$, respectively (Fig. 4).

The angiotensin II receptor antagonist, Sar^1-Leu^8-angiotensin II, reduced the contractile effect of angiotensin II on the intestine but was without effect on the contractile response to kallidin (Fig. 5).

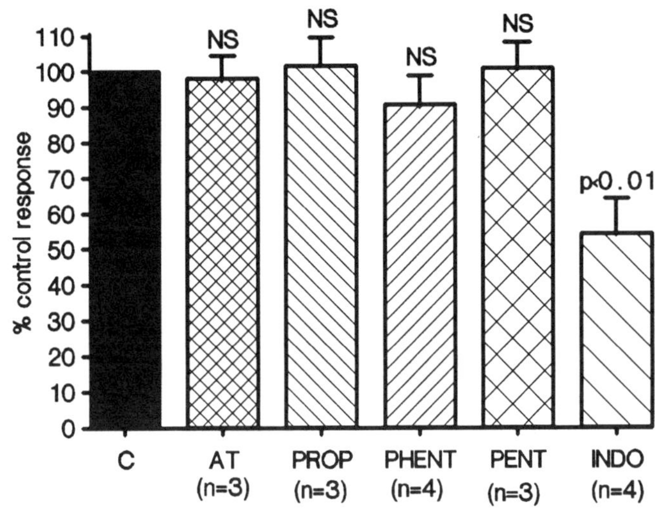

Figure 3. Effects of various drugs on the contractile response of the eel intestine to $10^{-7}M$ kallidin.

Results are expressed as percentages of the kallidin control response (100%). C : $10^{-7}M$ kallidin; AT : $10^{-7}M$ kallidin + $10^{-5}M$ atropine; PROP : $10^{-7}M$ kallidin + $4 \times 10^{-5}M$ propanolol; PHENT : $10^{-7}M$ kallidin + $10^{-5}M$ phentolamine; PENT : $10^{-7}M$ kallidin + $3 \times 10^{-5}M$ pentolinium; INDO : $10^{-7}M$ kallidin + $10^{-5}M$ indomethacin.

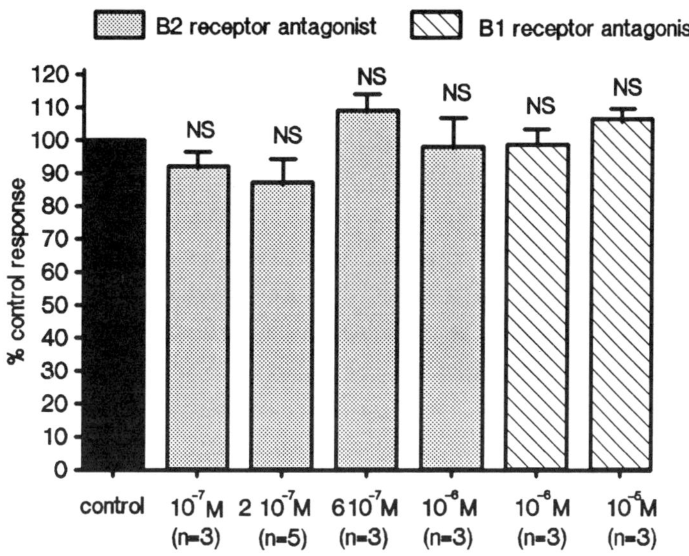

Figure 4. Effect of kinin receptor antagonists on the contractile action of 10^{-7}M kallidin on the eel intestine.

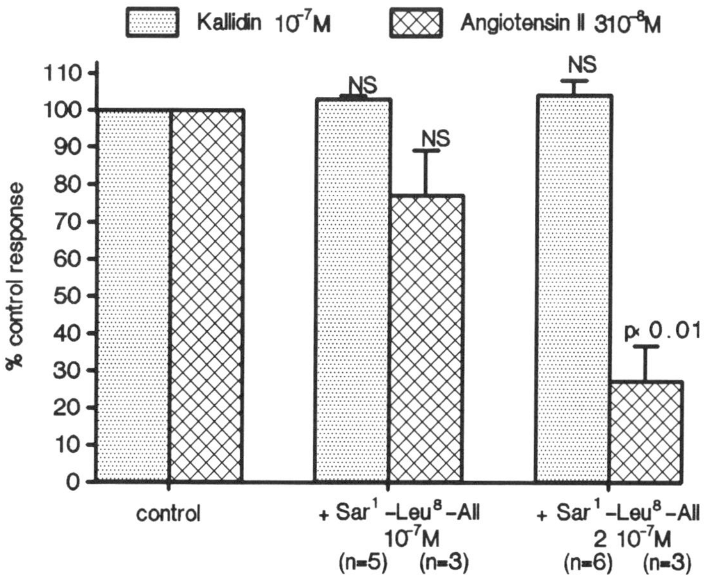

Figure 5. Effect of an angiotensin II antagonist on the contractile effect of 10^{-7}M kallidin on the eel intestine.

DISCUSSION

Previous observations [4] have been confirmed in that components of the plasma kallikrein-kinin system exist in teleost fish. However, methods to monitor eel bradykinin are critical since, for example rat bioassays may not always detect non-mammalian bradykinin analogues. Specific RIA methods and homologous bioassays are obviously more appropriate.

Previous investigations on the fish kallikrein-kinin system may be summarized:
-intravenous injections of bradykinin and kallidin do not affect the blood pressures of cartilagenous and teleost fish [7];
-fish plasma incubated with glass beads or trypsin has no effect on rat uterus;
-fish plasma incubated with hog pancreatic kallikrein contracts rat uterus [8];
-kinins [9], and kallikrein when the fish is pretreated with Captopril, a kininase II inhibitor [3], produce pressor responses *in vivo*;
-trout plasma incubated with porcine pancreatic glandular kallikrein generates a substance that, in trout, increases blood pressure by a mechanism in part mediated by catecholamines and the generated material displaces angiotensin II from its receptor [10].

The eel BK, compared with the mammalian peptide, has two amino acids substitutions : an as yet unidentified residue in position 5 and a leucine in position 8 substituted for the two phenylalanines. The amino acid at position 5 is unlikely to be phenylalanine as this is relatively easy to detect. However a single base change in the codon (UUU/UUC) could generate either cysteine (UGU/UGC) or serine (UCU/UCC). The latter was readily detected in the present study, whilst the former is notoriously difficult to determine but is the likely residue at position 5. Residues 5 and 8 are key elements in the interaction of bradykinin with its B_2 receptor and their substitution leads to full agonistic activity but with lower affinity for the receptor [1].

Receptors specific for kallidin seemed to be present in the eel intestine as anticholinergic, antiadrenergic and ganglion blocking drugs are without effect on the contraction. This receptor seems to be different from B_1 and B_2 receptors. Kallidin does not seem to interact with the angiotensin II receptor. This does not agree with other observations [3] showing that the generated peptide displaced angiotensin II from its receptor.

The physiological roles of kinins in fish are virtually unknown.

ACKNOWLEDGEMENTS

We would like to thank J.M. Conlon, Creighton University, Omaha, Nebraska, USA, for the generous gift of the antiserum.
This work was supported by EEC Grant SCI-0042C(GDF).

REFERENCES

1. Regoli D., Barabé J. Pharmacology of bradykinin and related kinins. Pharmacol. Rev. 1980; 32:1-46.

2. Margolis J. Activation of plasma by contact with glass: evidence for a common reaction which releases plasma kinin and initiates coagulation. J. Physiol. 1958; 144:1-22.

3. Lipke D.W., Olson K.R. Enzymes of the kallikrein-kinin system in rainbow trout. Am. J. Physiol. 1990b; 258:R501-506.

4. Cougnon N., Deacon C.F., Henderson I.W. J.Generation of a bradykinin-like peptide by contact with glass beads in the eel, *Anguilla anguilla*. Endocrinol. 1990; 127(suppl):74.

5. Conlon J.M., Hicks J.W., Smith D.D. Isolation and biological activity of a novel kinin ([thr^6]bradykinin) from the turtle, Pseudemys scripta. Endocrinol. 1990; 126:985-991.

6. Conover W.J. Practical Nonparametric Statistics 2nd edition, ed:John Wiley & Sons 1980; 229-233.

7. Vogel R., Schievelbein H., Lorenz W. and Werle E. Contributions to the evolution of blood pressure regulation. Part II : Evidence for the absence of Kinin-like polypeptides released by proteolytic enzymes for blood pressure regulation in fish. Z. Klin. Chem. u. Klin. Biochem. 1969; 7:S464-466.

8. Dunn R.S. and Perks A.M. Comparative studies of plasma kinins: the kallikrein-kinin system in poikilotherm and other vertebrates. Gen. Comp. Endocrinol. 1974; 26:165-178.

9. Lipke D.W., Oparil S., Olson K.R. Vascular effects of kinins in trout and bradykinin metabolism by perfused gill. Am. J. Physiol. 1990c; 258:R515-522.

10. Lipke D.W., Olson K.R. Generation of vasoactive substances in trout and rat plasma by trypsin and kallikrein. Am. J. Physiol. 1990a; 258:R507-513.

AAS 38/II
Recent Progress on Kinins
© 1992 Birkhäuser Verlag Basel

CHARACTERIZATION OF TWO DIFFERENT AFFINITY B2-KININ BINDING SITES IN RAT GLOMERULI

C. Emond, C. Pécher, J-L. Bascands, D. Regoli* and J-P. Girolami

INSERM U133, Institut Louis Bugnard, Faculté de Médecine Rangueil, 31062 Toulouse
Cédex France.
* Department of Pharmacology University of Sherbrooke, Québec, Canada

SUMMARY: We have recently characterized a bradykinin (BK) receptor in rat renal mesangial cells (1). Activation of this receptor is associated with PGE2 release and IP3 formation suggesting involvement in cell contraction which can be linked to the control of the glomerular filtration rate (2). Whether this mesangial BK receptor is the unique glomerular BK receptor remains to be elucidated. In an attempt to answer to this question, we performed binding studies using decapsulated isolated glomeruli.Scatchard analysis of the binding data obtained with this preparation revealed the presence of two distinct B2-kinin binding sites.However, a consistent difference was observed in both the affinity and the density. We further investigated the pharmacological binding profile after an initial step of solubilization. Several experiments were performed to establish optimal conditions of solubilization. For this, different detergents such as Triton X-100, CHAPS and n-octyl ß-D glucopyranoside were tested at various concentrations, durations and temperatures of incubation. The binding was performed with two different [^{125}I]-Tyr^0-BK concentrations (0.5 and 7 nM) with either untreated decapsulated glomeruli or solubilized preparation for 45 minutes at +4°C in the binding buffer containing a mixture of protease inhibitors. The greatest binding was achieved after treating glomeruli with 25 mM n-octyl ß-D glucopyranoside for 60 minutes at +4°C under constant shaking. Two B2-kinin receptors of different affinities were detected. The same binding characteristics were obtained both in the 12 000 x g and 100 000 x g supernatant. The soluble binding was still displaced by BK and HOE 140 but was not inhibited by des-Arg ^{9}-BK,captopril or phosphoramidon.These results demonstrate the presence of two B2-kinin binding sites for BK in rat glomeruli which can be solubilized in one step by n-octyl ß-D glucopyranoside without significant loss of specificity.

INTRODUCTION

Since the discovery of the nonapeptide bradykinin (BK), extensive studies have reported a wide variety of biological effects (3). Kinins appear as important mediators in inflammation, allergy and pain. They are also very potent natriuretic, diuretic and vasodilator agents and, because of these properties, a role in the regulation of blood pressure has been proposed. Finally, kinins are ubiquitous peptides whose wide variety of biological effects suggest a large family of receptors. *In vivo* and *in vitro*, pharmacological studies have established that kinins interact with, at least, two different classes of receptors named B1 and B2. Whereas the B2 receptor is the most prevalent under physiological conditions and demonstrates a specific affinity for bradykinin, the B1 receptor appears associated with stress and pathological situations showing a selective affinity for des-Arg^9-BK. However although the distinction between B1 and B2 receptors is well accepted, it also appears likely that the B2 class is not a uniform receptor family considering the wide tissue distribution and variety of biological effects. In the kidney, BK binding sites have been identified in cortical epithelial membranes (4) , interstitial medullary cells (5) and in the distal cells of the collecting duct (6). Recently, we demonstrated the presence of B2 receptor in glomerular membrane and localized this receptor in mesangial cells (1). This receptor is functionally associated with phospholipase C and A2 pathways (1-2). To further extend our knowledge of the glomerular B2 receptor and to investigate whether the mesangial BK receptor is the only glomerular BK receptor we undertook its solubilization.

MATERIALS AND METHODS

Glomerulus preparation
Male Sprague-Dawley rats (IFA Credo; mean body wt 240 ± 20 g, 12 weeks) were killed by decapitation and the kidneys were removed and immediately placed in cold saline. The cortex was dissected with scissors and the glomeruli were isolated by graded sieving. Briefly, the cortical tissue was extensively washed in cold saline and passed successively through 100 and 63 μm sieves. The glomeruli were collected on the last sieve, resuspended in cold saline and centrifuged at 600 x g for 5 minutes.The pellet was taken up again in the same solution. The glomeruli were decapsulated on passing through a syringe with a 0.6 x 25 mm needle and then centrifuged in the same conditions as previously described. By microscopic inspection, these preparations contained > 90-95 % glomeruli with < 5-10 % tubule fragments.

Conditions of solubilization
Glomerulus extract was treated with different conditions of temperature, duration and centrifugation in a buffered solution 20 mM Pipes pH 6.8 containing 0.1% bacitracine, 10 μM leupeptin, 2.5mM orthophenanthroline,5mM EDTA and various detergents at different concentrations under gentle rotative shaking. The supernatant obtained was used as solubilized extract for binding studies.The improvement of solubilization was monitored by the changes in percentage of specific binding. For this, the different fixed amounts of solubilized fractions (10 μg of protein) or untreated glomeruli (45 μg of protein) were incubated for 45 minutes at +4°C with two concentrations of [^{125}I] Tyr^{0}BK corresponding to the Kd determined for very-high and high affinity binding sites in Scatchard analysis of the binding data of untreated glomeruli (0.5 and 7 nM respectively). Values are expressed as a percent of the specific control BK binding measured in untreated glomeruli which was taken as 100 %.

Binding studies

For saturation studies, increasing concentrations (from 0.2 to 20 nM) of [^{125}I] Tyr^{0}BK were iodinated according to the chloramin-T method. It was immediately purified by HPLC and incubated with a fixed volume of untreated glomeruli (45 µg of protein) or solubilized fraction (10 µg of protein) for 45 min at +4°C in the following binding buffer: 5 mM potassium-phosphate pH 7.2 , 0.32 M sucrose, 10 µM leupeptine, 0.05% bacitracin, 1 mM benzamidine, 2 µM captopril, 0.2% bovine serum albumin (BSA).

For displacement studies, increasing concentrations of bradykinin agonist and antagonist (from 10^{-12} to 10^{-4} M) were incubated for 45 minutes at +4°C with 0.5±0.2 or 7±2.5 nM of radiolabelled ligand and fixed amount of either untreated glomeruli (45 µg of protein) or solubilized fraction (10 µg of protein). The two concentrations of radiolabelled ligand were chosen according to the Kd of the very-high and high affinity binding sites respectively.

In all these experiments the final assay volume was 0.4 ml. At the end of the incubation, 4 ml of washing buffer (5 mM phosphate buffer pH 7.2, 0.32 M sucrose) was added. The total volume was filtered through GF/C Whatman filters soaked in 0.1% polyethylenimine for at least 2 hours. The filter was washed four additional times with 4 ml of buffer.Filter-bound radioactivity was determined in a Crystal Multi RIA Packard gamma counter. Specific binding of [^{125}I] Tyr^{0}BK was defined as the difference in binding in the presence or absence of 10 µM unlabeled BK.

RESULTS
Conditions of solubilization

Different detergents such as Triton X-100, CHAPS and n-octyl-ß-D-glucopyranoside, dissolved in Pipes, were tested at various concentrations for their ability to solubilize bradykinin binding sites from rat glomeruli as illustrated in Fig.1.

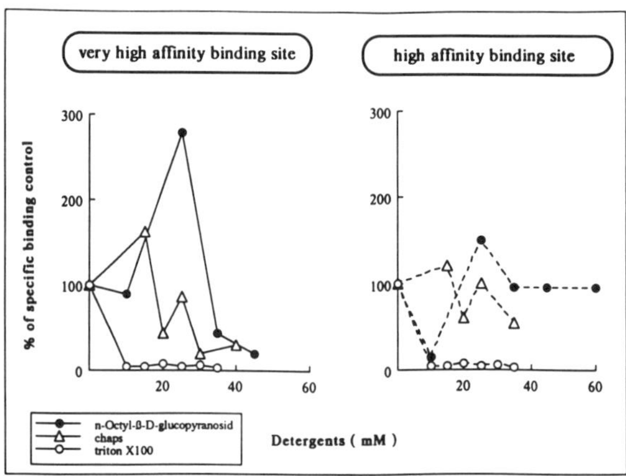

Figure 1.   Solubilization of BK-binding sites from rat glomeruli with increasing concentrations of different detergents.

The highest binding was achieved with 25 mM n-octyl ß-D-glucopyranoside which reached 279±20 and 150±8% of specific control binding for the very-high and high affinity binding sites respectively, whereas CHAPS allowed only 162±14 and 120±7% and TRITON X100 showed zero efficiency.

N-octyl ß-D glucopyranoside was retained for further studies. The most effective time of solubilization was about 60 minutes giving 430 and 226 % of specific control binding for the very-high and high affinity binding sites respectively (Fig. 2).

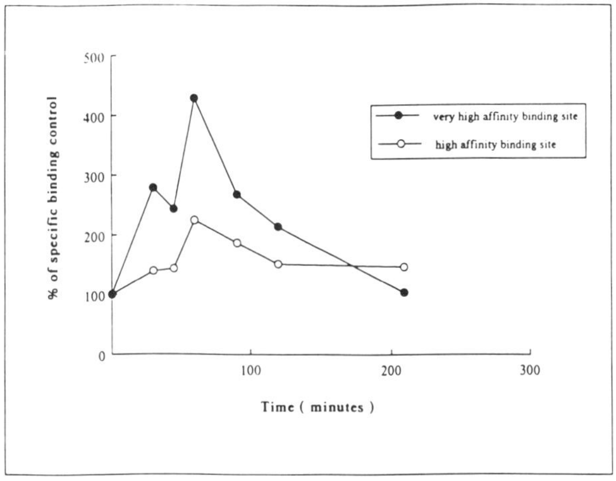

Figure 2.   Solubilization of BK-binding sites from rat glomeruli with 25 mM of n-Octyl-β-D-glucopyranosid at different times.

The glomeruli were incubated for 60 minutes under gentle rotative shaking at different temperatures with 25 mM Octyl ß-D glucopyranoside and then centrifuged for 15 minutes at either 12 000g or 100 000g at +4°C . The percentage of maximum specific control binding was achieved at +4°C and 12 000g : 366±32 and 212±19% for the very-high and high affinity binding sites respectively. Similar results were obtained at 100 000 g (364±33 and 227±20%) (Fig.3).

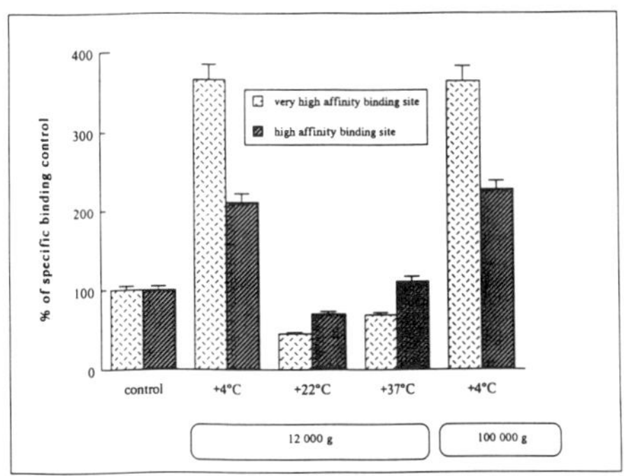

Figure 3.   Solubilization of BK-binding sites from rat glomeruli with 25 mM of n-Octyl-β-D-glucopyranosid at different temperatures.

The effect of increasing glomerular protein concentration on the efficiency of the solubilization step was then investigated. Maximal solubilized specific binding was obtained with a detergent/protein ratio of 8 with 45 µg of intact protein as starting material. In these conditions, a percentage of 22% solubilization is achieved (10µg of solubilized protein) (Fig.4).

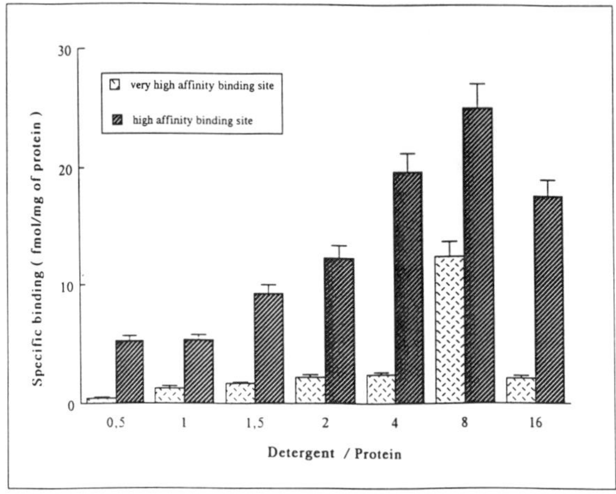

Figure 4.   Variation of specific binding with different detergent/protein ratio.

Binding studies

Specific BK binding of untreated and solubilized glomeruli was saturated at about 20 nM [^{125}I]-Tyr^0-BK. Scatchard analysis of both untreated glomeruli and solubilized extract revealed the existence of two populations of BK binding sites exhibiting similar affinity. The maximum number of binding sites was increased after solubilization (Fig.5-6).

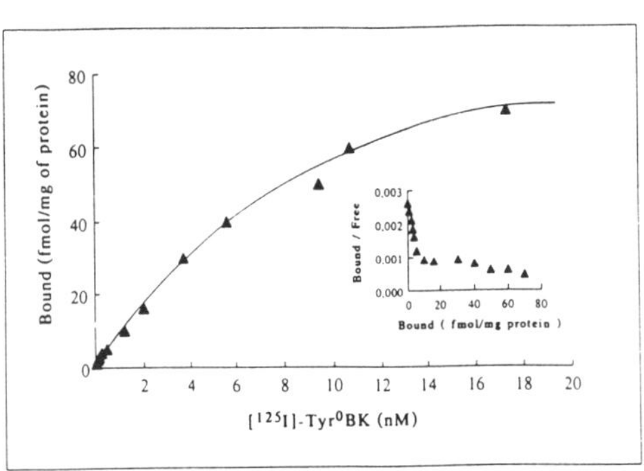

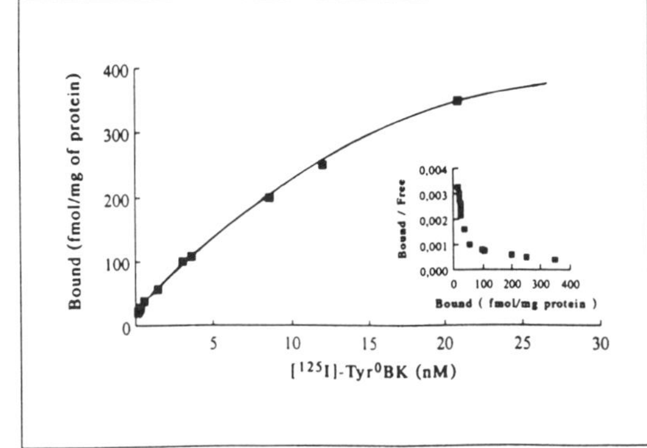

Figure 5.   Representative saturation-binding curve of an increasing amount of [^{125}I]-Tyr^{0}BK to untreated glomerular protein and Scatchard plot analysis.

Figure 6.   Representative saturation-binding curve of an increasing amount of [^{125}I]-Tyr^{0}BK to solubilized glomerular protein and Scatchard plot analysis.

The equilibrium dissociation constants (Kd) and maximum number of binding sites (Bmax) for the very-high and high affinity binding sites are summarized in table 1.

Table 1. Binding parameters of intact and solubilized glomeruli

Glomeruli	very-high affinity		high affinity	
	Kd (nM)	Bmax (fmol/mg protein)	Kd (nM)	Bmax (fmol/mg protein)
intact	0.44±0.2	11.7±2.3	6.3±2.5	112.3±11.6
solubilized	0.50±0.2	80.0±10.2	7.1±2.2	500.0±41.6

BK, HOE 140 (B2 antagonist) and des-Arg^9-BK (B1 agonist) were tested for their ability to compete with [^{125}I]-Tyr^0-BK for specific binding to intact and solubilized glomeruli. The pharmacological data are consistent with the characteristics expected from a B2 receptor : the binding of [^{125}I]-Tyr^0-BK to intact and solubilized glomeruli was inhibited by B2 antagonist and BK and not inhibited by B1 agonist (Fig.7-8). In any case the binding was not inhibited either by captopril or by phosphoramidon.

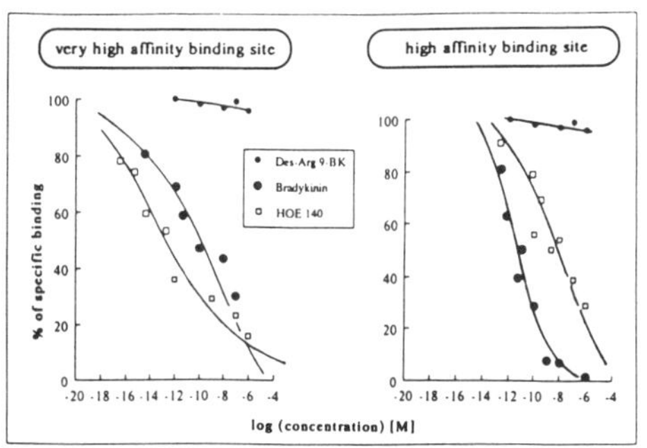

Figure 7.   Competition of [^{125}I]-Tyr^{0}BK binding to untreated glomeruli

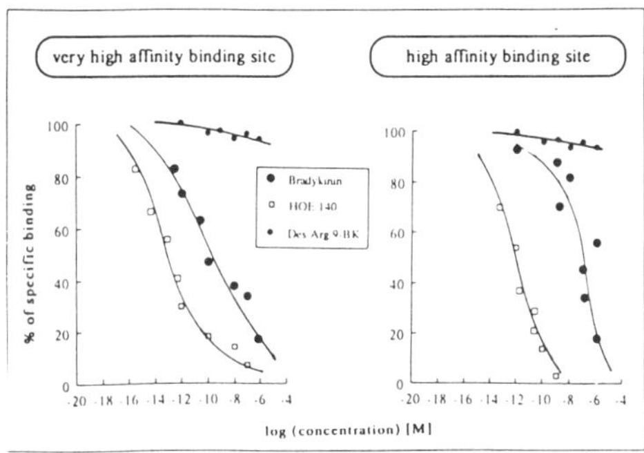

Figure 8.   Competition of [^{125}I]-Tyr^{0}BK binding to solubilized glomeruli

CONCLUSION

In this paper, we report the experimental conditions defined for the solubilization of BK binding activity from rat glomeruli in one step by n-octyl-ß-D-glucopyranoside. The established conditions preserve the specificity and activity of the binding. Furthermore, the density of binding sites was increased indicating a preferential solubilization of the receptor.

Recently, Roscher et al (7) solubilized B2 receptors from cultured human fibroblasts and Odya et al (8) from bovine uterine myometrium by CHAPS. In our system, CHAPS appears to be less effective than n-octyl-ß-D-glucopyranoside. Moreover, Webb et al (9) solubilized B2 receptors by digitonin from particular fractions of rat uterus and neuroblastoma cells or by digitonin combined with CHAPS from rat uterus only. This differential ability of detergents to solubilize seems to be tissue-specific. In fact, the lipid environment of these tissues could be variable making them the targets of specific detergents.However, the existence of various molecular forms of B2 receptors could be suggested.

The existence of a single affinity binding site has been reported for other tissues in several experiments. By using ^{3}H-BK, Roscher et al (7) demonstrated a single class of high affinity binding site in human fibroblasts with a dissociation constant of 1.68 ± 0.8 nM. In addition, Odya et al (8) revealed the presence of single site by the use of ^{125} ITyr^{1}Kallidin with a Kd of 0.35 nM. However, the solubilized site presents alterations of Kd and Bmax compared to intact preparations. A second higher affinity binding site in the pM range has been described by Roberts et al (10) and Liebmann et al (11). The Scatchard analysis of our soluble fraction reveals the presence of two binding sites with dissociation constants similar to those obtained with intact glomerulus preparations.The Kd of very-high and high affinity binding sites were respectively 0.5 ± 0.2 and 7.1 ± 2.2 nM for solubilized glomeruli, 0.44 ± 0.2 and $6.3\pm2,5$nM for intact glomeruli. The pharmacology of the solubilized BK-binding sites was characterized using B2 agonist and antagonist and B1 agonist. The results were compatible with B2 binding sites and are similar to those obtained with intact glomeruli.

In conclusion, we establish for the first time the presence of two B2 affinity binding sites in rat glomeruli and we show that the binding activity can be solubilized from glomeruli without any significant loss of specificity and with an increase in density which may be due to the properties of the detergent used. These results confirm the presence of two B2 binding sites in rat glomeruli.

Now, it will be of interest to determine the origin of these two sites : heterogenous B2 BK receptors or differences in the molecular forms of the receptor by coupling or uncoupling to G proteins. Indeed, this last possibility has recently been reported by Leeb-Lundberg et al (12). The comparison with a solubilized extract from mesangial cells could also be considered.

ACKNOWLEDGMENTS

HOE 140 was kindly provided by Hoescht.

REFERENCES

1. Emond C, Bascands JL, Pécher C, Cabos-Boutot G, Pradelles P, Regoli D, Girolami JP. Characterization of a B2-bradykinin receptor in rat renal mesangial cells. Eur J Pharmacol 1990 ; 190 : 381-392.

2. Bascands JL, Emond C, Pécher C, Regoli D, Girolami JP. Bradykinin stimulates production of inositol (1,4,5) trisphosphate in cultured rat mesangial cells via B2-kinin receptor. British J Pharmacol 1991 ; 102 : 962-916.

3. Regoli D, Barabé J. Pharmacology of bradykinin and related kinins. Pharmacol Rev 1980 ; 32 : 1-46.

4 Cox HM, Munday KA, Poat JA. Clin and Exp Theory and Practice A6, 1983.

5. Fredrick MJ, Abel FC, Righsel WA, Muirhead EE, Odya CE. B2-bradykinin receptor-like binding in rat renomedullary interstitial cells. Life Sci 1985 ; 37 : 331-338.

6. Tomita K, Pisano JJ. Binding of (3H) bradykinin in isolated nephron segments of the rabbit. Am J Physiol 1984 ; 246 : F732-F737.

7 Faußner A, Heinz-Erian P, Klier C, Roscher AA. Solubilization and characterization of B2 Bradykini receptors from cultured human fibroblasts. JBC 1991 ; 266 : 9442-9446.

8 Fredrick MJ, Odya CE. Characterization of soluble bradykinin receptor-like binding sites. Eur J Pharmacol 1987 ; 134 : 45-52.

9 Snell PH, Phillips E, Burgess GM, Snell C, Webb M. Characterization of bradykinin receptors solubilized from rat uterus and NG108-15 cells. Biochem Pharmacol 1990 ; 39 : 1921-1928.

10 Roberts RA, Gullick WJ. Bradykinin receptor number and sensitivity to ligand stimulation of mitogenesis is increased by expression of a mutant ras oncogene. J Cell Science 1989 ; 94 : 527-535.

11. Liebmann C, Offermanns S, Spicher K, Hinsch KD, Schnittler M, Morgat JL, Reissmann S, Schultz G, Rosenthal W. A high-affinity bradykinin receptor in membranes from rat myometrium is coupled to pertussis toxin-sensitive G-proteins of Gi family. BBRC 1990 ; 167 : 910-917.

12. Leeb-lundberg LMF, Mathis SA. Guanine nucleotide regulation of B2 kinin receptors.JBC 1990 ; 265 : 9621-9627.

AAS 38/II
Recent Progress on Kinins
© 1992 Birkhäuser Verlag Basel

MECHANISM OF THE RELAXANT RESPONSE OF THE RAT DUODENUM TO BRADYKININ

T. Feres, C.C.P. Funari, A.C.M. Paiva and T.B. Paiva

Department of Biophysics, Escola Paulista de Medicina,
04034 São Paulo, SP, Brazil

SUMMARY: Bradykinin (BK) did not increase cyclic AMP production in cultured rat duodenum smooth muscle cells. Its relaxant effect on the tissue was inhibited by apamin and potentiated by phorbol dibutyrate (PDBU). PDBU also caused a relaxation which was inhibited by apamin. BK's relaxant effect, and its potentiation by PDBU, are due to activation of Ca^{2+}-dependent K^+ channels.

INTRODUCTION

The response of the rat duodenum to bradykinin is diphasic, resulting from a balance between relaxant and contractile components which have been attributed, respectively, to subtypes of the B_2 and B_1 receptors (1). The contractile component, which is favoured by low Ca^{2+} concentration in the medium and by stretching (2), appears to be due to depolarization associated with a fall in membrane conductance, primarily due to the inhibition of a voltage-dependent K^+ current (3). The relaxant component, which is predominant under normal conditions, has been attributed to two different mechanisms. The finding that it is inhibited by apamin, a toxin that specifically blocks Ca^{2+}-dependent K^+ channels, indicates that the relaxation is caused by hyperpolarization due to activation of these channels (4). However, increased cAMP (cAMP) levels were found in duodenum strips treated with bradykinin, suggesting that stimulation of adenylylcyclase activity may be involved in the relaxant response (5).

To further investigate the mechanism of the relaxant property of bradykinin in the rat duodenum, we have measured the relaxant response of the tissue and cAMP production in cultured cells, and studied the effects of phorbol ester, apamin and low-Na^+ medium on these responses.

MATERIALS AND METHODS

Bradykinin was a synthetic product made in this laboratory. The inorganic salts were products of the highest analytical grade from Merck Darmstadt. Apamin, phorbol-12,13-dibutyrate (PDBU), isoproterenol, N-methyl-D-glucamine and theophylline were obtained from Sigma Chemical Co., St. Louis, MO. The [^{3}H] cAMP assay kit was obtained from Diagnostic Products Corporation, Los Angeles, CA, USA. Culture medium, supplements and fetal bovine serum were obtained from Gibco.

The isolated rat duodenum was prepared as previously described (2). The preparation was suspended in a 5-ml chamber containing Tyrode solution kept at 37°C and bubbled with a mixture of CO_2 (5%) and O_2 (95%). The composition of the Tyrode solution was (mM): NaCl 137, KCl 12.7, $CaCl_2$ 1.36, $MgCl_2$ 0.49, NaH_2PO_4 0.36, $NaHCO_3$ 11.9, glucose 5.0. The sodium-deficient solution (80 mM) was obtained by isosmotic replacement of the NaCl with N-methyl-D-glucamine. Isotonic recordings were made, under 1-g load, on smoked drums using frontal levers with 6-fold amplification, after a 60-min equilibration period. The concentration-response curves were obtained within the first 90 min after the end of the equilibration period. The drugs, in volumes not exceeding 0.2 ml, were added directly to the organ bath and the preparation was washed after 90-s contact. The interval between BK additions was 15 min. The relaxant component of the response was measured from the baseline to the deepest point of the recorded response. The dose-response curves were analyzed by linear regression of the double reciprocal plot, from which ED_{50} values were obtained.

Cultures of duodenal smooth muscle cells were prepared from enzymatically dispersed cells, and all procedures were carried out under sterile conditions. Wistar rats of either sex, weighing 190 to 220 g, were fasted for 24 h, then stunned by a blow to the head and decapitated. The duodenum was removed, washed and incubated for 10 min at 37°C in Ca^{2+} free physiological solution of the following composition (in mM): NaCl 132, KCl 5.9, $MgCl_2$ 1.2, HEPES 11.5 and glucose 11.5 (pH 7.2), containing 100 U/ml of penicillin and 100 µg/ml streptomycin. The piece of duodenum was stretched over a glass rod, the mesentery was cut away and lengths of longitudinal muscle were peeled from the underlying circular muscle by stroking with a moist wisp of cotton wool. After six washings, they were placed in 5 ml of Ca^{2+}-free physiological solution containing 0.1% collagenase, 0.1% soybean trypsin inhibitor and 0.2% bovine serum albumin (dispersal solution). After 5-min incubation at 37°C with mild agitation, the cells were centrifuged (1000 rpm, 8 min), and the incubation was repeated twice with fresh dispersal solution until a cloudy appearance of the solution was obtained. The solution was diluted twice with the culture medium, filtered through nylon mesh and the cells were collected by centrifugation and re-suspended in Dulbecco's modified Eagle's medium containing 10% fetal bovine serum, 0.03% glutamine, 100 U/ml of penicillin and 100 μg/ml of streptomycin. The viability of the cells was determined by the trypan blue exclusion method and was found to be higher than 90%. Because after inoculation the fibroblasts attach more rapidly to the bottom of the flask, the supernatant was removed and seeded in primary culture flasks (Falcon) or tissue culture plates (Primaria, 35-mm diameter) and left to grow in a humidified atmosphere of 5% CO_2-95% air. At 3-day intervals the medium was changed and the cells were confluent after approximately 10 days. Primary culture cells or subcultures (up to eight passages) were used. The identity and homogeneity of the cells were indicated by positive immunofluorescence with antibodies against myosin and actin (6).

For the cAMP assays (7,8), the culture medium of confluent cells (ca. 10^6 cells) was removed and the cells were rinsed at 37°C with Tyrode solution and then 1.0 ml of 1.0 mM theophylline was added. After equilibration for 30 min, the cells were incubated for the desired times with various test reagents. The reaction was terminated by aspirating off the assay medium and the cells in culture dishes were immediately frozen in an acetone-dry ice bath. The cAMP formed was extracted with the addition of 0.3% ice-cold perchloric acid, neutralized with 30% $KHCO_3$ and then measured by radioimmunoassay.

All tracings presented in the figures are representative of at least 4 replicate experiments and data are expressed as means ± standard errors, and were analyzed by Student's t test.

RESULTS AND DISCUSSION

In cultured duodenal smooth muscle cells, we did not detect an increase in cAMP in response to bradykinin concentrations above those known to cause maximum relaxant responses of the

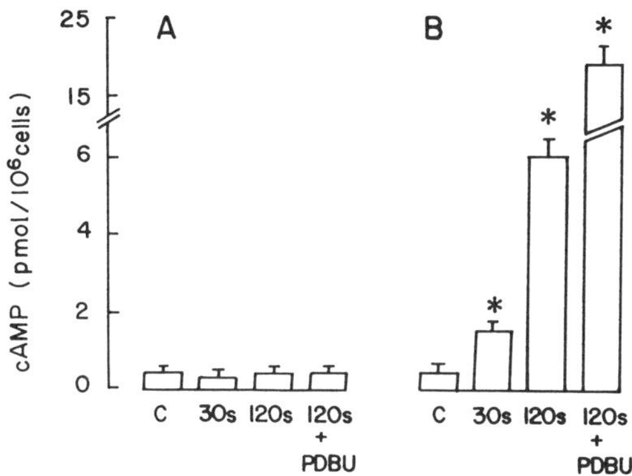

Figure 1. Effect of 10 nM bradykinin (A) and of 2 μM isoproterenol (B) on the cAMP content of cultured rat duodenum smooth muscle cells. cAMP was measured at times 0 s (C), 30 s and 120 s of incubation, in the absence and in the presence of PDBU (10^{-7} M). Values are means (± S.E.) of four experiments done in triplicate. *Significantly different from the respective controls (p < 0.05).

duodenum. Figure 1 shows that there was no change in the cAMP content of the cells incubated with 10 nM bradykinin, in contrast with the significant time-dependent increase seen after incubation with the β-adrenergic agonist isoproterenol. This increase was also observed in the presence of the phosphodiesterase inhibitor theophylline (1 mM, not shown).

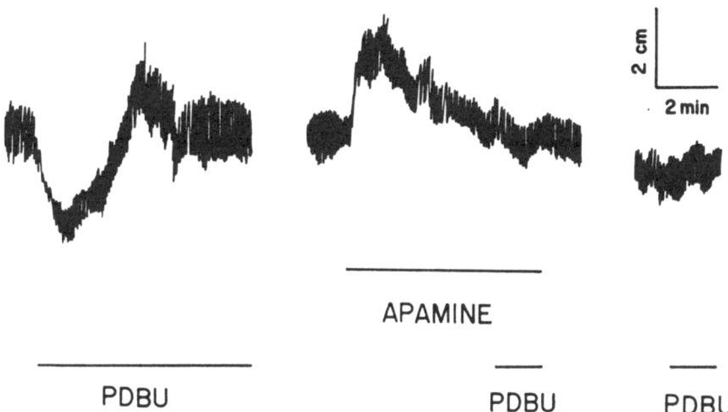

Figure 2. Effect of 10^{-7} M PDBU on the rat isolated duodenum, and its inhibition by 5 x 10^{-7} M apamin. Horizontal lines indicate presence of the drugs, and interruptions in the tracing represent 15-min intervals.

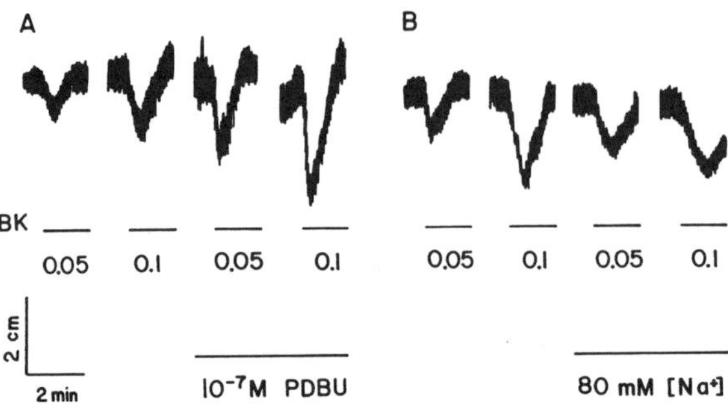

Figure 3. Effect of 10^{-7} M PDBU (A) and of low-sodium (80 mM) (B) medium on the responses of the isolated rat duodenum to bradykinin (nM).

Since phorbol esters enhance agonist-induced cAMP accumulation in vascular smooth muscle cells (9,10), we determined the effect of bradykinin and isoproterenol on cAMP levels of rat duodenum cells treated with phorbol dibutyrate (PDBU). A significant increase in cAMP accumulation was observed in the cultured cells incubated with isoproterenol, but not with bradykinin (Fig. 1). The contrast between these results and the previous finding of increased cAMP in rat duodena treated with bradykinin (5) may be due to the fact that we used only smooth muscle cells, whereas that report was based on whole duodenum strips, where cells other than smooth muscle are present. The mucosa was shown to accumulate cAMP under other stimuli (11), and the presence of these cells might influence the results obtained with the strips.

In the rat isolated duodenum preparation, the phorbol ester by itself produced a response. When added to the preparation, in concentrations that are known to activate protein kinase C in different systems, PDBU induced a transient relaxation followed by contraction (Fig. 2), similar to the response induced by bradykinin in this preparation (2). This diphasic response was abolished by apamin concentrations that were shown also to inhibit the response to bradykinin. This suggests that PDBU is able to activate Ca^{2+}-dependent K^+ channels, as was also proposed for the case of bradykinin (4).

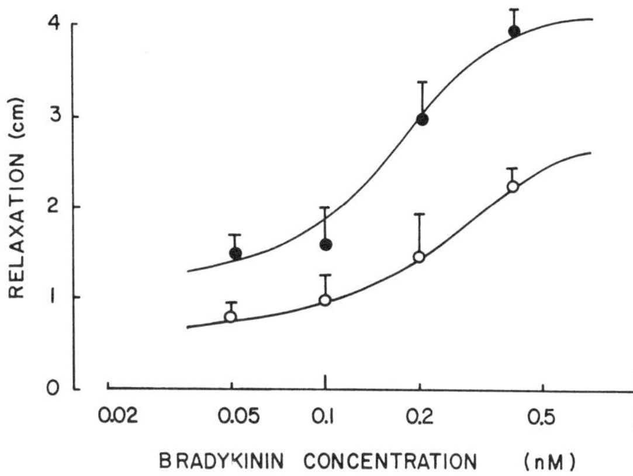

Figure 4. Concentration-response curves for the relaxant effect of bradykinin in the absence (○) and in the presence (●) of 10^{-7} M PDBU.

Figure 3A shows that in the presence of PDBU, and after its transient effect had subsided, the relaxation induced by bradykinin was potentiated. This potentiation cannot be attributed simply to an increase in the intracellular Ca^{2+} concentration by PDBU, since lowering of the external Na^+ concentration (which increases internal Ca^{2+} by inhibiting Na^+/Ca^2 exchange) (12) caused only a prolongation of the relaxation (Fig. 3B), in contrast with the increase in amplitude which was elicited by PDBU. It seems more probable that PDBU is acting through a direct effect on Ca^{2+}-activated K^+ channels, as proposed (13) for the case of neuroblastoma hybrid cells.

The effect of PDBU on the concentration-response curves for the relaxant effect of bradykinin is shown in Fig. 4, where it may be seen that the potentiation of the maximum effect was not accompanied by a change in the ED_{50} values. This suggests that activation of protein kinase C leads to an increase in the number of Ca^{2+}-activated K^+ channels, without affecting their affinity, as previously demonstrated in the case of cultured skeletal muscle cells (14).

CONCLUSION

Our results indicate that bradykinin's relaxant effect on the rat duodenum is due to activation of Ca^{2+}-dependent K^+ channels and not to cAMP accumulation. Potentiation of this effect by phorbol ester is not due to mediation by increased intracellular Ca^{2+}, but appears to involve a more direct action of phorbol on the Ca^{2+}-dependent K^+ channels.

REFERENCES

1.   Paiva, ACM, Paiva, TB, Pereira, CC, Shimuta, SI. Selectivity of bradykinin analogues for receptors mediating contraction and relaxation of the rat duodenum. Br J Pharmacol 1989; 98:206-210.

2.   Boschcov, P, Paiva, ACM, Paiva, T.B., Shimuta, SI. Further evidence for the existence of two receptor sites for bradykinin responsible for the diphasic effect in the rat isolated duodenum. Br Pharmacol 1984; 83:591-600.

3.   Higashida, H, Brown, DA. Bradykinin inhibits potassium (M) currents in N1E-115 neuroblastoma cells. FEBS Let 1987; 220:302-306.

4.   Hall, JM, Morton, IKM. Bradykinin B_2 receptor evoked K^+ permeability increase mediates relaxation in the rat duodenum. Eur J Pharmacol 1991; 193:231-238.

5.   Liebmann, C, Reissmann, S, Robbercht, P, Arold, H. Bradykinin action in the rat duodenum: Receptor binding and influence on the cyclic AMP system. Biomed Biochim Acta 1987; 46:469-478.

6.   Yamamoto, H, Kanaide, H, Nakamura, M. Metabolism of glycosaminoglycans of cultured rat aortic smooth muscle cells altered during subculture. Br J Exp Pathol 1983; 64:156-165.

7.   Gilman, AG. A protein binding assay for adenosine 3'5' cyclic monophosphate. Proc Natl Acad Sci US 1970; 67:305-312.

8.   Tovey, KC, Oldham, KG, Whelan, JAM. A simple direct assay for cyclic AMP in plasma and other biological samples using an improved competitive protein binding technique. Clin Chim Acta 1974; 56: 221-234.

9.   Nabika T, Nara, Y, Yamori, Y, Lovenberg, W, Endo, J. Angiotensin II and phorbol ester enhance isoproterenol- and vasoactive intestinal peptide (VIP)- induced cyclic AMP accumulation in vascular smooth muscle cells. Biochem Biophys Res Commun 1985; 131: 30-36.

10.   Phaneuf, S, Berta, P, Le Peuch, C, Haiech, J, Cavadore, JC. Phorbol ester modulation of cyclic AMP accumulation in a primary culture of rat aortic smooth muscle cells. J Pharmacol Exper Therap 1988; 245:1042-1047.

11.   Karlstrom, L. Mechanisms in bile-salt induced secretion in the small intestine. Acta Physiol Scand 1986; 126 Suppl 549:1-48.

12.   Smith, JB, Dwyer, SD, Smith, L. Decreasing extracellular Na^+ concentration triggers inositol polyphosphate production and Ca^{2+} mobilization. J Biol Chem 1989; 264:831-837.

13.   Higashida, H, Brown, DA. Ca^{2+}-dependent K^+ channels in neuroblastoma hybrid cells activated by intracellular inositol trisphosphate and extracellular bradykinin. FEBS Let 1988; 238:395-400.

14.   Navarro, J. Modulation of [^{3}H] dihydropyridine receptors by activation of protein kinase C in chick muscle cells. J Biol Chem 1987; 262:4649-4657.

AAS 38/II
Recent Progress on Kinins
© 1992 Birkhäuser Verlag Basel

DESARG^{10}[HOE 140] IS A POTENT B$_1$ BRADYKININ ANTAGONIST

K.J. Wirth, G. Wiemer and B.A. Schölkens

Hoechst AG, SBU Cardiovascular Agents, H 821, POB 80 03 20, W-6230 Frankfurt (Main) 80, FR Germany

SUMMARY: DesArg^{10}[Hoe 140] and Des(D-Arg^1,Arg^{10})[Hoe 140], desArg10-analogs of the potent and stable B$_2$ bradykinin (BK) receptor antagonist Hoe 140 were found to be potent and stable antagonists of the B$_1$ receptor in vitro and in vivo. They were, however, less selective than DesArg^9[Leu^8]BK, the metabolically unstable B$_1$ prototype antagonist. Surprisingly, Hoe 140, which behaved as a pure B$_2$ antagonist in several smooth muscle preparations, had a considerable inhibitory effect against the B$_1$ agonist DesArg^9-BK in bovine aortic endothelial cells. This finding for the first time suggests that B$_1$ receptors are heterogenous.

INTRODUCTION

Kinins act through at least two different receptors named B$_1$ and B$_2$ (1). This classification is based on agonist order of potency and on specific receptor antagonists. B$_1$ receptors are activated by the bradykinin fragment desArg^9-BK, which is more potent than bradykinin in contracting the rabbit aorta, the classical B$_1$ preparation. Most of the known effects of kinins are mediated by B$_2$ receptors whereas the in vivo function of B$_1$ receptors is not yet elucidated. Nevertheless, the idea of a pathophysiological role of B$_1$ receptors is supported by the observation that B$_1$ receptors are upregulated following some types of tissue injuries (2) and treatment of the rabbit with Lipopolysaccharide (LPS)

The prototype of the B$_1$ antagonists is desArg^9[Leu^8]BK. Although this compound lacks metabolic stability it helped to define the B$_1$ kinin receptor type. B$_1$ antagonists may possess a therapeutic potential. The evaluation of this potential, however, depends on the availability of more stable B$_1$ antagonists. With regard to B$_2$ receptors this problem has been overcome with the availabilty of the stable and potent B$_2$ antagonist Hoe 140 ((D-Arg[Hyp^3,Thi^5,D-Tic^7,Oic^8]BK) (3,4,5). In analogy to the agonists and yet described antagonists the analogs of HOE 140 without the C-terminal arginine might act as potent and stable B$_1$ receptor antagonists.

To test this hypothesis, the antagonistic potencies of Hoe 140, its desArg^{10}-analog (desArg^{10}[Hoe 140]) and the analog devoid of both terminal arginines (des(D-Arg^1,Arg^{10})[Hoe 140]) and the B$_1$-prototype antagonist desArg^9[Leu^8]BK were examined against the kinin agonists BK and desArg^9-BK in classical pure B$_1$ (rabbit aorta) or B$_2$ (ileum and pulmonary artery of the guinea pig) and mixed B$_1$/B$_2$ systems (rat duodenum, bovine endothelial cells and rabbit treated with LPS).

MATERIALS AND METHODS

<u>Comparison of potency in classical smooth muscle B$_1$ and B$_2$ preparation</u> (rabbit aorta versus ileum and pulmonary artery of the guinea pig) and rat duodenum (mixed B$_1$/B$_2$ system): Experiments in the pure B$_1$ and B$_2$ preparations (4) and the rat duodenum (6)were performed as described previously. The rat duodenum is a complex system and has two populations of BK receptors, B$_1$ and B$_2$. BK induces relaxation which is followed by contraction. By contrast, desArg^9-BK elicits only contraction. By increasing the BK concentration contraction becomes more and more predominant. Antagonists were tested against BK induced relaxation (10^{-9} M) and Des-Arg^9-BK induced contraction (2×10^{-7} M). Since all compounds devoid of the C-terminal arginine had considerable agonistic properties (as desArg^9-BK) the agonists were added 10 min after the test compounds when baseline levels were reached again.

<u>Comparison of stability in rabbit aorta</u>: Stability of desArg^{10}[Hoe 140] and desArg^9[Leu^8]BK was tested indirectly. Both compounds were incubated at 1 mM in rabbit plasma for 20 hours at room temperature and then used in the rabbit aorta at final bath concentrations of 10^{-5} M and 10^{-6} M for desArg^9[Leu^8]BK and desArg^{10}[Hoe140], respectively.

<u>LPS induced sensitivity to desArg^9-BK in rabbits</u>: Intraarterial injection of BK induces a vasodepressor effect in the non-treated rabbit whereas vasodepression to desArg^9-BK is normally absent. Sensitivity to desArg^9-BK was induced by intravenous injection of a nonlethal dose of 10 μg LPS from E.Coli 5 hours before the desArg^9-BK challenge (7). 2.5 μg desArg^9-BK and 100 ng BK lead to reproducible responses in the majority of the treated animals. Antagonists were either given as a bolus or by infusion. Challenges with BK and desArg^9-BK were performed alternatedly at intervals of at least two minutes to determine selectivity. Two to three rabbits were used for each dose.

<u>Bovine aortic endothelial cells</u>: Primary bovine aortic endothelial cells (BAEC) contain both B$_1$ and B$_2$ receptors. Experiments were performed as described previously (8). Stimulation of these cells by

both BK and desArg^9-BK leads to cyclic GMP increase, which was assessed with a radioimmunoassay. Hoe 140 and its desArg10-analog were tested against both BK and desArg^9-BK. Stimulatory agonist concentrations were used that gave maximal stimulation, 10^{-7}M for BK and 10^{-6}M for desArg^9-BK. Incubation time was one minute. Antagonists were added 5 min before the agonists. Results are the means of four independent assays including three wells of BAEC each determined in duplicate.

RESULTS AND DISCUSSION

<u>Smooth muscle preparations:</u> Comparison of potency in classical B$_1$ and B$_2$ preparations and rat duodenum.

In the B$_2$ systems of guinea pig ileum and pulmonary artery and the rat duodenum relaxed by BK, Hoe 140 was by far the most potent antagonist (Tab.1) and 2 to 3 orders of magnitude more potent than desArg^{10}[Hoe 140]. This underlines the importance of the C-terminal arginine for B$_2$-receptor occupancy. Whereas Hoe 140 was selective for B$_2$ and had no effect in the B$_1$ systems of the rabbit aorta and the rat duodenum stimulated by desArg^9-BK, desArg^9[Leu^8]BK had no effect at all in the B$_2$ systems. Both desArg10-analogs, however, were less selective.

Concerning potency on B$_1$, desArg^{10}[Hoe 140] was half to one order of magnitude more potent in the rabbit aorta but less potent in the rat duodenum than the B$_1$ prototype desArg^9[Leu^8]BK. In contrast to the latter compound, desArg^{10}[Hoe 140] seems to share the metabolic stability of Hoe 140 since after 20 hours of incubation in rabbit plasma desArg^{10}[Hoe 140] preserved still full inhibitory potency whereas desArg^9[Leu^8]BK was completely inactivated.

On B$_1$, des(D-Arg^1,Arg^{10})[Hoe 140] was weaker than desArg^{10}[Hoe 140], but still weaker on B$_2$ showing a certain selectivity for B$_1$. It can be speculated that the residual affinity of desArg^{10}[Hoe 140] to the B$_2$ receptors of the ileum and pulmonary artery of the guinea pig is due to the D-Arg residue. The N-terminal D-Arg seems to increase potency for both B$_1$ and B$_2$ receptors, and by that decreases selectivity.

The rat duodenum is a complex system and has two populations of BK receptors, B$_1$ and B$_2$. BK induces relaxation which is followed by contraction. By contrast, desArg^9-BK only elicits contraction. By increasing the BK concentration contraction becomes predominant. Both relaxation and contraction by BK were strongly inhibited by Hoe 140 (data not shown).

The B$_1$ antagonist desArg^9[Leu^8]BK acted as a strong contractant due to a residual B$_1$ agonism as did both desArg^{10}-analogs of Hoe 140 whereas Hoe 140 was devoid of any partial agonism. Because of this partial agonism BK-induced relaxation instead of constriction was used to compare the desArg^{10}-analogs with Hoe 140 as to their potency on B$_2$ because this enabled to use lower concentrations of the B$_1$ antagonists. Despite the complexity of this model we were able to confirm that the desArg^{10}-analogs had considerable activity on B$_1$ in the rat duodenum although their potency on B$_2$ was higher than in the ileum and pulmonary artery of the guinea pig and hence, they were less selective for B$_1$ than desArg^9[Leu^8]BK.

Table 1. Kinin antagonists in smooth muscle preparations (IC$_{50}$ values in M)

	Hoe 140	Des-Arg^{10} [Hoe 140]	Des-(D-Arg^1,Arg^{10}) [Hoe 140]	Des-Arg^9 [Leu^8]BK
[1]guinea pig pulm.art. (B$_2$)	5.4×10^{-9}	2.9×10^{-6}	25% at 10^{-4}	inactive at 10^{-4}
[2]guinea pig ileum (B$_2$)	1.1×10^{-8}	2.9×10^{-5}	N.D.	N.D.
[3]rat duodenum [a] (B$_2$)	3.8×10^{-9}	2.1×10^{-7}	1.1×10^{-6}	inactive at 10^{-4}
[b] (B$_1$)	inactive at 10^{-5}	4.9×10^{-8}	2.2×10^{-7}	8.2×10^{-9}
[4]rabbit aorta (B$_1$)	inactive at 10^{-5}	1.2×10^{-8}	6.6×10^{-8}	1.1×10^{-7}

[1] stimulated by BK 2×10^{-7} M; [2] BK 4×10^{-8} M; [3a] relaxation by BK 10^{-9} M; [3b] contraction by Des-Arg^9-BK 2×10^{-7} M; [4] Des-Arg^9-BK 3×10^{-7} M. Data were obtained from at least 9 determinations

LPS induced sensitivity to desArg^9-BK in rabbits: This model is the only established in vivo model for pharmacological testing of B$_1$ antagonists. Hoe 140 and desArg^9[Leu^8]BK showed selectivity for the respective agonists: Intravenous administration of Hoe 140 at a dose of 1 nmol/kg strongly inhibited BK induced vasodepression for more than 30 min whereas the response to desArg^9-BK was not at all affected (data not shown). The B$_1$ antagonist, desArg^9[Leu^8]BK, which had to be given by intravenous infusion due to metabolic instability, selectively inhibited desArg^9-BK at 100 nmol/kg/min.

1 μmol/kg of desArg^{10}[Hoe 140] given i.v. inhibited both desArg^9-BK and BK for more than 1 hour. Even at lower doses (10 nmol/kg) and infusion of low doses (1 nmol/kg/min) of this antagonist, or at a time after dosing when responses to the kinin agonists reappeared as a consequence of declining antagonist plasma levels the responses to BK and desArg^9-BK were always equally inhibited (data not shown). Thus, in rabbits, a relative selectivity for B$_1$ which could have

been anticipated from the comparison of potency in the rabbit aorta and pulmonary artery, and from BAEC (see below) but less from rat duodenum could not be found in this in vivo model.

Des(D-Arg^1,Arg^{10})[Hoe 140] which seemed to be more selective has not yet been tested. In summary desArg^9[Leu^8]BK and Hoe 140 are selective for their respective kinin receptors in this model whereas its desArg^{10}-analog seems to be a mixed type antagonist.

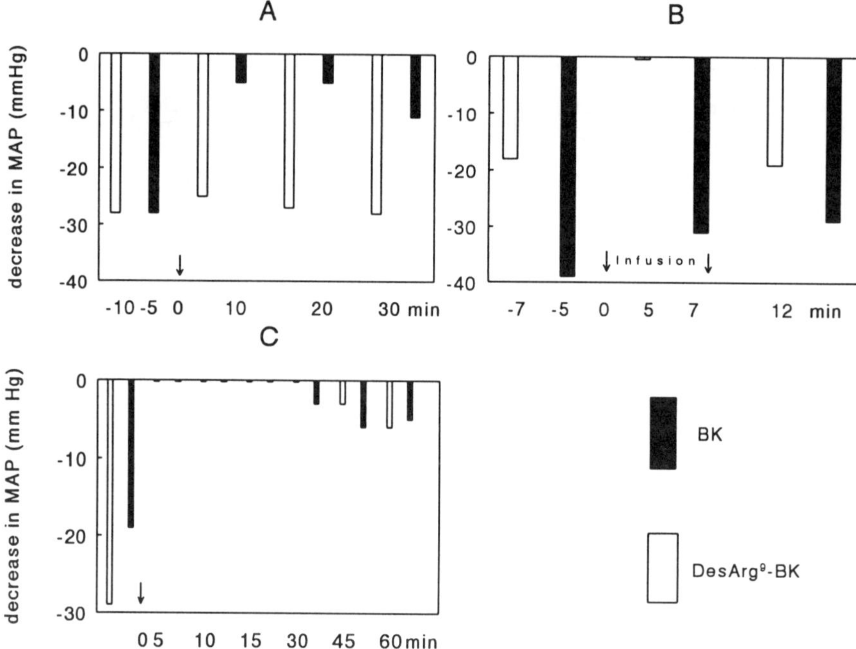

Figure 1. Effect of Hoe 140, 1 nmol/kg i.v. (panel A), DesArg^9[Leu^8]Bk infused at 100 nmol/kg/min (panel B) and DesArg^9[Hoe 140], 1 μmol/kg (panel C), on vasodepression induced by bradykinin and DesArg^9-BK in rabbits pretreated with a nonlethal dose of LPS. The first two columns are controls and show the effect of the kinin agonists before administration of test compounds. At time zero the compounds were given and the agonists were injected alternatedly.

<u>Primary bovine aortic endothelial cells (BAEC)</u>: Characterization of BK receptors is mainly based on isolated smooth muscle preparations. Therefore it is of interest to extend the scarce knowlegde of B$_1$ receptors to other in vitro systems. BAEC contain both B$_1$ and B$_2$ receptors. Stimulation of these cells by both BK and desArg^9-BK lead to cyclic GMP increased which could be abolished by LNNA, a specific inhibitor of NO synthase (data not shown). BK was about 6 fold stronger than desArg^9-BK in terms of EC$_{50}$ values but the same plateau was obtained for both kinin agonists (data not shown).

DesArg^{10}[Hoe 140] at 3×10^{-6} M was without any inhibitory effect on BK but abolished the effect of desArg^9-BK, and thus, demonstrated selectivity for B$_1$ receptors. As expected Hoe 140 at 10^{-7} M abolished the effect of BK. A similar inhibitory effect was achieved with 3×10^{-6} M of D-Arg-[Hyp^2,Thi$^{5.8}$,D-Phe^7]BK (9), a BK antagonist of the first generation.

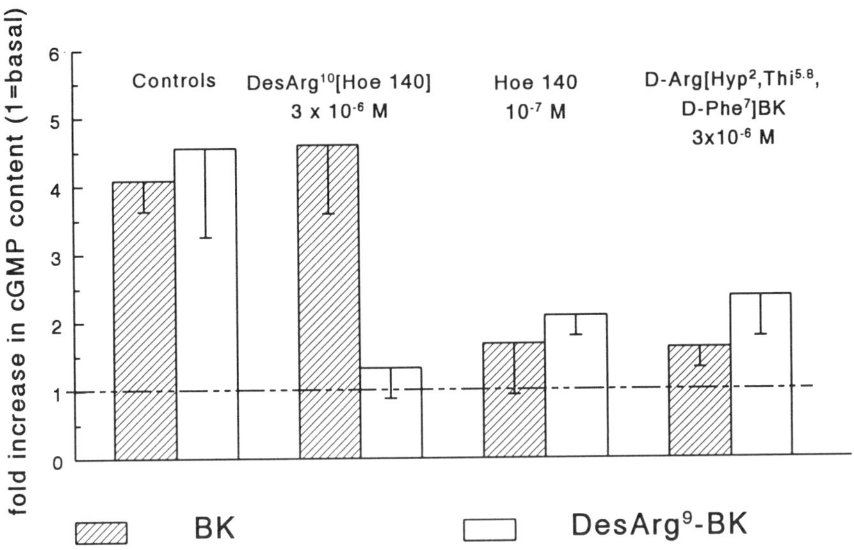

Figure 2. Effect of kinin antagonists on cGMP production of cultured primary bovine endothelial cells stimulated by either BK (10^{-7} M) or desArg^9-BK (10^{-6} M).

The most surprising result was that Hoe 140, which behaved as a pure B$_2$ antagonist in smooth muscle preparations, strongly inhibited the effect of desArg^9-BK in BAEC, at a concentration (10^{-7} M) which is not excessively high. 10^{-5} M of Hoe 140 were ineffective in rabbit aorta and rat duodenum against DesArg^9-BK. These experiments were repeated 4 times independently with the same result. The Stewart Compound also suppressed B$_1$. This is the first demonstration that Hoe 140 inhibits desArg^9-BK. The possibility that Hoe 140 is degraded to its desArg10-analog by carboxypeptidase and, by that, converted to a B$_1$ antagonist can be excluded since it has been shown to be resistant to degradation by carboxypeptidase (unpublished data). This obvious discrepancy suggests that the B$_1$ receptor in BAEC is different from the B$_1$ receptors in smooth muscle from rabbit aorta and rat duodenum where Hoe 140 had no inhibitory effect at all on desArg^9-BK. More research is needed including pA$_2$ determination to clarify this issue.

The original aim of these studies was to investigate whether desArg^{10}-analogs of Hoe 140 are potent and stable B_1 kinin antagonists. Indeed, our results demonstrate that DesArg^{10}-analogs of Hoe 140 are potent B_1 kinin receptor antagonists but in some systems they still inhibited B_2 effects although they were two to three orders of magnitude less potent than Hoe 140. They seemed to be rather selective for B_1 comparing rabbit aorta with guinea pig pulmonary artery but less selective in rat duodenum. DesArg^{10}[Hoe 140] seemed to be selective for B_1 in BAEC but nonselective in the LPS treated rabbit. The prototype B_1 antagonist DesArg^9[Leu^8]BK was the only antagonist completely selective for B_1. But this compound is metabolically unstable and has to be infused in vivo to be effective, in contrast to desArg^{10}[Hoe 140], which seems to share the metabolic stability of Hoe 140.

The complex picture emerging from the investigation of this potent class of compounds in different tissues and species was unexpected and probably reflects the complexity of kinin receptors. The different effects of these kinin antagonists in separate models in conjunction with the observation that Hoe 140 inhibited desArg^9-BK in bovine EC suggest that kinin receptors are heterogenous. As for B_2 receptors, heterogeneity has already been observed and discussed (10,11) but, as for the B_1 receptor, it is the first finding to suggest heterogeneity among this subtype of kinin receptors.

REFERENCES

1.   Regoli D, Barabe J. Pharmacology of bradykinin and related kinins. Pharmacol Rev 1980; 32:1-46.

2.   Marceau F, Lussier A., Regoli D, Giroud JP. Pharmacology of kinins: Their relevance to tissue injury and inflammation. Gen. Pharmacol 1983; 14: 209-229.

3.   Lembeck F, Griesbacher T, Eckhardt M, Henke S, Breipohl G, Knolle J. New, long-acting, potent bradykinin antagonists. Br J Pharmacol 1991; 102: 297-304.

4   Hock FJ, Wirth K, Albus U, Linz W, Gerhards G Wiemer, Henke St, Breipohl G, König W, Knolle J, Schölkens BA. Hoe 140 a new potent and long acting bradykinin- antagonist: in vitro studies. 1991; Br J Pharmacol 102: 769-773.

5.   Wirth K, Hock FJ, Albus U, Linz W, Alpermann HG, Anagnostopulos H, Henke St, Breipohl G, König W, Knolle J, Schölkens BA. Hoe 140 a new potent and long acting bradykinin-antagonist: in vivo studies. Br J Pharmacol 1991; 102: 774-777.

6.   Boschcov P, Paiva ACM, Paiva TB, Shimuta SI. Further evidence for the existence of two receptor sites for bradykinin responible for the diphasic effect in the rat isolated duodenum. Br J Pharamacol 1984; 83: 591-600.

7.   Regoli D, Marceau F, Lavigne J. Induction of B_1-receptors for kinins in the rabbit by a bacterial lipopolysaccharide. Eur J Pharmacol 1981; 71: 105-115.

8. Wiemer G, Schölkens BA, Becker RHA, Busse R. Ramiprilat enhances endothelial autacoid formation by inhibiting breakdown fo endothelium -derived bradykinin. Hypertension 1991; 18: 558-563.

9. Vavrek RJ, Stewart JM. Competitive antagonists of bradykinin. Peptides 1985; 6: 161-164.

10. Plevin R, Owen JP. Multiple B$_2$ kinin receptors in mamalian tissues. TIPS 1988; 9: 387-389.

11. Rifo J., Pourrat M., Vavrek RJ, Stewart JM, Huidobro-Toro JP. Bradykinin receptor antagonists used to characterize the heterogeneity of bradykinin-induced responses in rat vas deferens. Eur J Pharmacol 1987; 142: 305-312.

AAS 38/II
Recent Progress on Kinins
© 1992 Birkhäuser Verlag Basel

LACK OF SIGNIFICANT UNSPECIFIC EFFECTS OF HOE 140 AND OTHER NOVEL BRADYKININ ANTAGONISTS *IN VITRO* AND *IN VIVO*

F. Lembeck, T. Griesbacher, and F. J. Legat

Department of Experimental and Clinical Pharmacology, University of Graz,
Universitätsplatz 4, A-8010 Graz, Austria

SUMMARY: The novel, potent and long-acting bradykinin (BK) antagonists, HOE 140, compound II and compound III, slightly decreased blood pressure, but did not affect heart rate and respiration of rats. The antagonists did not cause bronchoconstriction in guinea-pigs. Neither HOE 140 nor BK released histamine from isolated perfused hindlegs of rats. The lack of significant unspecific side effects of the novel antagonists of effective doses will further increase the usefulness of these compounds for experimental and therapeutic purposes.

INTRODUCTION

Three Bradykinin (BK) analogues (HOE 140, compound II and compound III), containing the amino acids D-(1,2,3,4-tetrahydroisoquinolin-2-yl-carboxylic acid) (DTic) and L-[(3aS,7aS)-octahydroindol-2-yl-carboxylic acid] (Oic) in their amino acid sequence, proved to be potent BK antagonists both *in vitro* and *in vivo* [1, 2, 3, 4]. The long duration of action of these compounds is considered to be a valuable improvement because BK antagonists used before were subject to rapid enzymatic degradation [5]. Since BK is believed to play an important role in inflammation and inflammatory pain, the novel compounds may therefore be of interest as therapeutic agents. The most potent of the 3 antagonists, HOE 140, already is being tested in models involving the action of endogenous kinins [6, 7, 8].

It is important that receptor antagonists, employed as therapeutic agents, do not have any residual agonist effects or unspecific effects not related to specific receptors. We have investigated whether the 3 novel BK antagonists exhibit any such effects when used in high doses. A short-acting BK antagonist (compound IV) not containing DTic and Oic was used for comparison.

MATERIALS AND METHODS

Blood pressure, heart rate and respiration in rats. Sprague-Dawley rats (220-280 g) were pretreated with hyoscine butylbromide (40 mg kg^{-1}, s.c., 30 min before the experiment) and anaesthetized with pentobarbitone sodium (50 mg kg^{-1}, i.p.). One carotid artery was cannulated for measurement of arterial blood pressure with a Statham pressure transducer. The contralateral carotid artery was cannulated for retrograde i.a. injections of BK and the BK antagonists. The animals were injected i.v. with pancuronium bromide (3 μg kg^{-1}) and were ventilated artificially with air [5]. BK (0.4 nmol kg^{-1}) was injected i.a. at intervals of 10 min. The antagonists (1.2 or 4 nmol kg^{-1}) were administered i.a. as a short (3 min) infusion between the 2nd and 3rd BK injection. Control animals received an infusion of the solvent. The following BK injection was given 3 min after the end of this infusion.

In order to investigate whether the antagonists had an intrinsic effect of their own on respiration or heart rate, rats were operated as described above with the exception that the rats were not injected with pancuronium bromide and no artificial respiration was made. Respiratory flow was monitored in the tracheal cannula with a differential transducer. The heart rate was measured using a ramp recorder coupled to the pressure transducer which recorded the arterial blood pressure. The antagonists HOE 140, compound II and compound III were infused i.a. at a dose of 4 nmol kg^{-1} within 5 min.

Bronchoconstriction in guinea-pigs. Guinea-pigs (550-650 g) were anaesthetized with urethane (25% w/v, 6.5 ml kg^{-1}, i.p.). After cannulation of a jugular vein the animals were injected with pancuronium bromide (0.6 mg) and ventilated artificially (stroke volume 4 ml, 70 strokes min^{-1}). The pressure in the trachea was monitored in a side arm of the respiration system with a Statham pressure transducer. As a modification of the method described by Konzett and Rössler [8], a second side arm in the respiration system was connected to a glass tube which was inserted, vertically, 25 cm into water. The resulting registration is linear with respect to the air volume by-passing the lungs and thus allows the measurement of bronchoconstriction. The antagonists were injected i.v. in increasing doses (2-500 nmol kg^{-1}) at intervals of 10 min. At the end of each experiment, histamine (20-200 nmol kg^{-1}) was injected using the same dose intervals. For each antagonist, a separate group of 3 animals was used.

Histamine release from isolated perfused hindleg of rats. Sprague-Dawley rats (250-400 g) of either sex were injected with heparin (500 IU, i.p.) and anaesthetized with pentobarbitone sodium (60 mg kg^{-1}, i.p.). In both legs, the superficial epigastric arteries were ligated and the outer iliac arteries were cannulated. The legs were then separated from the body and perfused with Krebs solution (37°C, gassed with 5% CO_2 in O_2). The flow rate (2 ml min^{-1}) was kept constant using a roller pump. After an equilibration period of 30 min, the venous

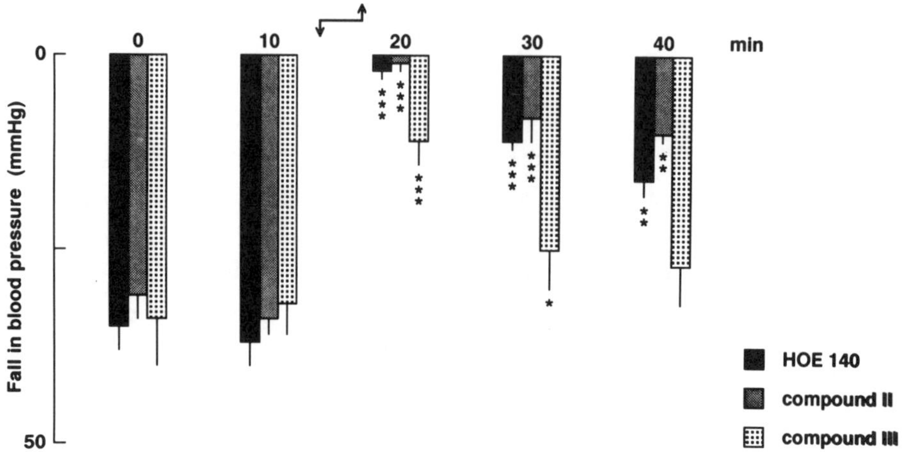

Figure 1. Fall in systemic arterial pressure (in mmHg) following i.a. injections of BK (0.4 nmol kg⁻¹) given at intervals of 10 min before and after the i.a. infusion (indicated by the arrows) of 4 nmol kg⁻¹ of the BK antagonists HOE 140, compound II or compound III. Significance of difference of to the effects observed before the antagonist infusion: $^*p < 0.05$, $^{**}p < 0.01$, $^{***}p < 0.001$ (Quade test). Means + SEM; $n = 5\text{-}8$.

effluent was collected in 10 consecutive 5 min periods. During the 3rd period, BK, HOE 140, or substance P were added to the perfusion at a final concentration of 3 μM. During the 8th period, compound 48/80 (3 μM) was infused to insure the viability of the organs. The samples of the venous effluent were acidified with perchloric acid (concentration in the sample 0.2 N) and the supernatant stored at -20°C until h.p.l.c. determination of histamine [9].

Substances. Bradykinin (BK) was obtained from Bachem (Switzerland). DArg-[Hyp³, Thi⁵, DTic⁷, Oic⁸]-BK (HOE 140), DArg-[Hyp³, DTic⁷, Oic⁸]-BK (compound II), [Arg(Tos)¹, Hyp³, Thi⁵, DTic⁷, Oic⁸]-BK (compound III) and DArg-[Hyp², Thi⁵,⁸, DPhe⁷]-BK (compound IV) were a gift from Hoechst A.G. (F.R.G.). Stock solutions were made in a 154 mM NaCl solution (saline) which contained 1 g l⁻¹ gelatine and 25 mg l⁻¹ cialit (sodium 2-ethylmercuriothio-benzoxazole-5-carboxylate, Asid-Institut, F.R.G.) to prevent adsorption to glass and bacterial growth. Substance P (Sigma, U.S.A.) was dissolved in 0.01 N acetic acid at a concentration of 6 mM, and dilutions were made with saline. Further substances used were: histamine dihydrochloride (Serva, F.R.G.), compound 48/80 (Wellcome, U.K.), hyoscine butylbromide (Buscopan^R, Boehringer Ingelheim, F.R.G.), pentobarbitone sodium (Nembutal^R, Ceva, F.R.G.), pancuronium bromide (Pavulon^R, Organon, Netherlands).

The composition of the Krebs solution was (in mM): NaCl 118.0, KCl 4.6, CaCl₂ 2.5, MgSO₄ 1.17, NaH₂PO₄ 25.0, D-glucose 10.1. All salts were of analytical grade and were obtained from Merck (F.R.G.).

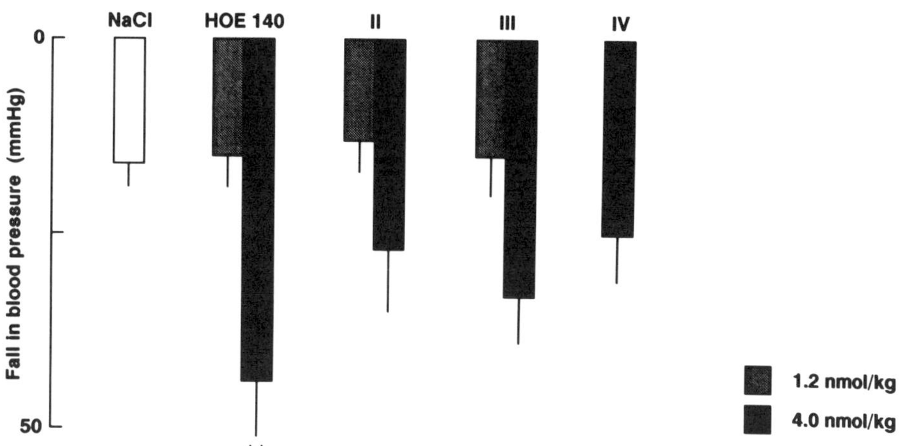

Figure 2. Fall in systemic arterial pressure (in mmHg) observed during a short (3 min) i.a. infusions of 1.2 or 4 nmol kg^{-1} of the BK antagonists HOE 140, compound II, compound III, and compound IV. Significance of difference to the effect of the infusion of a corresponding volume (1 ml) of the solvent: $^{**}p < 0.01$ (Dunnett's t test). Means + SEM; $n = 5$-8.

RESULTS

Rat blood pressure. Intraarterial retrograde injections of BK (0.4 nmol kg^{-1}) into a carotid artery led to a short-lasting fall in systemic arterial blood pressure by 35-45 mmHg. This effect was reproducible when BK was administered at dose intervals of 10 min. Following a 3 min i.a. infusion of the BK antagonists, the effect of subsequent injections of BK was significantly ($p < 0.001$) and dose-dependently inhibited by HOE 140, compounds II and III (Fig. 1 shows the results obtained with 4 nmol kg^{-1}). The BK effect returned to control values within 20 min after infusion of 1.2 nmol kg^{-1} of the novel antagonists. At this time point the effect of BK was still significantly reduced when 4 nmol kg^{-1} of HOE 140 or compound II had been administered (Fig. 1). Compound III was less active at both dose levels tested. Infusions of compound IV (4 nmol kg^{-1}) or of the solvent were completely inactive (not shown in Fig. 1).

The i.a. infusion of the BK antagonists (1.2 nmol kg^{-1}) was accompanied by a slight decrease in systemic arterial blood pressure as also evoked by the infusion of saline (Fig. 2). Infusions of 4 nmol kg^{-1} of the antagonists seemed to have a greater hypotensive effect. However, this was significant ($p < 0.01$) only for HOE 140. Blood pressure returned to baseline values within 3 min after the end of the antagonist infusion.

In spontaneously breathing anaesthetized rats, the i.a. infusion within 3 min of 5 nmol of the antagonists HOE 140, compound II and compound III also led to a similar fall in blood pressure during the time of infusion (3 min) comparable to that described above in ventilated

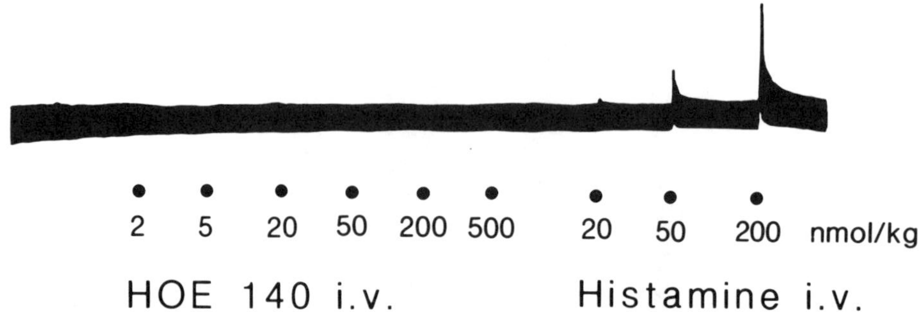

Figure 3. Ventilation pressure in artificially ventilated anaesthetized guinea-pigs. HOE 140 was injected i.v. at intervals of 10 min at increasing doses of 2-500 nmol kg^{-1}. Histamine (20-200 nmol kg-1) led to dose-dependent bronchoconstriction. The tracing is a representative of 3 experiments with HOE 140.

rats. However, the heart rate (180-230 min^{-1}) and the respiratory flow and respiration frequency (25-30 min^{-1}) remained unaltered.

Bronchoconstriction in guinea-pigs. Bronchoconstriction induced by i.v. injections of BK have been shown earlier to be blocked effectively by i.v. injections of low doses (about 2-4 nmol kg^{-1}) of the novel antagonists [1]. To investigate whether these antagonists had bronchoconstrictor effects on their own they were injected i.v. at doses up to 500 nmol kg^{-1}. Respiration was completely unaffected by HOE 140 (Fig. 3). Compound II and compound III also did not show any effect on respiration. Histamine produced short-lasting bronchoconstriction at doses of 20 nmol kg^{-1} and higher. Injections of 200 nmol kg^{-1} histamine elicited bronchoconstriction of about 80%.

Histamine release from isolated perfused rat hind legs. The i.a. infusion of SP (3 μM for 5 min) into the isolated perfused hindleg of rats caused the release of 867 $\pm$ 242 ng histamine within 25 min after the beginning of the infusion (Fig. 4A). Neither BK nor HOE 140, given at the same concentration as SP, caused any release of histamine exceeding basal levels (Fig. 4B-C). All preparations released comparable amounts of histamine (2-3 μg) during a 5 min infusion of compound 48/80 (3 μM) given at the end of each experiment (not shown in Fig. 4).

DISCUSSION

Kinins are thought to play an important role in a number of pathological conditions, such as inflammation and pain [see refs. 10, 11]. Increasing evidence has been found that it may also be involved in allergic diseases of the airways [see ref. 12]. Since the development of BK antagonists containing the unusual amino acids DTic and Oic resulted in compounds which

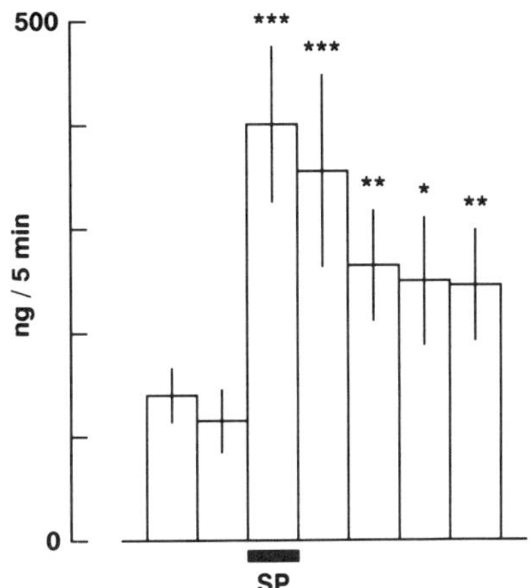
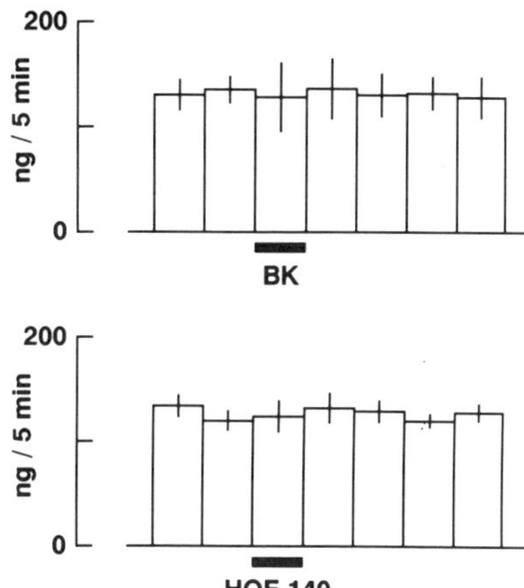

Figure 4. Release of histamine (in ng) from isolated perfused rat hindleg: The hindlegs were perfused with Krebs solution and the venous effluent was collected in fractions of 5 min for the determination of histamine. During the 3rd 5 min period, SP, BK or HOE 140 were added to the perfusion at a concentration of 3 μM. Significance of difference to basal values: $^*p<0.05$, $^{**}p<0.01$, $^{***}p<0.001$ (Quade test). Means $\pm$ SEM; $n = 6$-7.

showed a greatly enhanced potency and prolonged duration of action [1, 2, 3] it now may be feasible to use such compounds as therapeutic agents.

It is important that compounds which are candidates for clinical applications do not have any unspecific effects. In the case of receptor antagonists this includes also any residual agonist activities. Some of previously used BK antagonists showed effects of this kind [see ref. 13]. To date, no intrinsic agonist activity of the novel BK antagonists, HOE 140, compound II and compound III, was found on several smooth muscle preparations [1, 2]. In addition, the antagonists do not release prostaglandins [1] or catecholamines [14]. A weak agonist activity of very high doses of HOE 140 was found only in the plasma protein extravasation test in the rat [1] or on blood pressure in the dog [3].

A fall in blood pressure induced by a BK antagonist could be the effect of a residual intrinsic activity of the antagonist or it could be elicited by release of prostaglandins [15]. However, the novel antagonists did not release any prostaglandin E_2 from the isolated perfused rabbit ear [1]. The fall in blood pressure observed during the i.a. infusions of the BK antagonists (see Fig. 2) was not greater than the unspecific effect of the solvent. At a dose of 4 nmol kg^{-1}, only HOE 140 lowered the blood pressure significantly which might be regarded as a residual agonist activity. After i.v. administration of high doses of BK antagonists in rats, a transient rise in blood pressure, attributed to the blockade of the effects of endogenous kinins, has been reported [15, 16]. In the present experiments no such effect was found.

BK is a potent bronchoconstrictor substance acting both directly on the smooth muscles and indirectly via the release of other mediators or via neural mechanisms [17, 18]. Accumulating evidence has been found that BK is involved in the pathophysiological events in airway diseases, e.g. in asthma [see ref. 19]. Consequently, the development of potent BK receptor antagonists is of great interest for the treatment of these disorders. Although some short-acting BK receptor antagonists have only a weak potency [see ref. 20] they nevertheless are able to reduce responses in experimental models of asthma [21, 22]. BK-induced bronchoconstriction in guinea-pigs is inhibited by HOE 140 and the other novel BK antagonists with much higher potency and longer duration of action as compared to BK antagonists used until now [1, 3]. Results obtained with NPC 16731, a BK antagonist of a structure similar to HOE 140, already indicate that these antagonists may also be highly active in a model of asthma [12]. Therefore, antagonists of this kind will be much more suitable as therapeutic agents than previous compounds provided that they do not possess unspecific effects on the airways. HOE 140, compound II and compound III do not cause bronchoconstriction in guinea-pigs even when injected at doses up to 500 nmol kg^{-1} (see Fig. 3). This concentration is more than 100 times greater than that which effectively blocks BK-induced bronchoconstriction for at least 1 h [1, 3]. Undesirable effects of HOE 140, compound II or compound III in the airways are, thus, not to be expected.

A number of biologically active peptides, including BK and some of its analogues, are able to release histamine from mast cells [23, 24]. In the case of compounds that might be suitable for clinical applications such an action would clearly be undesirable. The mode of action does not include the activation of specific receptors but apparently relies on the number of basic, especially aromatic, residues in the amino acid sequence of the peptides [23, 24]. SP potently released histamine from isolated perfused hindlegs of rats as has been described before [25, 26]. No histamine was released from this preparation by BK, whereas, at concentrations much higher than those required with other peptides, BK liberated histamine from isolated mast cells [23]. Human histamine-containing cells do not release histamine in response to challenge with BK [27]. Nevertheless, even a single amino acid substitution in the sequence of BK can result in analogues which are potent secretagogues for mast cells [24]. HOE 140, the most potent of the novel BK antagonists, is also a compound which, due to its amino acid composition, would be the most likely candidate to have such an effect. The fact that no histamine release was induced by HOE 140 (see Fig. 4) further demonstrates that this compound will be a suitable candidate for clinical trials.

CONCLUSION

The novel BK analogues HOE 140, compound II and compound III again proved to be potent antagonists of the actions of exogenously applied BK. An unspecific effect of

HOE 140, the most potent of these compounds, was observed only after i.a. administration of doses by far exceeding those that effectively block BK. Compound II and compound III were only slightly less potent as BK antagonists and did not show any unspecific effects at all.

ACKNOWLEDGEMENTS

The investigation was supported by the Pain Research Commission of the Austrian Academy of Sciences.

REFERENCES

[1]   Lembeck F, Griesbacher T, Eckhardt M, Henke S, Breipohl G, Knolle J. New, long-acting, potent bradykinin antagonists. Br J Pharmacol 1991; 102: 297-304.

[2]   Hock FJ, Wirth K, Albus U, Linz W, Gerhards HJ, Wiemer G, Henke S, Breipohl G, König W, Knolle J, Schölkens BA. Hoe 140 a new potent and long acting bradykinin-antagonist: in vitro studies. Br J Pharmacol 1991; 102: 769-773.

[3]   Wirth K, Hock FJ, Albus U, Linz W, Alpermann HG, Anagnostopoulos H, Henke S, Breipohl G, König W, Knolle J, Schölkens BA. Hoe 140 a new potent and long acting bradykinin-antagonist: in vivo studies. Br J Pharmacol 1991; 102: 774-777.

[4]   Griesbacher T, Lembeck F. Analysis of the antagonistic actions of HOE 140 and other novel bradykinin analogues on the guinea-pig ileum. Eur J Pharmacol 1992; in press.

[5]   Griesbacher T, Lembeck F, Saria A. Effects of the bradykinin antagonist B4310 on smooth muscles and blood pressure in the rat, and its enzymatic degradation. Br J Pharmacol 1989; 96: 531-538.

[6]   Martorana PA, Kettenbach B, Breipohl G, Linz W, Schölkens BA. Reduction of infarct size by local angiotensin-converting enzyme inhibition is abolished by a bradykinin antagonist. Eur J Pharmacol 1990; 182: 395-396.

[7]   Heapy GG, Farmer SG, Shaw JS. The inhibitory effect of HOE 140 in mouse abdominal constriction assays. Br J Pharmacol 1991; 104 (Proc Suppl): 455P.

[8]   Beresford IJM, Birch PJ. Antinociceptive activity of the bradykinin antagonist HOE-140 in rat and mouse. Proc Br Pharmacol Soc, London, 17-19 December 1991, abstract P6.

[8]   Konzett H, Rössler R. Versuchsanordnung zu Untersuchungen an der Bronchial-muskulatur. Arch Exp Pathol Pharmakol 1940; 195: 71-74.

[9]   Skofitsch G, Donnerer J, Petronijevic S, Saria A, Lembeck F. Release of histamine by neuropeptides from the perfused rat hindquarter. Naunyn-Schmiedeberg's Arch Pharmacol 1983; 322: 153-157.

[10] Marceau F, Lussier A, Regoli D, Giraud GP. Pharmacology of kinins: their relevance to tissue injury and inflammation. Gen Pharmacol 1983; 14: 209-229.

[11] Ness TJ, Gebhart GF. Visceral pain: a review of experimental studies. Pain 1990; 41: 167-234.

[12] Farmer SG, Meeker SN, Wilkins DE. Effects of bradykinin receptor antagonists on antigen-induced airway hyperresponsiveness. FASEB J 1991; 5: A1242 (abstract 5056).

[13] Plevin R, Owen PJ. Multiple B_2 kinin receptors in mammalian tissues. Trends Pharmacol Sci 1988; 9: 387-389.

[14] Bao G, Quadri F, Stauss B, Stauss H, Gohlke P, Unger T. HOE 140, a new highly potent and long-acting bradykinin antagonist in conscious rats. Eur J Pharmacol 1991; 200: 179-182.

[15] Carbonell LF, Carretero OA, Madeddu P, Scicli AG. Effects of a kinin antagonist on mean blood pressure. Hypertension 1988; 11 (Suppl I): I-84-I-88.

[16] Benetos A, Gavras I, Gavras H. Hypertensive effect of bradykinin antagonist in normotensive rats. Hypertension 1986; 8: 1089-1092.

[17] Kaufman MP, Coleridge HM, Coleridge JCG, Baker DG. Bradykinin stimulates afferent vagal C-fibres in intrapulmonary airways of dogs. J Appl Physiol 1980; 48: 511-517.

[18] Abraham WM, Ahmed A, Cortes A, Soler M, Farmer SG, Baugh LE, Harbeson SL. Airway effects of inhaled bradykinin, substance P, and neurokinin A in sheep. J Allergy Clin Immunol 1991; 87: 557-564.

[19] Farmer SG. Role of kinins in airway diseases. Immunopharmacology 1991; 22: 1-20.

[20] Farmer SG, Burch RM. Airway bradykinin receptors. Ann New York Acad Sci 1991; 629: 237-249.

[21] Soler M, Sielczak M, Abraham WM. A bradykinin antagonist blocks antigen-induced airway hyperresponsiveness and inflammation in sheep. Pulm Pharmacol 1990; 3: 9-15.

[22] Abraham WM, Burch RM, Farmer SG, Sielczak MW, Ahmed A, Cortes A. A bradykinin antagonist modifies allergen-induced mediator release and late bronchial responses in sheep. Am Rev Respir Dis 1991; 143: 787-796.

[23] Lagunoff D, Martin TW. Agents that release histamine from mast cells. Ann Rev Pharmacol Toxicol 1983; 23: 331-351.

[24] Burch RM, Farmer SG, Steranka LR. Bradykinin receptor antagonists. Med Res Rev 1990; 10: 237-269.

[24] Lawrence ID, Warner JA, Cohan VL, Lichtenstein LM, Kagey-Sobotka A, Vavrek RJ, Stewart JM, Proud D. Induction of histamine release from human skin mast cells by bradykinin analogs. Biochem Pharmacol 1989; 38: 227-233.

[25] Erjavec F, Lembeck F, Florjanc-Irman T, Skofitsch G, Donnerer J, Saria A, Holzer P. Release of histamine by substance P. Naunyn-Schmiedeberg's Arch Pharmacol 1981; 317: 67-70.

[26] Holzer-Petsche U, Schimek E, Amann R, Lembeck F. In vivo and in vitro actions of mammalian tachykinins. Naunyn-Schmiedeberg's Arch Pharmacol 1985; 330: 130-135.

[27] Cohan VL, MacGlashan DW, Warner JA, Lichtenstein LM, Proud D. Mechanisms of mediator release from human skin mast cells upon stimulation by the bradykinin analog, [DArg^0-Hyp^3-DPhe^7]bradykinin. Biochem Pharmacol 1991; 41: 293-300.

KININ CONTRIBUTION TO CHRONIC ANTIHYPERTENSIVE ACTIONS OF ACE-INHIBITORS IN HYPERTENSIVE RATS

G. Bao, P. Gohlke, and Th. Unger

Department of Pharmacology and German Institute for High Blood Pressure Research, University of Heidelberg, Im Neuenheimer Feld 366, W-6900 Heidelberg, Germany

SUMMARY: The contribution of endogenous bradykinin to the chronic antihypertensive actions of the ACE-inhibitor, ramipril, was investigated in 2-kidney 1 clip (2K1C) hypertensive kinin-deficient Brown Norway Katholieke rats (BN-K) and 2K1C hypertensive Wistar rats (WI) as well as in spontaneously hypertensive rats (SHR). Treatment with ramipril plus the BK B_2-receptor antagonist HOE 140 for 6 weeks significantly attenuated the antihypertensive effects of the ACE-inhibitor in 2K1C hypertensive WI rats, but not in 2K1C hypertensive BN-K rats and in SHR.
Our data support the hypothesis that potentiation of endogenous kinins contributes to the chronic antihypertensive actions of ACE-inhibitors in experimental renal hypertension. Whether this holds also true for other forms of hypertension remains to be answered.

INTRODUCTION

Angiotensin converting enzyme (ACE), also known as kininase II, catabolizes bradykinin (BK) to inactive fragments (1). A potentiation of endogenous BK has, therefore, been implicated in the antihypertensive action of ACE-inhibitors. However, attempts to determine the contribution of endogenous kinins to the various cardiovascular actions of ACE-inhibitors have yielded equivocal results (2). The apparent discrepancies in the literature are partly due to methodological difficulties, since kinin concentrations in blood and urine could not be readily measured in the past, and tools to antagonize the actions of kinins, such as BK receptor antagonists, were lacking. This situation has now improved considerably with the introduction of reliable kinin assays (3) as well as the development of potent and specific bradykinin antagonists (4-5). Among those, the newly developed BK antagonist, HOE 140 (D-Arg-[Hyp^3, Thi^5, D-Tic^7, Oic^8]-bradykinin), is characterized by high potency and specificity as well as a long half-life (6-8). With this new tool it is now possible to study the effects of chronic BK receptor blockade on the antihypertensive actions of ACE-inhibitors.

Brown Norway rats of the Katholieke strain (BN-K) completely lack the high molecular weight kininogen and are further deficient in low molecular weight kininogen (9-12) as well as plasma prekallikrein (9, 13, 14). This kinin-deficient strain lends itself to evaluate the role of endogenous kinins in the cardiovascular actions of ACE-inhibitors.

In spontaneously hypertensive rats (SHR) ACE-inhibitors are very effective in lowering blood pressure despite normal or low plasma renin levels, suggesting that mechanisms other than the suppression of the renin-angiotensin system alone are involved in the antihypertensive actions of these drugs.

In the present study, we investigated the effect of chronic BK B_2-receptor blockade on the blood pressure lowering actions of the ACE-inhibitor, ramipril, in 2-kidney 1 clip (2K1C) hypertensive kinin-deficient BN-K compared with those in 2K1C hypertensive Wistar (WI) rats and SHR, using the BK B_2-receptor antagonist HOE 140.

MATERIALS AND METHODS

Male BN-K rats originally obtained from the Katholieke Universiteit of Leuven, Heverlee, Belgium, are now bred at the Department of Pharmacology, University of Heidelberg. WI rats and SHR (300±25 g) were purchased from Dr. K. Thomae GmbH, Biberach, Germany, and Møllegaard Ltd., Skensved, Denmark, respectively. Animals were housed under conditions of constant temperature with a 12-hour light/dark cycle and had free access to tap water and rat chow.

Renal hypertension was induced by placing a solid silver clip with a 0.2 mm aperture on the left renal artery (two-kidney one clip hypertension). Six to eight weeks after the surgery, systolic blood pressure (SBP) was measured by tail plethysmography under light ether anesthesia. Rats with a SBP level of 190 mmHg or more were used for the experiments.

Experimental protocol:

After the measurement of SBP, 2K1C hypertensive rats of BN-K (n=16) and WI (n=21) strains as well as SHR (n=26) were cannulated with a femoral artery catheter. One day after the surgery, mean arterial blood pressure (MAP) and heart rate (HR) were recorded in conscious unrestrained rats over a 60-min period via the arterial catheter. MAP and HR were measured directly using a Statham P23Db pressure transducer, amplified by a Gould Brush pressure processor (both Gould Inc., Oxnard, Calif., USA). Data were recorded on-line by a PC-AT computer with specifically developed software that was also used for data calculation.

Rats of each strain were then divided randomly into two groups. Group 1 (BN-K, n=8; WI, n=11; SHR, n=14) was treated with ramipril (1 mg/kg/d, orally) plus HOE 140 (500 µg/kg/d, s.c. via osmotic minipumps) for 6 weeks, group 2 (BN-K, n=8; WI, n=10; SHR, n=12) with ramipril plus physiological saline (s.c. via osmotic minipumps) for 6 weeks as control. Osmotic minipumps (model 2002, Alza Corp., Palo Alto, Calif., USA) filled with the BK antagonist, HOE 140, or physiological saline were implanted s.c. for 2 weeks and renewed every 2 weeks. Ramipril and HOE 140 were provided by Hoechst AG, Frankfurt/M, Germany. SBP was measured weekly by tailplethysmography during the 6-week treatment period. At the end of the 6-week treatment, MAP and HR were measured again as described above. Means±SEM are reported. Data were subjected to analysis of variance (ANOVA) followed by multiple pairwise comparisons (Bonferroni) as appropriate. Differences were considered significant if p<0.05.

RESULTS

Six-week oral treatment with ramipril plus physiological saline significantly reduced blood pressure in all three rat strains. However, the depressor effect of the ACE-inhibitor was different between strains. SBP was lowered by 96 mmHg (from 218±5 to 122±7 mmHg) in 2K1C hypertensive WI rats, by 62 mmHg (from 208±7 to 146±3 mmHg) in

Table 1. Direct Measurement of MAP before and after 6-week Treatment with Ramipril (1 mg/kg/day p.o.) + HOE 140 (500 µg/kg/day s.c.) or Ramipril + Physiological Saline (Vehicle) in 2K1C Hypertensive Wistar (WI), 2K1C Hypertensive Brown Norway Katholieke (BN-K) Rats and Spontaneously Hypertensive Rats (SHR)

Group	Treatment	Before MAP (mmHg)	6 weeks After MAP (mmHg)
WI	Vehicle	180.1±8.1	105.4±4.8 ⎤
	HOE 140	180.3±4.1	124.4±4.2 ⎦ *
BN-K	Vehicle	179.3±3.9	114.4±6.4
	HOE 140	180.5±3.0	110.4±7.7
SHR	Vehicle	160.3±3.2	129.9±3.5
	HOE 140	163.0±3.0	132.8±2.4

Means ± SEM are reported. MAP, mean arterial pressure; p.o., per oral; s.c., subcutaneous; BK, bradykinin; 2K1C, two-kidney one clip. * p<0.05.

2K1C hypertensive BN-K rats and by 38 mmHg (from 196±3 to 158±6 mmHg) in SHR (Figure 1). After co-administration of ramipril and HOE 140, the reduction in SBP was attenuated in the WI rats. The difference between the HOE 140- and the saline-treated groups became significant after 1 week of treatment (149±4 mmHg vs 128±8 mmHg) and remained significant during the experiment (146±4 mmHg vs 122±7 mmHg after 6 weeks). HOE 140 did not affect the antihypertensive effects of ramipril in 2K1C

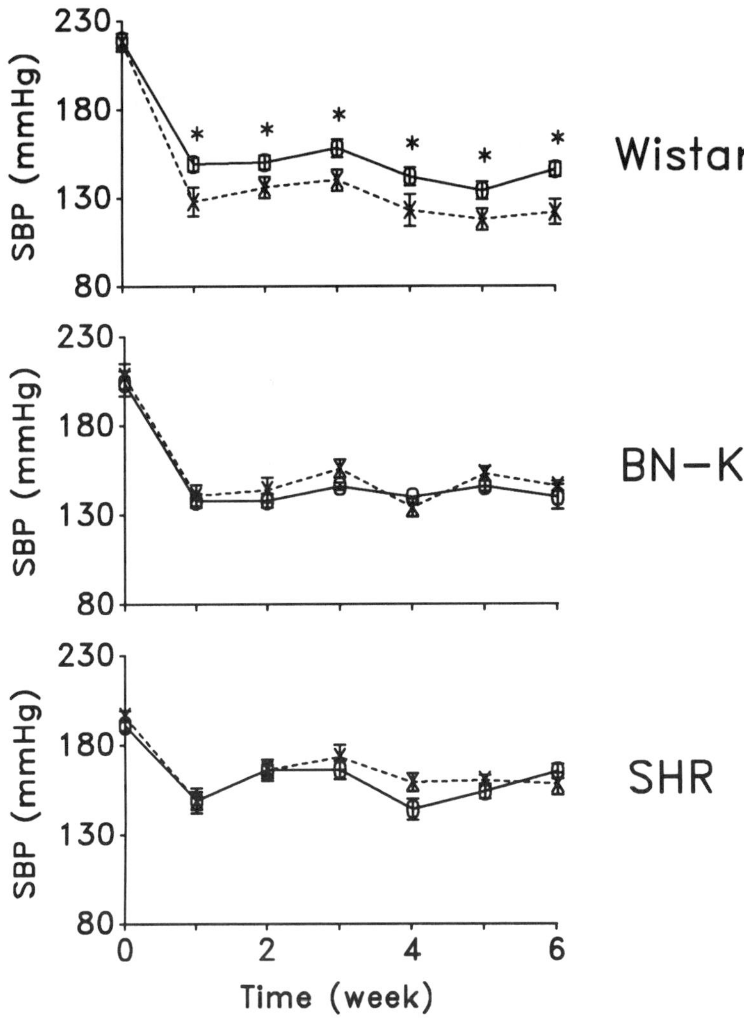

Figure 1. Effect of chronic bradykinin B_2-receptor blockade on blood pressure lowering actions of ramipril in kinin-deficient 2K1C hypertensive Brown Norway rats (BN-K), 2K1C hypertensive Wistar rats and spontaneously hypertensive rats (SHR). Rats of each strain were treated with either ramipril (1 mg/kg/day p.o.) plus the BK antagonist HOE 140 (500 µg/kg/day s.c., solid lines) or ramipril plus physiological saline (dashed lines) as control. SBP, systolic blood pressure. * p<0.05.

hypertensive BN-K rats (140 ± 7 vs 146 ± 3 mmHg after 6 weeks) and in SHR (165 ± 4 vs 158 ± 6 mmHg after 6 weeks, Figure 1). These results were confirmed by direct measurement of MAP at the end of the treatment (Table 1). A significant difference in MAP between the HOE 140- and the vehicle-treated group was only observed in 2K1C hypertensive WI rats, but not in 2K1C hypertensive BN-K rats and in SHR. Heart rate remained unchanged in all three strains.

DISCUSSION

Chronic oral treatment with the ACE-inhibitor, ramipril, lowered blood pressure to a greater extent in 2K1C hypertensive WI rats than in 2K1C hypertensive BN-K rats or in SHR. Additional chronic blockade of BK B_2-receptors by HOE 140 attenuated the antihypertensive effect of ramipril in the WI rats. In kinin-deficient 2K1C hypertensive BN-K rats, the antihypertensive effects of ramipril were much lower than those observed in the WI rats, although both of them had a similar SBP at the beginning of the experiment. Furthermore, chronic BK receptor blockade did not affect the antihypertensive actions of ramipril in the BN-K rats.

Our data are in agreement with the results from acute studies obtained from our laboratory using the BK antagonist B4146 in 2K1C hypertensive WI and BN-K rats (15), by Carretero et al. (16) using captopril and antibodies to kinins and with those reported by Benetos et al. (17), who used enalapril and the BK antagonist B4146 in renovascular hypertension. Similar findings were also obtained by Carbonell et al. (18), who used enalapril and the BK antagonist B4146 in severely hypertensive rats with aortic ligation between both renal arteries, and by Seino et al. (19), who used captopril and the BK antagonist B4147 in anesthetized normotensive rats.

In the SHR used in this study, SBP was not quite as high as in other two strains prior to the experiment. The blood pressure reduction was least after 6-week ramipril plus saline treatment. Similar to the BN-K rats, chronic BK blockade did not attenuate the depressor effect of ramipril.

Interestingly, as demonstrated here and in other studies, BK antagonists seem to be particularly effective in renovascular models of hypertension of kinin replete animals associated with a stimulated renin-angiotensin system, but less effective in genetic hypertension with normal or suppressed plasma renin such as in SHR, although one might have expected the opposite, i.e. that kinin potentiation by ACE inhibitors would be more effective in non-renin dependent hypertension. At this point we can only speculate on the reasons underlying this phenomenon. First, the kallikrein-kinin system in SHR may be

                                                    G. Bao et al.

deficient. There are a few studies showing that the kallikrein-binding protein in SHR is significantly lower than in Wistar Kyoto rats (WKY) (20) and the kallikrein mRNA levels in kidneys of adult SHR were found to be less than those in WKY (21). Second, early-induced changes in blood vessels of SHR such as vascular hypertrophy could inhibit the production of kinins and vasodilating actions of kinins against hypertension, and vascular as well as cellular damage may reduce the reactivity to kinins and other vasodilators in these animals. Finally, endogenous kinins may gain importance for blood pressure regulation in cases where elevated blood pressure is maintained by circulatory pressor agents such as angiotensin II (22). Under these conditions, BK could contribute to the endothelial production of relaxing factors such as nitric oxide (NO) to counteract the pressor actions of angiotensin II. ACE inhibitors could then potentiate the NO generating vasodilator action of BK as has most recently been demonstrated in vitro (23). The question as to whether or not the potentiation of endogenous kinins also contributes to the antihypertensive actions of ACE inhibitors in non-renin dependent hypertension remains a challenging question to be addressed in future studies.

REFERENCES

1. Erdös EG. Angiotensin I converting enzyme. Circ Res 1975; 36:247-255.

2. Unger Th, Gohlke P, Gruber MG. Converting enzyme inhibitors, in Ganten D, Mulrow PJ (eds): Handbook of experimental Pharmacology, Pharmacology of antihypertensive Therapeutics. Heidelberg/New York, Springer-Verlag, 1990, pp377-481.

3. Bönner G, Iwersen D, Shimamoto K. The analytical value of kinin concentration in blood dependents on the antiserum used in the bradykinin radioimmunoassay. J Clin Chem Clin Biochem 1987; 25:39-43.

4. Vavrek RJ, Stewart JM. Development and modification of competitive antagonists of bradykinn, in Deber CM, Hruby VL, Kopple KD (eds): Peptides - Structure and function. Proceedings 9th American Peptide Symposium. Rockford, Ill, Piece Chem Co, 1985, pp 655-658.

5. Benetos A, Gavras I, Gavras H. Hypertenisve effect of a bradykinin antagonist in normotensive rats. Hypertension 1986; 8:1089-1092.

6. Hock FJ, Wirth K, Linz W, Gerhards HJ, Wiemer G, Henke St, Breipohl G, König W, Knolle J, and Schölkens BA. Hoe 140 a new potent and long acting bradykinin-antagonist: in vitro studies. Br. J Pharmacol 1991; 102:769-773.

7. Wirth K, Hock FJ, Albus U, Linz W, Anagnostopoulos H, Henke St, Breipohl G, König W, Knolle J, and Schölkens BA. Hoe 140 a new potent and long acting bradykinin-antagonist, in vivo studies. Br. J Pharmacol 1991; 102:774-777.

8. Bao G, Qadri F, Stauss H, Gohlke P, and Unger Th. HOE 140, a highly potent and long-acting bradykinin antagonist in conscious rats. Eur. J. Pharmacol 1991; 200:179-182.

9. Damas J, Adam A. Congenital deficiency in plasma kallikrien and kininogens in the Brown Norway rat. Experientia 1980; 36:586-587.

10. Hayashi I, Ino T, Kato H, Iwanaga S, Nakano T, Oh-ishi S. Demonstration of the third kininogen in high and low molecular weight kininogens-deficient Brown Norway Katholiek rat. Thromb Res 1984; 36:509-516.

11. Suzuki H, Bouhnik J, Alhenc.Gelas F, Corvol P, Menard J. Direct radioimmunoassay for rat high molecular weight kininogen-Measurement of immunoreactive high molecular weight kininogen in normal and kininogen deficient plasma. Vasodepressor Hormones 1987; AAS 22:277-287.

12. Reis ML, Alhenc-Gelas F, Alhenc Gelas M, Allegrini J, Kerbiriou-Nabias D, Corvol P, Menard J. Rat high-molecular-weight kininogen: Purification, production of antibodies and demonstration of lack of immunoreactive kininogen in a strain of Brown Norway rats. Biochem Biophys Acta 1985; 831:106-113.

13. Damas J, Remacle-Volon, Adam A. Inflammation in the rat paw due to urate crystals ——Involvement of the kinin system. Naunyn-Schmiedeberg's Arch Pharmacol 1984; 325:76-79.

14. Oh-ishi S, Satoh K, Hayashi I, Yamazaki K, Nakano T. Differences in prekallikrein and high molecular weight kininogen levels in two strains of Brown Norway rat (Kitasato strain and Katholiek strain). Thromb Res 1982; 28:143-147.

15. Danckwardt L, Shimizu I, Bönner G, Rettig R, and Unger Th. Converting enzyme inhibition in kinin-deficient Brown Norway rats. Hypertension 1990; 16:429-435.

16. Carretero OA, Miyazaki S, Scicli AG. Role of kinins in the acute antihypertenisve effects of the converting enzyme inhibitor, captopril. Hypertension 1981; 3:18-22.

17. Benetos A, Gavras H, Stewart JM, Vavrek RJ, Hatinoglou S, Gavras I. Vasodepressor role of endogenous bradykinin assessed by a bradykinin antagonist. Hypertension 1986; 8:971-974.

18. Carbonell LF, Carretero OA, Stewart JM, Scicli AG. Effect of a kinin antagonist on the acute antihypertenisve activity of enalaprilat in severe hypertension. Hypertenison 1988; 11:239-243.

19. Seino M, Abe K, Nushiro N, Omata K, Yoshinaga J. Role of endogenous bradykinin in the acute depressor effect of angiotensin converting enzyme inhibitor captopril ——Assessed by a competitive antagonist of bradykinin. Clin Exp Hypertens 1989; A11:35-43.

20. Murray SR, Chao Julie, Lin FK, and Chao L. Kallikrein multigene families and the regulation of their expression. J Cardiovasc Pharmacology 1990; 15 (suppl 6):S7-S16.

21. Goud DH, Oza NB and Levinsky NG. Renal kallikrein in spontaneously hypertensive rats (abstract). FASEB J 1991; 5:6048.

22. Aubert JF, Waeber B, Nussberger J, Vavrek R, Stewart JM, Brunner HR. Influence of endogenous bradykinin on acute blood pressure response to vasopressors in normotensive rats assessed with a bradykinin antagonist. J Cardiovasc Pharmacol 1988; 11:51-55.

23. Wiemer G, Schölkens BA, Becker RHA, Busse R. Ramipril enhances endothelial autocoid formation by inhibiting breakdown of endothelium-derived bradykinin. Hypertenison 1991; 18:558-563.